Aneuploidy in Health and Disease
Edited by Zuzana Storchova

Published by InTech
Janeza Trdine 9, 51000 Rijeka, Croatia

Publishing Process Manager Jana Sertic

Technical Editor Teodora Smiljanic

Cover Designer InTech Design Team

Additional hard copies can be obtained from orders@intechopen.com

Aneuploidy in Health and Disease, Edited by Zuzana Storchova
p. cm.
ISBN 978-953-51-0608-1

For EU product safety concerns:
IN TECH d.o.o., Prolaz Marije Krucifikse Kozulić 3, 51000 Rijeka, Croatia,
info@intechopen.com or visit our website at intechopen.com.

Meet the editor

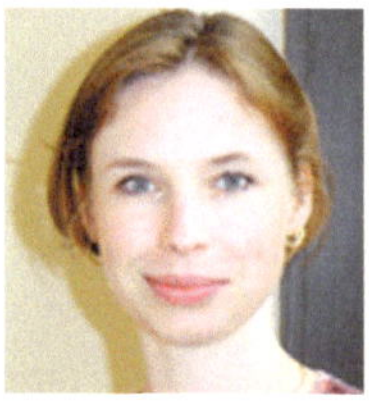

Dr Zuzana Storchova received her Ph.D. in Molecular Genetics at the Charles University in Prague, Czech Republic. She than continued working on mechanisms of DNA repair at the University of Zurich, Switzerland, in the laboratory of Prof. J. Jiricny. Her postdoctoral work in the laboratory of Prof. D. Pellman at the Dana-Farber Cancer Institute/Harvard Medical School in Boston, USA, focused on the consequences of polyploidy in budding yeast. Zuzana Storchova joined the Max Planck Institute of Biochemistry in Martinsried, Germany, in 2008. There she established a research group with the main focus on uncovering the causes and consequences of polyploidy and aneuploidy in yeast and human cells.

Contents

Preface XI

Section 1 Causes and Consequences of Aneuploidy 1

Chapter 1 **The Causes and Consequences of Aneuploidy in Eukaryotic Cells 3**
Zuzana Storchova

Chapter 2 **Uncover Cancer Genomics by Jointly Analysing Aneuploidy and Gene Expression 23**
Lingling Zheng and Joseph Lucas

Chapter 3 **Sister Chromatid Cohesion and Aneuploidy 41**
Erwan Watrin and Claude Prigent

Chapter 4 **Mouse Models for Chromosomal Instability 59**
Floris Foijer

Section 2 The Impact of Aneuploidy on Human Health 79

Chapter 5 **Aneuploidy and Epithelial Cancers: The Impact of Aneuploidy on the Genesis, Progression and Prognosis of Colorectal and Breast Carcinomas 81**
Jens K. Habermann, Gert Auer, Madhvi Upender, Timo Gemoll, Hans-Peter Bruch, Hans Jörnvall, Uwe J. Roblick and Thomas Ried

Chapter 6 **Aneuploidy and Intellectual Disability 107**
Daisuke Fukushi, Seiji Mizuno, Kenichiro Yamada, Reiko Kimura, Yasukazu Yamada, Toshiyuki Kumagai and Nobuaki Wakamatsu

Chapter 7 **Sex Chromosome Aneuploidies 123**
Eliona Demaliaj, Albana Cerekja and Juan Piazze

Chapter 8 **Human Male Meiosis and Sperm Aneuploidies 141**
María Vera, Vanessa Peinado, Nasser Al-Asmar, Jennifer Gruhn, Lorena Rodrigo, Terry Hassold and Carmen Rubio

Chapter 9 **Morphology and Aneuploidy of *in vitro* Matured (IVM) Human Oocytes 163**
Lidija Križančić Bombek, Borut Kovačič and Veljko Vlaisavljević

Chapter 10 **Comparing Pig and Amphibian Oocytes: Methodologies for Aneuploidy Detection and Complementary Lessons for MAPK Involvement in Meiotic Spindle Morphogenesis 193**
Michal Ješeta and Jean-François L. Bodart

Chapter 11 **The Role of Aneuploidy Screening in Human Preimplantation Embryos 217**
Christian S. Ottolini, Darren K. Griffin and Alan R. Thornhill

Preface

Genetic information is physically carried on large DNA strings that are organized into chromosomes. Each species is characterized by a chromosome set that carry the information necessary and sufficient for its development and survival. Eukaryotic organisms are mostly diploid, containing two sets of chromosomes with each pair carrying nearly identical genetic information. Occasionally, exceptions to this rule are found, such as haploid yeast (with only one set of chromosomes) or polyploid ferns and frogs (with multiple sets). Nevertheless, the composition of chromosome set remains identical within a species.

Aneuploidy describes exceptions from this rule. Some organisms or individual cells might contain an extra chromosome or two, some might have lost a chromosome arm. These alterations might be rare in normal, healthy organisms, but are often found under pathological conditions. Years of research uncovered a multitude of mechanisms and defects in cellular pathways that can lead to aneuploidy, and the list is still growing. Recent analysis shed first light on the effects that aneuploidy instigates upon cells. Only slowly we start to untangle the intricate relationship between chromosome numbers and structure and cell physiology.

Part of the urge to study aneuploidy is triggered by the clear association of aneuploidy with various pathologies. In humans, aneuploidy is the most frequent cause of spontaneous abortions as it severely impairs embryo development. A handful of aneuploidies compatible with survival leads to newborns with variable handicaps and a limited life span. The majority of malignant tumors consists of cells with an aneuploid karyotype. The relationship of tumorigenesis and aneuploidy remains enigmatic despite growing scientific interest. Recently, novel observations suggest that aging and, in particular, neurodegeneration might be associated with aneuploidy as well.

Aneuploidy means anything that is not euploid, anything that stands outside the norm. Thus, aneuploidy takes numerous variable features and is remarkably demanding to study. Two particular characteristics make the studies of aneuploidy challenging. First, it is often hard to distinguish what is a cause and what is a consequence. Was aneuploidy first and then the pathological conditions came? Or is aneuploidy itself a consequence of a gene mutation or other cellular changes? The progress in long term imaging techniques as well as the techniques enabling to generate artificially aneuploid cells expand our experimental tools to address these questions. Secondly, aneuploidy is often associated with chromosomal instability, a persistent defect of the cellular ability to equally distribute genetic information into daughter cells. Thus, working with aneuploid, chromosomally unstable cells means to analyze an ever changing creature and capture the features that persist. The hopes are high that new genome-wide systems biology approaches will help to identify the patterns shared among aneuploid cells and organisms.

This book attempts to map our current knowledge on aneuploidy from the basic research view on the causes and consequences of aneuploidy, covered in Part I, to the medical relevance of aneuploidy in cancer research, reproductive biology and stem cell research, which is addressed in Part II. The multitude of covered topics reflects the variability of aneuploid cells as well as the broad extent of methods applied in aneuploidy research. I would like to thank the authors for the broad and at the same time deep review of their topics, and the editors for the support that enabled to produce the book in your hands.

Dr. Zuzana Storchová
Max Planck Institute of Biochemistry
Martinsried, Germany

Section 1

Causes and Consequences of Aneuploidy

1

The Causes and Consequences of Aneuploidy in Eukaryotic Cells

Zuzana Storchova
Max Planck Institute of Biochemistry
Germany

1. Introduction

Correct transfer of genetic information to daughter cells is essential for successful propagation of any organism. Three processes are involved in maintenance and propagation of genetic information: DNA replication, DNA damage repair and chromosome segregation. Error in any of these processes might result in cell death, or, in another scenario, in survival of cells with altered genetic information. This might be reflected either by single nucleotide changes as well as small insertions and deletions; or it might lead to larger alterations in the structure and number of chromosomes, together called aneuploidy. In this chapter, our current knowledge on causes and consequences of aneuploidy in human cells and relevant model organisms will be summarized.

2. What is aneuploidy?

Aneuploidy describes any karyotype that differs from a normal chromosome set (called euploidy) and its multiples (called polyploidy). Aneuploidy can occur either by chromosome gains and losses due to chromosome segregation errors, a so called "whole chromosomal" aneuploidy, or due to rearrangements of chromosomal parts, often accompanied by their deletion and amplification, that is referred to as a "structural" or "segmental" aneuploidy (Fig. 1). Frequently, a combination of both structural and numerical chromosomal changes can be found, in particular in cancer cells (composite aneuploidy). Aneuploidy and its link to various pathologies has been known for more than a century.

Aneuploidy often reflects chromosomal instability (CIN), which is an ongoing defect in faithful transmission of chromosomes [1, 2]. Chromosomally instable cells accumulate new karyotype alterations as they proliferate and they are always aneuploid. In contrast, not every aneuploidy is linked to CIN, some cells can remain in a stable aneuploid status for multiple generations. This is well documented by the fact that patients with trisomy syndrome (e.g. trisomy of chromosome 21 in Down syndrome) usually show stable karyotype [3]. CIN, and consequently aneuploidy levels are often elevated in high-grade tumors and can be considered a reliable marker of high malignancy and drug resistance at least in some cancer types [4] [5].

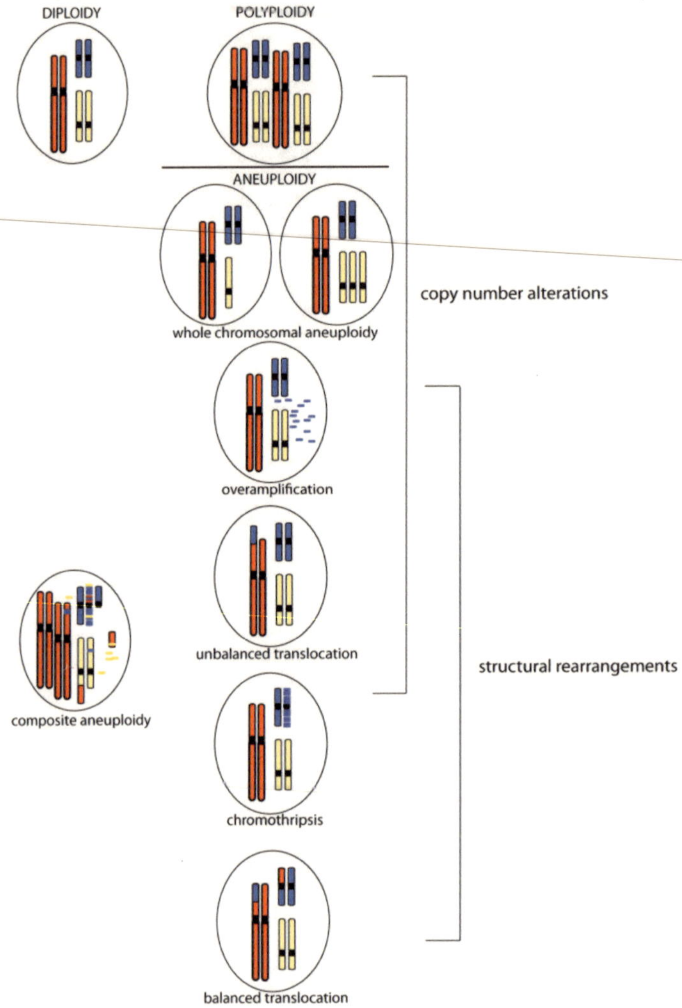

Fig. 1. Types of aneuploidy and copy number changes in eukaryotic cells.

2.1 Whole chromosomal aneuploidy

Whole chromosomal aneuploidies might arise due to random and sporadic chromosome missegregation events that occur with low frequency during any cell division. The missegregation levels range from 1/1000 to 1/10000 for human cells, and 1/10000 - 1/100000 for budding yeast in laboratory conditions and can increase in response to endogenous and exogenous agents that impair mitotic functions. The frequency of aneuploidy *in vivo* is difficult to estimate and likely depends on the type of tissue, but it might be as high as 1-2% abnormal numbers per chromosome.

Missegregation errors can occur also in germline cells. Aneuploid germinal cells that arise due to a chromosome segregation error in meiosis give rise to aneuploid embryos that show significant defects and frequently die during embryonic development. In fact, a whole chromosome aneuploidy is one of the major causes of spontaneous miscarriages [6]. There are only few types of aneuploidies that are compatible with survival. Various aneuploidies of sex chromosomes usually do not interfere with the survival and manifest with rather mild growth alterations, mild mental disability and infertility [7]. The effect of sex chromosome abnormalities is relatively low and does not interfere with viability due to the small genetic contribution of chromosome Y and due to X chromosome silencing via an epigenetic mediated pathway [8].

Autosomal trisomies have a much larger effect and only trisomy of chromosome 13 (Edwards syndrome), trisomy of chromosome 18 (Pateu syndrome) and trisomy of chromosome 21 (Down syndrome) are compatible with survival [9]. In all cases the presence of an extra chromosome copy results in a complex pathologic phenotype (for example there is up to different 72 pathological features linked to trisomy 21) that often severely impair quality of life. Down syndrome with mental disability, frequent heart defects, multiple facial and dactylic alterations and early onset lymphomas (among other pathologic features) is the only trisomy compatible with survival untill adulthood. The reasons for the dramatic effect of the trisomies as well as the molecular mechanisms underlying the phenotypes are not fully understood [10]. Accordingly, no targeted therapy is available for trisomy syndrome patients despite several decades of intense research.

Congenital trisomy leads to embryonic death also in mice, indicating that whole chromosomal aneuploidy is generally not well tolerated and leads to detrimental changes in organism physiology. In some cases, mosaic aneuploidy or aneuploidy only within a part of a tissue can be identified suggesting that low levels of aneuploidy might be better tolerated or even beneficial.

2.2 Structural aneuploidy

Recent large-scale screens of the human genome by deep sequencing, single nucleotide polymorphism analysis (SNP) and comparative genomic hybridization (CGH) revealed a fascinating and dynamic genomic landscape with multiple copy number changes of various chromosome regions. In principal there are two major types of copy number changes that usually cover a sequence from approximately one kilobase to several megabases.

First, copy number variations (CNV) describe congenital abnormalities in gene copy numbers that usually affect segments of individual chromosomes. Their identification suggests an unanticipated plasticity of the human genome and it has been proposed that CNVs represent an important factor that affects the outcome of complex, multifactorial genetic traits ([11], for review see [12]). Many of the subchromosomal CNVs identified so far are functionally linked to various pathological phenotypes that are frequently related to neurological defects. The second type of structural changes called somatic copy number alterations (SCNA) was uncovered by large scale deep sequencing that revealed a puzzling dynamic landscape of copy number changes of human genome and reflects the variability within somatic cells of a single individual [13]. SCNAs are found in both normal tissues and, at much higher frequency in human cancers, in particular in leukaemias and lymphomas.

3. Causes of aneuploidy

As aneuploidy describes broad spectra of numerical and structural chromosome changes, multiple different mechanisms may lead to the emergence of aneuploid karyotypes.

3.1 Whole chromosome aneuploidy

Whole chromosome aneuploidy results mostly from chromosome segregation errors, thus generating daughter cells that have lost or gained an individual chromosome (or few of them). This can occur even during normal unpertubed cell division or after an exposure to endogenous or exogenous damaging agents. Live cell microscopy of cells missegregating their chromosomes suggests that spontaneously arising aneuploid cells often die or arrest in a p53 dependent manner [14]. Even if the aneuploids survive, they are likely outgrown by fitter euploid cells (see below).

The frequency of aneuploidy is significantly enhanced by gene mutations that impair chromosome segregation. Such a mutation leads to both aneuploidy as well as to a general chromosomal instability phenotype (CIN). This has been observed for mutations of genes that affect cell cycle regulation, mitotic spindle checkpoint and sister chromatid cohesion. Increased frequency of cells with abnormal karyotype and CIN phenotype might be also due to mutations that disrupt the capacity of cells to activate the p53 pathway or to undergo apoptosis. However, this is likely not sufficient as a knock out of p53 does not increase aneuploidy and chromosome instability in human cells [15].

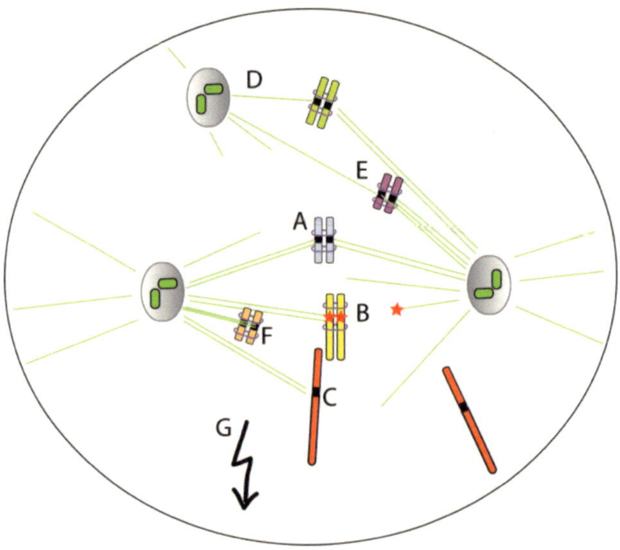

A. Normal, amphitelic attachment, B. Kinetochore or microtubule defect that interferes with correct attachment, C. Defect in sister chromatid cohesion hinders correct attachment, D. multiple centrosomes lead to formation of multipolar spindles, which in turn interferes with normal chromosome segregation, E. merotelic attachments are not recognized by spindle assembly checkpoint and often remain uncorrected, resulting in lagging chromosomes and aneuploidy, F. syntelic attachments lead to incorrect chromosome segregation, G. defects in SAC interfere with error recognition and repair.

Fig. 2. Schematic depicting the mitotic spindle defects that lead to whole chromosomal aneuploidy

The most obvious triggers of chromosome missegregation are defects of the spindle. During cell division, the genetic information carried on chromosomes is equally divided into the two daughter cells. The elaborate mitotic spindle consists of microtubules emanating from the spindle poles formed by microtubule organizing centers (called centrosomes in mammalian cells and spindle pole bodies in yeast) that attach to a proteinaceous structure, so called kinetochore, that forms at the centromeric DNA of each chromosome. Defects in kinetochore composition, microtubule dynamics or in spindle pole function lead to increased frequency of chromosome segregation errors (Fig. 2). Correct chromosome segregation is surveyed by complex machinery called spindle assembly checkpoint (SAC). Components of SAC, such as Bub1, Bub3, BubR1, Mad1, Mad2, Mad3, Mps1 and CENP-E, recognize incorrectly attached or empty kinetochores and trigger cell cycle delay until all chromosomes are properly attached to microtubules and aligned at the metaphase plate [16]. The cell cycle delay is executed via inhibition of the anaphase promoting complex-cyclosome (APC/C), whose activity is required for the metaphase-to-anaphase progression [17]. Defects in SAC lead inevitably to high chromosome missegregation levels both *in vitro* and *in vivo* and thus to aneuploidy.

Besides mutations in spindle assembly checkpoint and in mitotic spindle genes, aneuploidy is also increased in cells that carry mutant alleles of genes important for sister chromatid cohesion. Sister chromatid cohesion is maintained by evolutionary conserved cohesin rings that hold the two newly replicated chromatids together until they are separated during mitosis. Cohesion is essential for the maintenance of structural integrity of chromosomes and for proper attachment of chromosomes to the mitotic apparatus [18, 19]. The functional relevance of sister chromatid cohesion and aneuploidy has been underscored by finding that age-dependent defects in sister chromatid cohesion lead to increased frequency of aneuploid oocytes in older women, thus decreasing the chances of conceiving a healthy embryo [20, 21]. Recently, it was shown that inactivation of STAG2, which codes one of the cohesin subunits, leads to aneuploidy in human cells [22].

The widespread aneuploidy in cancer suggests that the majority of cancer cells should carry a mutation that compromises maintenance of chromosomal stability. There is over a hundred of genes identified in budding yeasts in screens aimed to identify factors avoiding CIN, most of them conserved and with multiple human orthologues. Yet mutations in these genes are not very frequent in tumors. Thus, it is possible that aneuploidy might be triggered by other events as well. Recent observations suggest that increased ploidy instigates chromosomal instability in both budding yeast [23] and human cells [24]. The hypothesis that tetraploidy facilitates CIN and subsequently tumorigenesis is supported by several *in vivo* data such as the observation that early pre-malignant stages of several tumors are characterized by increased levels of tetraploid cells [25].

Tetraploidy can arise spontaneously, by a sporadic cytokinesis error or due to cell-cell fusion induced by viral activity [26]. The list of mutations and defects that trigger formation of tetraploid cells has continuously increased in the past years. For example, telomere shortening most likely enhances the aneuploidy levels also via promoting tetraploidy as it has been shown that progressive telomere shortening leads to the accumulation of tetraploid cells in p53 deficient cell lines. It remains to be addressed in future experiments whether these mechanisms indeed contribute to the occurrence of aneuploid cells and potentially to tumorigenesis in humans.

3.2 Causes of structural aneuploidy

Whereas whole chromosomal instability and whole chromosomal aneuploidy are mostly linked to the defects in mitotic spindle function, the structural aneuploidy is generally viewed as a consequence of DNA breakage. The inherited CNVs are likely generated through meiotic unequal crossing over or nonallelic homologous recombination (NAHR) mediated by flanking repeated sequences or segmental duplications [27]. The somatic SCNA may arise by multiple mechanisms acting on a primary DNA damage. This might lead to the breakage-fusion-bridge cycle, where the broken chromosomes can join, thus forming a bi-centric chromosome that will be inevitable exposed to massive pulling forces upon attachment to microtubules during mitosis. The opposing pulling forces cause a chromosome breakage, thus providing new DNA break points for yet another fusion. Hence, once destabilized, the genome may undergo several rounds of structural changes.

The priming DNA breakage can occur by multiple mechanisms, but the relative importance remains unclear. The identified brake sites are both recurrent, e.g. they occur at specific hotspots, or random, thus suggesting a nonspecific mechanism of DNA damage (oxidative free radicals, ionizing radiation, or spontaneous DNA backbone hydrolysis). The non-random DNA breaks can arise near telomeres, as the DNA ends get exposed due to telomere attrition and become free for the double strand break repair, mostly via non-homologous end joining with another chromosome, thus generating a bi-centric chromosome. However, it should be noted that telomere shortening is not the only factor in genomic instability and tumor formation[28]. The primary break can be also formed at chromosome fragile sites, where DNA fork is frequently posing during replication stress and might eventually disassemble, thus exposing vulnerable DNA [29]. Surprisingly, the breakpoints identified at sites of copy number changes in cancer cells mostly do not overlap with the mapped fragile sites, thus suggesting other factors influencing the DNA strand breaks. The increasingly detailed map of human DNA will certainly bring new insight into the possible links between DNA secondary structure and sites of DNA breaks [13]. For example, recent large-scale genome profiling studies of breakpoints in cancer cells identified spatial clusters that are significantly enriched for potential G-quadruplex-forming sequences [30].

Recently, occurrence of DSBs in a close vicinity of centromeric DNA has been observed during mitosis in human cells *in vitro*. These pericentromeric breaks occur due to the merotelic attachments, where one kinetochore attaches to microtubules emanating from both spindle poles, thus exposing a chromatid to opposing pulling forces[31]. Similar pericentromeric breaks were observed also in tumor cells *in vivo*, and whole arm changes that could result from this type of breaks are frequently found in cancerous genomes. Furthermore, it has been suggested that lagging chromosomes can be damaged when the lagging DNA gets trapped within the cleavage furrow and brakes due to the forces of the actomyosin ring during cytokinesis [32]. Further research will be required to address how frequently these mitotic DNA breaks occur *in vivo* and whether they can explain the chromosomal rearrangements observed in tumors.

The lagging chromosomes are often left behind the main chromosome mass during cell division. These chromosomes, even if segregated properly, often form a micronucleus surrounded by its own nuclear envelope, hence isolated from the main nucleus. Recently, it has been shown that the replication of DNA trapped in the micronuclei is often defective, most likely due to the unbalanced sources of DNA replication machinery [33]. In several cases, a total "pulverization" of such a chromosome or chromosome part can be observed (called chromothripsis). The chromosome can get again reassembled and joins with the main chromosome mass during the next mitosis. Such abnormally reassembled chromosomes are observed in some specific tumor types at low frequency[34], and might also lead to copy number alterations, as some parts of the chromosome are lost or amplified.

4. Consequences of aneuploidy

The severe consequences of abnormal chromosome numbers in trisomy syndromes as well as the link of aneuploidy to cancer clearly suggest remarkable effects of aneuploidy on the physiology of eukaryotic cells. Recently, several model systems have been carefully analyzed in respect to the consequences of copy number changes. This research brought a plethora of observations of the phenotypes of aneuploid cells, but so far only a little understanding about the underlying molecular mechanisms.

4.1 Growth defect of aneuploid cells

Whole chromosomal aneuploidy has a detrimental effect in nearly all organisms analyzed so far, which is most frequently manifested by the remarkably slow growth or even cell death. Various developmental abnormalities and growth defects have been shown in many different organisms starting from *Schizosaccharomyces pombe* [35], *Saccharomyces cerevisiae* [36], Drosophila [37], *Caenorhabditis elegans* [38], mouse [39] and human [9]. This is in particular remarkable in response to monosomy, where one homologous chromosome is missing. Monosomy is nearly non-existent in normal, non-cancerous human cells, most likely due to a frequent haploinsufficiency of many human genes. In contrast, diploid budding yeasts cells with monosomy can survive, as there are only few haploinsufficient genes [40]. Yet, even in this case a population of cells with a normal diploid karyotype will be quickly selected [41]. Cancerous cells often show a monosomic pattern for individual chromosomes. However, as monosomy in tumor cells is often accompanied by multiple additional changes within their composite karyotype, we can assume that the haploinsufficiency is compensated for by other genomic changes.

Not only a loss of chromosomes detrimental; a presence of extra chromosomes impairs cell growth as well. The first studies linking aneuploidy to the decreased fitness of eukaryotic cells were conducted in primary fibroblasts from Down syndrome patients that were shown to proliferate more slowly than euploid control cells *in vitro* [42]. Moreover, aneuploid embryos are often characterized by slow intrauterinal growth and a lower birth weight. Similarly, trisomic human cells generated *in vitro* by a single chromosome transfer show frequently a slow growth, which is also observed in mouse trisomic cells obtained by selection of cells after Robertsonian translocation [39]. Experimentally generated disomic budding yeasts show a significant growth delay as well [36].

What exactly causes the growth defect that is often observed in cells with an extra chromosome remains an open question. It has been shown that it is not simply the presence of extra DNA, as an artificial chromosome engineered from non-transcribed human DNA does not cause a growth delay in budding yeasts [36]. Thus, an increased expression of the extra genes is necessary to trigger the detrimental effect. There are at least two principal possibilities. First, the phenotypic changes might be due to an effect of individual de-regulated gene(s) that affect pathways important for cell survival. As an example, disomy of chromosome 6 in budding yeast is not viable, whereas other disomies are, and the likely explanation is the increased expression of *TUB2* and *ACT1*, which were previously shown to interfere with cell viability [36]. Further lines of evidence support this idea. For example, some regions of the genome are rarely amplified, which might be due to the presence of a gene whose over-expression would not be compatible with survival. Addition of an extra chromosome might be also advantageous, if for example a specific gene supporting proliferation is carried on the extra chromosome.

The second possibility is that the defect of aneuploid cells is due to a cumulative effect of low but chronic overexpression of many genes. For example, over-expression of up to a few thousands of genes on a single human chromosome might bring the cellular homeostasis out of balance. It has been found that the gene expression analyzed on the level of mRNA roughly corresponds to the gene copy numbers in most of the organisms analyzed so far. This suggests that all the genes of the extra chromosome are transcribed and likely also translated, thus leading to the presence of extra proteins. One of the current models hypothesizes that the overexpression of extra copies of specific genes might lead to accumulation of useless proteins that impair general cellular proteostasis. This interesting option is discussed in more details below.

4.2 Protein homeostasis in aneuploids

The hypothesis of impaired protein homeostasis in aneuploid cells originates mostly from recent analysis of artificially prepared haploid yeast strains with a single disomic chromosome. The presence of an extra chromosome significantly decreases the growth rates and renders the cells sensitive to drugs that target transcription, translation and protein degradation via the proteasome. Thus, it was proposed that the presence of an extra chromosome leads to imbalances in protein composition that might be partially compensated for by increased protein degradation. This conclusion is further supported by the fact that disomic budding yeasts that evolved to improve their growth rates often acquired mutations in Ubp6 gene [43]. This gene encodes a ubiquitin-specific protease that removes ubiquitin from ubiquitin chains and negatively regulates proteasomal degradation. Thus, increased permissivity of the proteasome improves the growth of artificially prepared disomic budding yeast [43]. Rapid development in proteomics enabled analysis of protein levels in budding yeast cells. Interestingly, using the model disomic cell lines, Torres et al. [43] showed that although the transcript levels correspond to the copy number changes, the corresponding protein levels are partially compensated, that means expressed at levels more similar to the abundance identified in normal haploid cells. This compensatory effect was observed in approximately 20 % of proteins and significantly more often for subunits of multimolecular complexes. However, it remains unclear whether the increased proteasome activity improves the cellular growth by enhancing the compensatory effect, or rather by a more general increase of turnover of cellular proteins. Moreover, no similar compensatory effects were detected by analysis of aneuploid budding yeasts with a more complex karyotype [44], leaving the question whether the compensation of protein levels occurs and affects growth of aneuploid cells open for future experiments.

Using Drosophila as another excellent model for analysis of the effects of aneuploidy, recent research revealed a significant buffering of genes in aneuploid regions [45, 46]. The authors also identified that the buffering is more efficient for differentially expressed genes than for genes that are expressed ubiquitously. Remarkably, the buffering of copy number changes on both autosomes and sex chromosomes occurs on the transcriptional level, making the Drosophila model significantly different from mammalian and yeast model systems. Further research will be required to confirm the buffering on transcriptional level in Drosophila (and the lack thereof in yeasts and mammalian cells) and to identify the reasons of the differences.

4.3 Global response to aneuploidy

One of the interesting questions is whether aneuploidy elicits a specific physiological response in eukaryotes, or whether its effects depend on the extra chromosomes due to a deregulation of cellular pathways depending on the specific karyotype combination. Addressing this question is important as the existence of a specific response to aneuploidy, or the identification of essential adaptations that are required for survival of aneuploid cells might provide new targets for therapy of aneuploid tumors.

The most comprehensive analysis so far was performed in two different models of budding yeast aneuploids. Microarray analysis of haploid disomic budding yeasts shows a common gene expression pattern [36] that was identified previously as the environmental stress response (ESR) signature [47]. Moreover, an increased expression of ribosomal biogenesis and nucleic acid metabolism genes and down-regulation of carbohydrate energy metabolism genes were determined under growth conditions that normalized the growth differences between euploid and aneuploid strains [36]. Using budding yeast with complex aneuploidies that originated from aberrant meiosis of polyploid cells, Pavelka et al. revealed the ESR expression pattern in three out of five analyzed strains, but only when the highest stringency analysis was applied [44]. No other specific pathway deregulations were identified. Thus, although it appears that the rather general stress response is often activated in disomic budding yeast, no clear expression pattern shared by different types of aneuploid cells was identified. The differences in the two studies might be explained by the a difference between disomic and complex aneuploidies. Moreover, possible genome instability of aneuploid cells [48] might mask gene expression patterns.

There is only limited data regarding the effects of aneuploidy on gene expression in other eukaryotes. Using model trisomic human cells that were created by transfer of individual chromosomes into both normal and transformed human cells, no specific pathway deregulation was identified [49], although it should be noted that the complex pattern of transcriptional deregulation was not analyzed in detail. Another study used trisomic mouse embryonic fibroblasts (MEFs) harboring an extra chromosome 1, 13, 16, or 19 [39]. Similarly, microarray analysis of mRNA levels revealed a gene-dosage dependent increase of mRNA levels of genes encoded on the extra chromosomes, as well as other deregulations, but no specific expression pattern in these trisomic MEFs [39]. Analysis of transcriptional data from Drosophila cells with various segmental and chromosomal aneuploidies identified no general response to the chromosome number changes [45, 46]. Thus, further research will be required to address the question whether all eukaryotic cells show a unified response to aneuploidy, or whether this is something to be observed only in budding yeast.

Recent results obtained from a drug sensitivity screen using the above mentioned MEF cells suggest that there is a common defect in aneuploid cells. The authors tested approximately 20 drugs inducing genotoxic, proteotoxic as well as energy stress; most of them showed no specific effect except for AICAR, chloroquine and 17-AAG [50]. AICAR induces energy stress, leading to the activation of the AMP-activated protein kinase AMPK1, whereas 17-AAG is a derivative of Geldanamycin, which inhibits the heat shock responsive chaperone Hsp90. Chloroquine, also used as an anti-malaric drug, was found to inhibit autophagy, a protein degradation pathway. These results correspond with the previously observed changes in energy metabolism and protein homeostasis in aneuploid budding yeast, thus pointing out these molecular processes as the possible pitfalls of aneuploidy. The authors also showed that these three identified compounds inhibit growth of aneuploid cancer cell lines significantly more than the growth of euploid cancer cell lines [50]. Thus, the drugs that inhibit growth of trisomic cells might potentially be useful for treatment of highly aneuploid cancer types. Indeed, autophagy inhibiting drugs are currently tested for cancer treatments.

4.4 Benefits of aneuploidy

Aneuploidy can also provide benefits to the cells as is documented by the fact that aneuploidy conveys resistance to antimycotic drugs in the human pathogene *Candida albicans* [51]. Aneuploid and polyploid strains of budding yeast *Saccharomyces cerevisiae* can be frequently found in nature, and multiple laboratory strains, in particular the ones that contain various deletions, show some degree of aneuploidy [52]. The association with a deletion mutation suggests that aneuploidy arises as a consequence of these mutations or that it might provide some compensation of the effect of specific mutations.

The decision whether aneuploidy will be beneficial or detrimental is likely influenced by the type of aneuploidy and the type of selection imposed by the environment. Experimentally created budding yeast cells that contain one extra chromosome show a significant growth impairment and increased sensitivity to numerous drugs [36], however, *in vitro* evolution lead to selection of fast growing cell populations adapted to disomy [43]. Aneuploid budding yeasts that arose via meiosis of triploid parents do not show a remarkable growth defect, and their karyotype confers an increased phenotypic variability, as assessed by altered sensitivity to multiple drugs in comparison to the original euploid wild type [44]. The sporulation efficiency of triploid parents is very low and thus likely only karyotype combinations with the least detrimental effect on viability survive. The various compositions arising from the meiosis could lead to chromosome combinations that provide a compensation of the imbalances. Moreover, aneuploid cells might be chromosomally unstable, thus allowing continuous "reinvention" of the karyotype composition during various drug treatments, a phenomenon that resembles the enhanced resistance acquisition in chromosomally unstable composite aneuploid cancer cells [5] [53]. Further investigations should address the mechanisms of the increased fitness in aneuploid cells.

How can aneuploidy be advantageous? One can envision that an addition of a single chromosome triggers a stress response, as it has been shown in budding yeast. Activation of a stress response to one stress factor can potentially protect cells against another stress factors. Another possibility is that aneuploidy increases chromosomal instability and thus accelerates evolution of a clone with a karyotype that provides an advantage under specific conditions. A recent study revealed that aneuploid fission and budding yeasts indeed display an increased level of chromosome missegregation, DNA damage and mitotic recombination, compared to haploid yeast [35, 48]. Similarly, aneuploid MEF cells were able to immortalize faster than normal diploid MEFs [39]. Since immortalization is an event that requires multiple mutations of various genes leading to increased proliferation, this finding could be due to an increased mutation rate as it was observed for aneuploid yeasts. Taken together, the observations so far suggest that despite the adverse effects of addition of a single (or few) chromosome, the aneuploid cells can adapt to the situation and these adaptations may provide new characteristics that may be advantageous under specific conditions. It will be interesting to investigate what molecular mechanisms are responsible for the increased genome instability in aneuploid cells and how this can contribute to increased fitness.

5. Aneuploidy and cancer

The vast majority of cancer cells contain abnormal chromosome numbers (Fig. 3) - approximately 75 % of heamatopoietical cancers and 90% of solid tumors consists of cells with abnormal chromosome numbers [26]. Recently, a comprehensive analysis of somatic copy number alterations across human cancers revealed that nearly a quarter of the entire genome of cancer cells is affected by a whole arm or a whole chromosome copy number changes, whereas approximately 10 % shows small, site specific change, so called focal SCNAs [13]. Many of these changes are non-random, with strong preferences across cancer lineages, thus implying that selection plays an important role. The remarkable prevalence of aneuploidy in cancer has been noticed already at the end of the 19th century and aneuploidy was even proposed to trigger tumorigenesis [54]. However, with discoveries of tumor-suppressor genes and oncogenes, another view won appreciation that aneuploidy is rather a side-effect of gene mutations that are the real triggers of malignancy [25].

One of the major obstacles in causatively linking CIN and aneuploidy with tumorigenesis was the lack of evidence that mutations triggering CIN are also causing cancer. For example, mutations in SAC components clearly show a CIN phenotype, and although mutations in SAC genes can be found in chromosomally unstable colon cancers, the frequency is very low [55]. Recently, an interesting link was found by identification of the causal mutations of a congenital syndrome called Mosaic Variegated Aneuploidy. MVA is a rare recessive constitutional mosaicism of chromosomal aneuploidy caused by a germline mutation in BUB1B, which encodes BubR1, a key SAC protein [56]. Approximately 25 % of cells from MVA patients carry variable monosomies and trisomies, with multiple different chromosomes involved. Importantly, the syndrome is associated with a 50% risk of early childhood cancer.

Only recently the hypothesis that aneuploidy triggers cancer could be tested more rigorously. Several mouse models have been developed to address the question whether altered chromosome numbers can trigger tumorigenesis. Most of these mouse models carry a mutation in one of the SAC genes, thus reducing the ability of cells to avoid incorrect chromosome segregation. Depending on the type of mutation, this leads to variable levels of chromosome missegregation, resulting in ongoing chromosome instability and increased frequency of cells with variable karyotypes. Indeed, many of these mouse models carrying either a deletion of one of the gene copies (as deletion of both copies is usually embryonic lethal) or a hypomorphic allele (labeled H), are more tumor-prone than the wild type

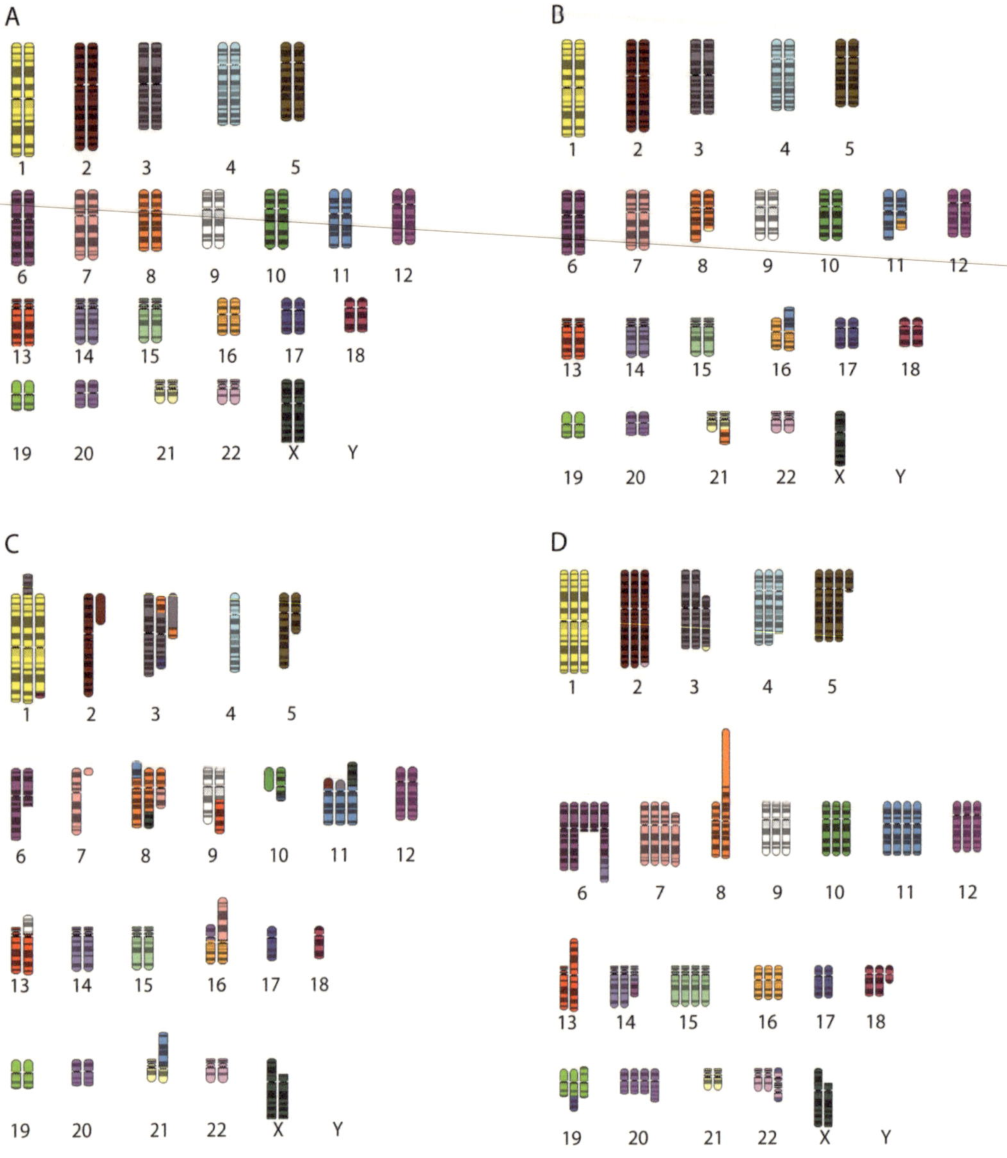

Skygrams (graphical depiction of spectral karyotyping) of normal human tissue (A); cancerous cells from acute myeloid leukemia (B), ovarian adenocarcinoma (C) and from colorectal cancer (D). Mitelman Database of Chromosome Aberrations and Gene Fusions in Cancer (http://cgap.nci.nih.gov/Chromosomes/Mitelman).

Fig. 3. Variable karyotypes in cancer cells.

mouse, in particular when exposed to carcinogen. Several of the mouse models show an increased tumor incidence per se, in particular defects in Bub1, Mad1, Mad2 and others (for an excellent review on the mouse models, see [57]). Interestingly, there is no direct correlation between the probability of cancer development and the degree of aneuploidy. For example, $Bub1^{-/H}$ and $Bub1^{H/H}$ mouse models show similar levels of aneuploidy [58] as

Rae2$^{+/-}$ -Bub3$^{+/-}$ [59] or Rae2$^{+/-}$-Nup98$^{+/-}$ [60] double heterozygous mice, yet the latter ones do not show any increase in spontaneous tumorigenesis. Moreover, not all tissues are comparably prone to aneuploidy-associated tumorigenesis. Additionally, some mutations in spindle-assembly checkpoint genes were shown to prevent or at least delay the occurrence of tumors in some tissues. For example, in Cenp-E heterozygous mice the levels of spontaneous liver tumor formation are much lower than in the controls [61].

Not only gene mutations that impair the protein function, but also changing the expression levels can lead to aneuploidy and tumorigenesis. Transgenic mice engineered to overexpress Mad2 have cells with widespread chromosomal instability and develop various types of neoplasms. Interestingly, continued overexpression of Mad2 is not required for tumor maintenance, suggesting that whereas the chromosomal instability was important for initiating carcinogenesis, it is dispensable for maintaining the neoplastic phenotype [57]. Other genes were associated with cancer formation and triggering chromosomal instability as well. For example, constitutive expression of cyclin E results in karyotypic instability in mammalian cells [62] and high levels of cyclin E are correlated to breast, endometrial and skin cancers, that also show increased aneuploidy [63]. However, it should be noted when using model systems with gene mutations, it is often difficult to distinguish whether the observed effects are indeed due to chromosomal instability or due to as yet unknown function of the analyzed factor. Thus, to address the question whether tumorigenesis can be triggered by chromosomal instability and aneuploidy, it would be necessary to develop a model lacking any initial mutation, yet showing high chromosomal instability and aneuploidy.

So far only one experimental set up fulfils this condition. In this model, p53 deficient tetraploid mouse mammary epithelial cells were subcutaneously injected into a nude mouse. Tetraploid cells are inherently instable and the frequency of chromosome missegregation is significantly increased in comparison to diploids in many models analyzed so far [25]. Thus, tetraploidy alone can facilitate aneuploidy. Whereas none of the mice injected with isogenic diploid cells developed tumors, 10 out of 39 mice injected with tetraploid cells did [24]. The tumors were near-tetraploid showing multiple chromosome re-arrangements. Taken together, it appears plausible that aneuploidy and chromosomal instability itself can facilitate tumorigenesis, most likely by providing a variability that serves as a material for selection. It will be interesting to uncover the molecular mechanisms underlying chromosomal instability of aneuploid and tetraploid cells and how exactly this facilitates tumorigenesis.

6. Role of aneuploidy in neurodegeneration and aging

Recent discoveries that abnormal chromosome numbers impact on protein homeostasis has pointed out a possible link to neurodegenerative diseases and instigated the interest in the association of aneuploidy and neuropathologies. Neurons might be particularly sensitive to random genetic changes: diploid population cannot outgrow cells with abnormal karyotypes because neurons are mostly postmitotic.

Interestingly, an increasing body of evidence indicates that the adult brain cells show low levels of aneuploidy (0.5 - 0.7%) and might be viewed as a mosaic of cells with variable genotypes [64]. The level of chromosomal aneuploidy correlates with diseases affecting the brain [65]. In particular, the percentage of aneuploid cells is higher in brains from patients with Alzheimer disease (AD) than in the healthy population. This is likely not restricted to neuronal tissues as lymphocytes and splenocytes from the AD patients are aneuploid as well and exhibit defects in mitosis and chromosomal segregation [66]. It should be noted that the the fluorescence *in situ* hybridization (FISH) of interphase cells that is used for aneuploidy evaluation in tissues of dominantly postmitotic cells is particularly prone to artifacts. So far, detailed data are lacking about the effects of the aneuploidy on neuronal cells, but the cells appear to be fully functional and the expression levels are altered according to the copy number changes [67]. The frequent occurrence of aneuploidy in the brain raises an attractive possibility that aneuploidy is required for neuronal functions, for example by contributing to the functional variability of neuronal types. On the other hand, the association of increased aneuploidy levels with AD suggests pathological effects of abnormal karyotypes in neurons.

Aneuploidy and genome instability, in particular DNA damage, are also linked to aging, as is supported by the observation that the frequency of chromosomal aberrations in senescence-accelerated strains of mice increases [68]. Similarly, frequency of aneuploidy increases with age in fibroblasts taken at successive times from the same donors as part of the Baltimore Longitudinal Study of Aging [69]. Similarly as for cancer, it remains a matter of debate whether increased levels of DNA damage and aneuploidy might be a primary trigger of cellular aging, or whether they are mere consequences of other age-associated changes. Lushnikova et al. demonstrated that aging increased specific forms of genomic instability, and proposed that the probability of accumulation of certain chromosomal abnormalities linked to cancer development might increase with aging [70].

An interesting supporting evidence of the link between aneuploidy and aging came recently from a different model. Mouse model expressing low levels of spindle assembly checkpoint protein kinase BubR1 develop progressive aneuploidy, no significant cancer increase and multiple aging-associated phenotypes [71]. Although the authors suggest that BubR1 might regulate aging, another attractive hypothesis is that aneuploidy in these cells accelerates the onset of aging.

7. Aneuploidy in stem cells

An emerging importance of aneuploidy in embryonic stem cells (ESCs) research is substantiated by two interesting phenomena. First, it was observed that the early human and mouse embryos contain remarkable numbers of chromosomally aberrant cells. Second, *in vitro* cultivation of both embryonic and adult stem cells leads to the accumulation of chromosomal abnormalities. As the usage of stem cells for human therapies is accompanied by great expectations, the causes and consequences of aneuploidy in stem cells become a subject of intense research.

Eukaryotic cells maintain genomic integrity through control checkpoint mechanisms, but ES cells differ significantly in the mechanism of cell cycle regulation and it's link to checkpoints [72]. This is most likely due to the requirement for rapid cell divisions during the early development, which is achieved by relaxing the cell cycle control and uncoupling the checkpoint control from apoptosis. The control systems are activated later, when differentiation begins [73]. The ES cells compensate the lack of checkpoint coupling to cell cycle and apoptosis by increased repair efficiency after DNA damage [74]. Nevertheless, the lack of the checkpoint control leads to a high frequency of chromosomal mosaicism (as high as 50 %) in normal human preimplantation embryos, as was revealed by fluorescence in situ hybridization (FISH). Upon differentiation, the efficient checkpoint control and the coupling to apoptosis are established [75]. This ensures that after the cleavage stage, embryos undergo a selection that prefers euploidy, which results in lower aneuploidy levels [76] [77]. How exactly this selection occurs and what is the effect on the efficiency of the early embryonic survival remains poorly understood.

For use in therapies, large amounts of stem cells need to be prepared *in vitro*. Remarkably, stem cells acquire chromosomal aberrations in culture in a process known as culture adaptation [78] [79]. These aberrations may increase the tumorigenicity of the ES cells [80] and impair their differentiation capacity, rendering the stem cells dangerous and ineffective for therapy. Previously, it has been already shown that transplantation of human adult stem cells may result in tumor formation [81], possibly due to the chromosomal aberrations. Thus, validating the genomic integrity and developing culturing strategies that would minimize the occurrence of aneuploidy in stem cells is essential for future development of their therapeutic potential.

8. Closing remarks

More than a hundred years ago, abnormal karyotypes were suggested to have a detrimental effect on cellular physiology and ultimately to cause cancer. Now, we slowly collect information that suggest indeed abnormal chromosome number, even so minimal such as gain or loss of a single chromosome, remarkably alter physiology of eukaryotic cells. They can lead to imbalance of protein homeostasis, changes in genome stability and altered growth characteristics. To what degree these physiological changes are responsible for aneuploidy linked diseases such as Down syndrome or multiple variegated aneuploidy remains to be addressed by future experiments. The emerging association of aneuploidy with cancer and with neuropathologic diseases might provide novel opportunities for developing efficient treatments of these diseases.

9. References

[1] Ono S (1971) Genetic implication of karyological instability of malignant somatic cells. *Physiological reviews* 51, 496-526.

[2] Lengauer C, Kinzler KW and Vogelstein B (1998) Genetic instabilities in human cancers. *Nature* 396, 643-649.

[3] Thomas P, Harvey S, Gruner T and Fenech M (2008) The buccal cytome and micronucleus frequency is substantially altered in Down's syndrome and normal ageing compared to young healthy controls. *Mutation Research/Fundamental and Molecular Mechanisms of Mutagenesis* 638, 37-47.

[4] Walther A, Houlston R and Tomlinson I (2008) Association between chromosomal instability and prognosis in colorectal cancer: a meta-analysis. *Gut* 57, 941-950.

[5] McClelland SE, Burrell RA and Swanton C (2009) Chromosomal instability: A composite phenotype that influences sensitivity to chemotherapy. *Cell Cycle* 8, 3262-3266.

[6] Hassold T, Hall H and Hunt P (2007) The origin of human aneuploidy: where we have been, where we are going. *Human Molecular Genetics* 16, R203-208.

[7] Lenroot RK, Lee NR and Giedd JN (2009) Effects of sex chromosome aneuploidies on brain development: evidence from neuroimaging studies. *Dev Disabil Res Rev* 15, 318-327.
[8] Prestel M, Feller C and Becker P (2010) Dosage compensation and the global re-balancing of aneuploid genomes. *Genome Biology* 11, 216.
[9] Hassold T, Abruzzo M, Adkins K, Griffin D, Merrill M, Millie E, Saker D, Shen J and Zaragoza M (1996) Human aneuploidy: incidence, origin, and etiology. *Environ Mol Mutagen* 28, 167-175.
[10] Hassold T, Hall H and Hunt P (2007) The origin of human aneuploidy: where we have been, where we are going. *Hum Mol Genet* 16 Spec No. 2, R203-208.
[11] Iafrate AJ, Feuk L, Rivera MN, Listewnik ML, Donahoe PK, Qi Y, Scherer SW and Lee C (2004) Detection of large-scale variation in the human genome. *Nat Genet* 36, 949-951.
[12] Girirajan S, Campbell CD and Eichler EE (2011) Human copy number variation and complex genetic disease. *Annu Rev Genet* 45, 203-226.
[13] Beroukhim R, Mermel CH, Porter D, Wei G, Raychaudhuri S, Donovan J, Barretina J, Boehm JS, Dobson J, Urashima M, Mc Henry KT, Pinchback RM, Ligon AH, Cho YJ, Haery L, Greulich H, Reich M, Winckler W, Lawrence MS, Weir BA, Tanaka KE, Chiang DY, Bass AJ, Loo A, Hoffman C, Prensner J, Liefeld T, Gao Q, Yecies D, Signoretti S, Maher E, Kaye FJ, Sasaki H, Tepper JE, Fletcher JA, Tabernero J, Baselga J, Tsao MS, Demichelis F, Rubin MA, Janne PA, Daly MJ, Nucera C, Levine RL, Ebert BL, Gabriel S, Rustgi AK, Antonescu CR, Ladanyi M, Letai A, Garraway LA, Loda M, Beer DG, True LD, Okamoto A, Pomeroy SL, Singer S, Golub TR, Lander ES, Getz G, Sellers WR and Meyerson M (2010) The landscape of somatic copy-number alteration across human cancers. *Nature* 463, 899-905.
[14] Thompson SL and Compton DA (2010) Proliferation of aneuploid human cells is limited by a p53-dependent mechanism. *J Cell Biol* 188, 369-381.
[15] Bunz F, Fauth C, Speicher MR, Dutriaux A, Sedivy JM, Kinzler KW, Vogelstein B and Lengauer C (2002) Targeted inactivation of p53 in human cells does not result in aneuploidy. *Cancer Res* 62, 1129-1133.
[16] Musacchio A and Salmon ED (2007) The spindle-assembly checkpoint in space and time. *Nat Rev Mol Cell Biol* 8, 379-393.
[17] Nilsson J, Yekezare M, Minshull J and Pines J (2008) The APC/C maintains the spindle assembly checkpoint by targeting Cdc20 for destruction. *Nat Cell Biol* 10, 1411-1420.
[18] Guacci V, Koshland D and Strunnikov A (1997) A direct link between sister chromatid cohesion and chromosome condensation revealed through the analysis of MCD1 in S. cerevisiae. *Cell* 91, 47-57.
[19] Michaelis C, Ciosk R and Nasmyth K (1997) Cohesins: chromosomal proteins that prevent premature separation of sister chromatids. *Cell* 91, 35-45.
[20] Lister LM, Kouznetsova A, Hyslop LA, Kalleas D, Pace SL, Barel JC, Nathan A, Floros V, Adelfalk C, Watanabe Y, Jessberger R, Kirkwood TB, Hoog C and Herbert M (2010) Age-related meiotic segregation errors in mammalian oocytes are preceded by depletion of cohesin and Sgo2. *Curr Biol* 20, 1511-1521.
[21] Chiang T, Duncan FE, Schindler K, Schultz RM and Lampson MA (2011) Evidence that weakened centromere cohesion is a leading cause of age-related aneuploidy in oocytes. *Curr Biol* 20, 1522-1528.

[22] Solomon DA, Kim T, Diaz-Martinez LA, Fair J, Elkahloun AG, Harris BT, Toretsky JA, Rosenberg SA, Shukla N, Ladanyi M, Samuels Y, James CD, Yu H, Kim J-S and Waldman T (2011) Mutational Inactivation of STAG2 Causes Aneuploidy in Human Cancer. *Nature* 333, 1039-1043.

[23] Storchova Z, Breneman A, Cande J, Dunn J, Burbank K, O'Toole E and Pellman D (2006) Genome-wide genetic analysis of polyploidy in yeast. *Nature* 443, 541-547.

[24] Fujiwara T, Bandi M, Nitta M, Ivanova EV, Bronson RT and Pellman D (2005) Cytokinesis failure generating tetraploids promotes tumorigenesis in p53-null cells. *Nature* 437, 1043-1047.

[25] Storchova Z and Pellman D (2004) From polyploidy to aneuploidy, genome instability and cancer. *Nat Rev Mol Cell Biol* 5, 45-54.

[26] Storchova Z and Kuffer C (2008) The consequences of tetraploidy and aneuploidy. *J Cell Sci* 121, 3859-3866.

[27] Stankiewicz P and Lupski JR (2010) Structural variation in the human genome and its role in disease. *Annu Rev Med* 61, 437-455.

[28] Desmaze C, Soria J-C, Freulet-MarriÃ¨re M-A, Mathieu N and Sabatier L (2003) Telomere-driven genomic instability in cancer cells. *Cancer Letters* 194, 173-182.

[29] Debatisse M, Le Tallec Bt, Letessier A, Dutrillaux B and Brison O (2011) Common fragile sites: mechanisms of instability revisited. *Trends in Genetics* 28, 22-32.

[30] De S and Michor F (2011) DNA secondary structures and epigenetic determinants of cancer genome evolution. *Nat Struct Mol Biol* 18, 950-955.

[31] Guerrero AA, Gamero MC, Trachana V, Futterer A, Pacios-Bras C, Diaz-Concha NP, Cigudosa JC, Martinez AC and van Wely KH (2010) Centromere-localized breaks indicate the generation of DNA damage by the mitotic spindle. *Proc Natl Acad Sci U S A* 107, 4159-4164.

[32] Janssen A, van der Burg M, Szuhai K, Kops GJ and Medema RH (2011) Chromosome segregation errors as a cause of DNA damage and structural chromosome aberrations. *Science* 333, 1895-1898.

[33] Crasta K, Ganem NJ, Dagher R, Lantermann AB, Ivanova EV, Pan Y, Nezi L, Protopopov A, Chowdhury D and Pellman D (2011) DNA breaks and chromosome pulverization from errors in mitosis. *Nature* 482, 53-58.

[34] Stephens PJ, Greenman CD, Fu B, Yang F, Bignell GR, Mudie LJ, Pleasance ED, Lau KW, Beare D, Stebbings LA, McLaren S, Lin ML, McBride DJ, Varela I, Nik-Zainal S, Leroy C, Jia M, Menzies A, Butler AP, Teague JW, Quail MA, Burton J, Swerdlow H, Carter NP, Morsberger LA, Iacobuzio-Donahue C, Follows GA, Green AR, Flanagan AM, Stratton MR, Futreal PA and Campbell PJ (2011) Massive genomic rearrangement acquired in a single catastrophic event during cancer development. *Cell* 144, 27-40.

[35] Niwa O, Tange Y and Kurabayashi A (2006) Growth arrest and chromosome instability in aneuploid yeast. *Yeast* 23, 937-950.

[36] Torres EM, Sokolsky T, Tucker CM, Chan LY, Boselli M, Dunham MJ and Amon A (2007) Effects of aneuploidy on cellular physiology and cell division in haploid yeast. *Science* 317, 916-924.

[37] Lindsley DL, Sandler L, Baker BS, Carpenter ATC, Denell RE, Hall JC, Jacobs PA, Miklos GLG, Davis BK, Gethmann RC, Hardy RW, Hessler A, Miller SM, Nozawa

H, Parry DM and Gould-Somero M (1972) Segmental aneuploidy and the genetic gross structure of the Drosophila genome. *Genetics* 71, 157-184.
[38] Hodgkin J (2005) Karyotype, ploidy, and gene dosage. *WormBook*, 1-9.
[39] Williams BR, Prabhu VR, Hunter KE, Glazier CM, Whittaker CA, Housman DE and Amon A (2008) Aneuploidy affects proliferation and spontaneous immortalization in mammalian cells. *Science* 322, 703-709.
[40] Deutschbauer AM, Jaramillo DF, Proctor M, Kumm J, Hillenmeyer ME, Davis RW, Nislow C and Giaever G (2005) Mechanisms of Haploinsufficiency Revealed by Genome-Wide Profiling in Yeast. *Genetics* 169, 1915-1925.
[41] Reid RJD, Sunjevaric I, Voth WP, Ciccone S, Du W, Olsen AE, Stillman DJ and Rothstein R (2008) Chromosome-Scale Genetic Mapping Using a Set of 16 Conditionally Stable Saccharomyces cerevisiae Chromosomes. *Genetics* 180, 1799-1808.
[42] Segal DJ and McCoy EE (1974) Studies on Down's syndrome in tissue culture. I. Growth rates and protein contents of fibroblast cultures. *J Cell Physiol* 83, 85-90.
[43] Torres EM, Dephoure N, Panneerselvam A, Tucker CM, Whittaker CA, Gygi SP, Dunham MJ and Amon A (2010) Identification of aneuploidy-tolerating mutations. *Cell* 143, 71-83.
[44] Pavelka N, Rancati G, Zhu J, Bradford WD, Saraf A, Florens L, Sanderson BW, Hattem GL and Li R (2010) Aneuploidy confers quantitative proteome changes and phenotypic variation in budding yeast. *Nature* 468, 321-325.
[45] Stenberg P, Lundberg LE, Johansson A-M, RydÃ©n P, Svensson MJ and Larsson J (2009) Buffering of Segmental and Chromosomal Aneuploidies in Drosophila melanogaster. *PLoS Genet* 5, e1000465.
[46] Zhang Y, Malone JH, Powell SK, Periwal V, Spana E, MacAlpine DM and Oliver B (2010) Expression in Aneuploid <italic>Drosophila</italic> S2 Cells. *PLoS Biol* 8, e1000320.
[47] Gasch AP, Spellman PT, Kao CM, Carmel-Harel O, Eisen MB, Storz G, Botstein D and Brown PO (2000) Genomic Expression Programs in the Response of Yeast Cells to Environmental Changes. *Mol Biol Cell* 11, 4241-4257.
[48] Sheltzer JM, Blank HM, Pfau SJ, Tange Y, George BM, Humpton TJ, Brito IL, Hiraoka Y, Niwa O and Amon A (2011) Aneuploidy Drives Genomic Instability in Yeast. *Science* 333, 1026-1030.
[49] Upender MB, Habermann JK, McShane LM, Korn EL, Barrett JC, Difilippantonio MJ and Ried T (2004) Chromosome transfer induced aneuploidy results in complex dysregulation of the cellular transcriptome in immortalized and cancer cells. *Cancer Res* 64, 6941-6949.
[50] Tang YC, Williams BR, Siegel JJ and Amon A (2011) Identification of aneuploidy-selective antiproliferation compounds. *Cell* 144, 499-512.
[51] Selmecki A, Forche A and Berman J (2006) Aneuploidy and isochromosome formation in drug-resistant Candida albicans. *Science* 313, 367-370.
[52] Hughes TR, Roberts CJ, Dai H, Jones AR, Meyer MR, Slade D, Burchard J, Dow S, Ward TR, Kidd MJ, Friend SH and Marton MJ (2000) Widespread aneuploidy revealed by DNA microarray expression profiling. *Nat Genet* 25, 333-337.
[53] Lee AJ, Endesfelder D, Rowan AJ, Walther A, Birkbak NJ, Futreal PA, Downward J, Szallasi Z, Tomlinson IP, Howell M, Kschischo M and Swanton C (2011)

Chromosomal instability confers intrinsic multidrug resistance. *Cancer Res* 71, 1858-1870.

[54] Boveri T (1902) Ueber mehrpolige Mitosen als Mittel zur Analyse des Zellkerns. *Verh. Ges. Wurzburg (n. f.)* xxxv, pp. 67-90.

[55] Cahill DP, Lengauer C, Yu J, Riggins GJ, Willson JKV, Markowitz SD, Kinzler KW and Vogelstein B (1998) Mutations of mitotic checkpoint genes in human cancers. *Nature* 392, 300-303.

[56] Hanks S, Coleman K, Reid S, Plaja A, Firth H, Fitzpatrick D, Kidd A, Mehes K, Nash R, Robin N, Shannon N, Tolmie J, Swansbury J, Irrthum A, Douglas J and Rahman N (2004) Constitutional aneuploidy and cancer predisposition caused by biallelic mutations in BUB1B. *Nat Genet* 36, 1159-1161.

[57] Ricke RM, van Ree JH and van Deursen JM (2008) Whole chromosome instability and cancer: a complex relationship. *Trends Genet* 24, 457-466.

[58] Jeganathan K, Malureanu L, Baker DJ, Abraham SC and van Deursen JM (2007) Bub1 mediates cell death in response to chromosome missegregation and acts to suppress spontaneous tumorigenesis. *J Cell Biol* 179, 255-267.

[59] Babu JR, Jeganathan KB, Baker DJ, Wu X, Kang-Decker N and van Deursen JM (2003) Rae1 is an essential mitotic checkpoint regulator that cooperates with Bub3 to prevent chromosome missegregation. *J Cell Biol* 160, 341-353.

[60] Jeganathan KB, Malureanu L and van Deursen JM (2005) The Rae1-Nup98 complex prevents aneuploidy by inhibiting securin degradation. *Nature* 438, 1036-1039.

[61] Weaver BA, Silk AD, Montagna C, Verdier-Pinard P and Cleveland DW (2007) Aneuploidy acts both oncogenically and as a tumor suppressor. *Cancer Cell* 11, 25-36.

[62] Spruck CH, Won KA and Reed SI (1999) Deregulated cyclin E induces chromosome instability. *Nature* 401, 297-300.

[63] Dutta A, Chandra R, Leiter LM and Lester S (1995) Cyclins as markers of tumor proliferation: immunocytochemical studies in breast cancer. *Proc Natl Acad Sci U S A* 92, 5386-5390.

[64] Rehen SK, Yung YC, McCreight MP, Kaushal D, Yang AH, Almeida BSV, Kingsbury MA, Cabral KtMS, McConnell MJ, Anliker B, Fontanoz M and Chun J (2005) Constitutional Aneuploidy in the Normal Human Brain. *The Journal of Neuroscience* 25, 2176-2180.

[65] Iourov IY, Vorsanova SG, Lichr T, Kolotii AD and Yurov YB,2009). Vol. 18 2656-2669

[66] Petrozzi L, Lucetti C, Scarpato R, Gambaccini G, Trippi F, Bernardini S, Del Dotto P, Migliore L and Bonuccelli U (2002) Cytogenetic alterations in lymphocytes of Alzheimer's disease and Parkinson's disease patients. *Neurological Sciences* 23, s97-s98.

[67] Kaushal D, Contos JJA, Treuner K, Yang AH, Kingsbury MA, Rehen SK, McConnell MJ, Okabe M, Barlow C and Chun J (2003) Alteration of Gene Expression by Chromosome Loss in the Postnatal Mouse Brain. *The Journal of Neuroscience* 23, 5599-5606.

[68] Nisitani S, Hosokawa M, Sasaki MS, Yasuoka K, Naiki H, Matsushita T and Takeda T (1990) Acceleration of chromosome aberrations in senescence-accelerated strains of mice. *Mutat Res* 237, 221-228.

[69] Mukherjee AB and Thomas S (1997) A Longitudinal Study of Human Age-Related Chromosomal Analysis in Skin Fibroblasts. *Experimental Cell Research* 235, 161-169.

[70] Lushnikova T, Bouska A, Odvody J, Dupont WD and Eischen CM (2011) Aging mice have increased chromosome instability that is exacerbated by elevated Mdm2 expression. *Oncogene* 30, 4622-4631.

[71] Baker DJ, Jeganathan KB, Cameron JD, Thompson M, Juneja S, Kopecka A, Kumar R, Jenkins RB, de Groen PC, Roche P and van Deursen JM (2004) BubR1 insufficiency causes early onset of aging-associated phenotypes and infertility in mice. *Nat Genet* 36, 744-749.

[72] Ambartsumyan G and Clark AT (2008) Aneuploidy and early human embryo development. *Human Molecular Genetics* 17, R10-R15.

[73] Mantel C, Guo Y, Lee MR, Kim MK, Han MK, Shibayama H, Fukuda S, Yoder MC, Pelus LM, Kim KS and Broxmeyer HE (2007) Checkpoint-apoptosis uncoupling in human and mouse embryonic stem cells: a source of karyotpic instability. *Blood* 109, 4518-4527.

[74] Maynard S, Swistowska AM, Lee JW, Liu Y, Liu S-T, Da Cruz AB, Rao M, de Souza-Pinto NC, Zeng X and Bohr VA (2008) Human Embryonic Stem Cells Have Enhanced Repair of Multiple Forms of DNA Damage. *STEM CELLS* 26, 2266-2274.

[75] Lin T, Chao C, Saito Si, Mazur SJ, Murphy ME, Appella E and Xu Y (2005) p53 induces differentiation of mouse embryonic stem cells by suppressing Nanog expression. *Nat Cell Biol* 7, 165-171.

[76] Frumkin T, Malcov M, Yaron Y and Ben-Yosef D (2008) Elucidating the origin of chromosomal aberrations in IVF embryos by preimplantation genetic analysis. *Molecular and Cellular Endocrinology* 282, 112-119.

[77] Fragouli E and Wells D (2011) Aneuploidy in the human blastocyst. *Cytogenet Genome Res* 133, 149-159.

[78] Baker DEC, Harrison NJ, Maltby E, Smith K, Moore HD, Shaw PJ, Heath PR, Holden H and Andrews PW (2007) Adaptation to culture of human embryonic stem cells and oncogenesis in vivo. *Nat Biotech* 25, 207-215.

[79] Mayshar Y, Ben-David U, Lavon N, Biancotti J-C, Yakir B, Clark AT, Plath K, Lowry WE and Benvenisty N (2010) Identification and Classification of Chromosomal Aberrations in Human Induced Pluripotent Stem Cells. *Cell Stem Cell* 7, 521-531.

[80] Ben-David U and Benvenisty N (2011) The tumorigenicity of human embryonic and induced pluripotent stem cells. *Nat Rev Cancer* 11, 268-277.

[81] Amariglio N, Hirshberg A, Scheithauer BW, Cohen Y, Loewenthal R, Trakhtenbrot L, Paz N, Koren-Michowitz M, Waldman D, Leider-Trejo L, Toren A, Constantini S and Rechavi G (2009) Donor-derived brain tumor following neural stem cell transplantation in an ataxia telangiectasia patient. *PLoS Med* 6, e1000029.

2

Uncover Cancer Genomics by Jointly Analysing Aneuploidy and Gene Expression

Lingling Zheng and Joseph Lucas
Duke University
USA

1. Introduction

Human cancers are heterogeneous due to combined effects of genetic instability and selection, where the accumulation of the most advantageous set of genetic aberrations results in the expansion of cancer cells (Pinkel & Albertson, 2005). There are many different types of instability that occurs during tumor development, such as point mutation, alteration of microsatellite sequences, chromosome rearrangements, DNA dosage aberrations and epigenetic changes such as methylation. These abnormalities acting alone or in combination alter the expression levels of mRNA molecules. However, the genetic history of tumor progression is difficult to decipher. Because it is only a sufficiently protumorigenic aberration or obligate products of a crucial alteration that results in tumor development (Pinkel & Albertson, 2005).

Genomic DNA copy number variations (CNVs), kilobase- or megabase-sized duplications and deletions, are frequent in solid tumors. It has been shown that CNVs are useful diagnosis markers for cancer prediction and prognosis (Kiechle et al., 2001; Lockwood et al., 2005). Therefore, studying the genomic causes and their association with phenotypic alterations is emergent in cancer biology. The underlying mechanism of CNV related genomic instability amongst tumors includes defects in maintenance/manipulation of genome stability, telomere erosion, chromosome breakage, cell cycle defects and failures in DNA repairs (Albertson, 2003). Consequential copy number aberrations of the above mentioned malfunctions will further change the dosage of key tumor-inducing and tumor-suppressing genes, which thereby affect DNA replication, DNA damage/repair, mitosis, centrosome, telomere, mRNA transcription and proliferation of neoplastic cells. In addition, microenvironmental stresses play a role in exerting strong selective pressure on cancer cells with amplification/deletion of particular regions of the chromosome (Lucas et al., 2010). Recently, high-throughput technologies have mapped genome-wide DNA copy number variations at high resolution, and discovered multiple new genes in cancer. However, there is enormous diversity in each individual's tumor, which harbors only a few driver mutations (copy number alterations playing a critical role in tumor development). In addition, CNV regions are particularly large containing many genes, most of which are indistinguishable from the passenger mutations (copy number segments affecting widespread chromosomal instability in many advanced human tumors) (Akavia et al., 2010). Thus analysis based on CNV data alone will leave the functional importance and physiological impact of genetic alteration ineluctable on the tumor. Gene expression has been readily available for profiling many tumors, therefore, how to incorporate it with CNV data to identify key drivers becomes an important problem to uncover cancer mechanism.

This chapter is laid out as follows: Section 2 covers a variety of CNV data topics, starting with a range of different CNV measurement techniques, which includes a brief discussion of the data format. Practical examples are used to show collecting, generating and assessing data, plus several ways to manipulate data for normalization. In the end, different computational approaches are introduced for analyzing CNV data. Section 3 focuses on an algorithm for integrating CNV with mRNA expression data, which can be potentially extended to incorporate multiple genomic data. Basic concepts of Bayesian factor analysis are briefly mentioned. Case studies then provide detailed description for this particular approach. Section 4 provides a brief wrap-up of the main ideas in the chapter. It illustrates the advantage of our statistical models on studying cancer genomics, and discusses the significance of the approach for clinical application.

2. Copy number analysis

2.1 Copy number analyses techniques

Comparative genome hybridization (CGH) is a recently developed technology and profiles genome-wide DNA copy number variations at high resolution. It has been popular for molecular classification of different tumor types, diagnosis of tumor progression, and identification of potential therapeutic targets (Jonsson et al., 2010; McKay et al., 2011). The use of CGH array offers many advantages over traditional karyotype or FISH (fluorescence *in situ* hybridization). It can detect microduplications/deletions throughout genome in a single experiment.

BAC Array

The CGH array using BAC (bacterial artificial chromosome) clones has been widely used. The spotted genomic sequences are inserted BACs: two DNA samples from either subject tissue (target sample) or control tissue (reference sample) are labeled with different fluorescent dyes–for example, with the test labeled in green and reference in red. The mixture is hybridized to a CGH array slide containing hundreds or thousands of defined DNA probes. The probes targeting regions of the chromosome that are amplified turn predominantly green. Conversely, if a region is deleted in the test sample, the corresponding probes become red. However, given the resolution limitation on the order of 1Mb and array size of 2400 to $\sim$30000 unique elements, the BAC array data is relatively low density.

cDNA/oligonucleotide Array

cDNA and oligonucleotide arrays are designed to detect complementary DNA "targets" derived from experiments or clinics. It allows greater flexibility to produce customized arrays, and reduces the cost for each study. Since commercial arrays are often more expensive and contain a large number of genes that are not of interest to the researchers. The shorter probes spotted on these new arrays are less robust than large segmented BACs. But they provide higher resolution in the order of 50-100kb, where oligonucleotide array is a particular case.

Tiling Array

Tiling arrays are available now for finer resolution of specific CNV regions. These arrays are designed to cover the entire genome or contiguous regions within the genome. Number of elements on the array ranges from 10000 to over 6000000. This relatively high resolution technique allows the detection of micro-amplifications and deletions.

SNP Array

SNP (single nucleotide polymorphism) arrays are a high-density oligonucleotide-based array that can be used to identify both loss of heterozygosity (LOH) and CNVs. LOH is the loss of one allele of a gene, which can lead to functional loss of normal tumor suppressor genes, particularly if the other copy of the gene is inactive. LOH is quite common in malignancies. Therefore, utilization of SNP arrays to detect LOH provides great potential for cancer diagnosis.

Array CGH

Array comparative genomic hybridization (array CGH, or aCGH) is a high-resolution technique for genome-wide DNA copy number variation profiling. This method allows identification of recurrent chromosome changes with microamplifications and deletions, and detects copy number variations on the order of 5-10kb DNA sequences. In the rest of this chapter, we will use the CNV data generated from the general Agilent Human Genome CGH microarray 244A.

2.2 Array CGH data

The CNV data is obtained from The Cancer Genome Atlas (TCGA) project. TCGA is a joint effort of the National Cancer Institute and the National Human Genome Research Institute (NIHGRI) to understand genomic alterations in human cancer. It aims to study the molecular mechanisms of cancer in order to improve diagnosis, treatment and prevention. The importance of DNA copy number variations has been demonstrated in many tumors. TCGA targets to perform high-resolution CNV profiling in a large-scale study, using diverse tumor tissues and across different institutes. In this section, we will show an example from TCGA project.

Sample collection

Biospecimens were collected from newly diagnosed patients with ovarian serous cystadenocarcinoma (histologically consistent with ovarian serous adenocarcinoma confirmed by pathologists), who had not received any prior treatment, including chemotherapy or radiotherapy. Technical details about sample collection and quality control are described in (*Integrated genomic analyses of ovarian carcinoma*, 2011). Raw copy number data was generated at two centers, Brigham and Women's Hospital of Harvard Medical School and Dana Farber Cancer Institute, using the Agilent Human Genome Comparative Genome Hybridization 244A platform.

Data process

After the array CGH is constructed and tumor DNA samples hybridized to the platform, several steps need to be completed for detecting regions of copy number gains or losses: image scanning, image analysis (including gridding, spot recognition, segmentation and quantification, and low-intensified feature removal or mark), background noise subtraction, spot intensity ratio determination, log-transformation of ratios, signal normalization and quality control on the measured values. For Agilent 244K array, there are specific details on the data generation (*Comprehensive genomic characterization defines human glioblastoma genes and core pathways*, 2008). First of all, the raw signal is obtained by scanning images using Agilent Feature Extraction Software (v9.5. 11), followed by image analysis steps mentioned above. *Background correction:* The background corrected intensity ratios for both channels are calculated by subtraction of median background signal values (median pixel intensities in the predefined background area surrounding the spot) of each channel from the median signal values (median pixel intensities computed over the spot area) of each probe in the corresponding channel. Since there are multiple copies of probes on an array, the final background corrected values are computed by taking the median across the duplicated probes. The $\log_2$ ratios of the above results are then estimated based on the background corrected values of sample channel over that of the reference channel. *Normalization of logarithmic ratio:* The normalization procedure involves the application of LOWESS (locally weighted regression and scatterplot smoothing) algorithm on $\log_2$ ratio data. This method assumes that the majority of probe $\log_2$ ratios do not change, and are independent of background corrected intensities of the probes. To develop the LOWESS model, a 21-probe window is applied for smoothing process after sorting the chromosome positions. It corrects the $\log_2$ ratio data so that the corresponding central tendency after normalization lies along zeros, assuming an equal number of up- and down- regulated features in any given intensity range. In addition, the artifact of the difference in the probe GC content on $\log_2$ ratios is considered for correction, in which case, the probe GC%, regional GC % (GC% of 20KB of genome sequence containing the probe sequence) and $\log_2$ ratio are used in the LOWESS model. *Quality control:* There are several criterions taken into account for quality assurance at various stages. 1) Probes that are flagged (marking spots of poor quality and low intensity) or saturated by the Agilent feature extraction software are eliminated; 2) Screening of the array image is conducted to exclude probes whose median signal values are lower than that of the background intensity; 3) Arrays with over 5% probes flagged out or being faint are considered as low quality; 4) The square root of the mean sum squares of variance in $\log_2$ ratio data between consecutive probes are calculated for quality assessment. Arrays with the value over 0.3 are considered as low quality.

The final result after these processes forms a data set containing 227614 probes with normalized $\log_2$ ratio values for every sample. The logarithmic ratios are computed as $\log_2(x) - \log_2(2)$, where x is the copy number inferred by the chip. Thus, ratios should be 0 for double loss, $\frac{1}{2}$ for a single loss, 1 for the normal situation, $\frac{3}{2}$ for a single gain, and $\frac{n}{2}$ for n copies. TCGA provides an Array Design Format file with annotation data, including information on chromosomal location and gene symbol for each probe.

Algorithms for CNVs detection

The main biomedical question for studying CNVs and downstream research is to accurately identify genomic/chromosomal regions that show significant amplification or deletion in DNA copy number. Satisfactorily solving this problem requires a method that reflects the underlying biology and key features of the technological platform. The array CGH data has particular characteristics: The status of DNA copy number remains stable in the contiguous loci, and the copy number of a probe is a good predictor for that of the neighboring ones, whereas for probes located far apart, it provides less information to predict the likely state of its neighboring probes (Rueda & Díaz-Uriarte, 2007). However, widely used array CGH platforms, such as cDNA/oligonucleotide arrays, do not have equally spaced probes, making it less informative based on consecutive probes. Furthermore, the identification of disease causal genes sometimes requires examining the amplitude of CNVs, especially when high-resolution technologies are available, it can be valuable to distinguish between moderate copy number gains and large copy number amplification.

A number of well-known methods have been developed to carry out automatic identification of copy number gains/loss, and correlate that with diseases. These approaches are designed to estimate the significance level and location of CNVs. Models differ in distribution assumption and incorporation of penalty terms for parameter estimation. Subsequently, smoothing algorithms were derived for denoising and estimating the spatial dependence, such as wavelets (Hsu et al., 2005) and lowess methods (Beheshti et al., 2003; Cleveland, 1979). Later on, a binary segmentation approach, called circular binary segmentation (CBS) (Olshen et al., 2004), was proposed that allows segments in the aCGH data in each chromosome, and computes the within-segment means. CBS recursively estimates the maximum likelihood ratio statistics to detect the narrowed segment aberrations. A more complicated likelihood function was used with weights chosen in a completely data adaptive fashion (Adaptive weights smoothing procedure, AWS) (Hup et al., 2004). A different kind of modeling approach involves the hidden Markov model (HMM) (Fridlyand, 2004), which assigns hidden states with certain transition probabilities to underlying copy numbers. Thus, it adequately takes advantage of the physical dependence information of the nearby fragments. However, questions arise on how to appropriately select the number of hidden states. The sticky hidden Markov model with a Dirichlet distribution (sticky DD-HMM) (Du et al., 2010) was then developed to infer the number of states from data, while also imposing state persistence. Alternatively, the reversible jump aCGH (RJaCGH) (Rueda & Díaz-Uriarte, 2007) was introduced to fit the model with varying number of hidden states, and allow for transdimensional moves between these models. It also incorporates interprobe distance.

3. Joint analysis on copy number variation and gene expression

3.1 Overview

With the increasing availability of concurrently generating multiple different types of high throughput data on single samples, there is a lot of interest to jointly analyze this information and refine the generation of relevant biological hypotheses. This will lead to a greater, more integrated understanding of cellular mechanism, and will allow the identification of genomic regulators as well as suggest potentially synergistic drug targets for those regulators, which will lead to potential combination therapies for the treatment of human cancer. A number of approaches have demonstrated an ability to select specific genes from joint analysis and test specific hypotheses regarding the regulation of cellular responses, which is a tremendous advantage over the pathway analyses that can be obtained from gene expression or CNVs alone.

Recently, there are publications that highlight the impact of combining other types of DNA modification and gene expression. (Parsons et al., 2008) have identified a number of potential driver mutations in Glioblastoma through an analysis of mutation, copy number variation and gene expression. Their approach is designed around the use of currently available methods for the analysis of individual data types to create a compressed set of features which are then used independently in predictive models. They utilize tree models, however the compressed features are independent variables that can, in principle, be used in any type of predictive model. The approach does make use of correlation within each type of data, but not across different data types.

A similar approach to the integration of disparate types of data is outlined in (Lanckriet et al., 2004), but in this case features are compressed through the use of kernel functions. These must be predefined for each data type, but once that is done all of the different data types are mapped to the same vector space allowing joint analysis. The approach is particularly suited to the use of support vector machines, rather than tree models, for the generation of models from all of the different data types. The approach is remarkably general in that almost any type of data may be incorporated, and in the paper they include compelling examples of the integration of expression and protein sequence data. It, however, does suffer from the same flaws as (Parsons et al., 2008) in that there is no provision for dealing with correlation across data types.

Another approach to integrative analysis is through the use of data from different assays to filter lists of genes sequentially. (Garraway et al., 2005) describe such an approach, in the context of the identification of MITF as a genomic determinant in malignant melanoma. The algorithm first identifies genomic regions that show copy number variation in the condition of interest, and then searches for genes that are significantly over or under expressed in samples that have duplications or deletions in that region. This is a very powerful approach in cases where there are few genes that pass the filtering criteria and where the relationship between gene expression and CNV is direct. Through our own experimentation, we find that there are often many genes that pass both filtering criteria. Additionally, the approach is dependent on the order in which the data types are used to perform the filtering. This is because the filtering criterion on the second data set is determined by the behavior observed on the first.

The version of integrative genomic analysis that is most similar to our own proposal is CONEXIC, detailed in (Akavia et al., 2010). CONEXIC is based on gene modules, which was initially developed for the analysis of gene expression data in isolation. Gene modules consist of groups of genes that are coexpressed, and these are embedded as leaves in a binary tree structure where the nodes are populated by putative gene expression regulators. In its original incarnation, the approach was intended to identify important regulators of groups of genes in the context of experimental interventions. As such, expression is assumed to be constant within any particular experimental group. Also, the original approach depends on a list of putative regulators, which can be tricky to generate. With CONEXIC, the identification of lists of potential regulators is generated from regions of the genome that demonstrate consistent copy number variation, and the gene module algorithm is largely retained. Fundamental to a binary tree model is the assumption that the expression pattern of a leaf, conditional on the expression pattern of its parent node, is independent of all other elements in the tree. This is a shortcoming of the CONEXIC approach. It is quite reasonable to expect that there are many ways that a cell has available to control the expression of a particular gene, including CNV, methylation, inactivation of promoters, and RNA interference, and multiple different regulators may combine to ultimately regulate gene expression. Because each node of the tree contains only one putative regulator, the model assumes that only one regulator is responsible for the observed expression pattern of a module.

3.2 Bayesian factor analysis

Bayesian factor analysis is a dimension reduction method to decompose variability among observations into a lower number of unobserved, uncorrelated factors. It has been widely applied in microarray analysis (Carvalho et al., 2008; Lucas et al., 2009), where the data usually comes with a much higher dimension than the number of observed samples. Therefore, it is desirable to select important genes that should bear some biological meanings. Recent developments in Bayesian multivariate modeling has enabled the utility of sparsity induced structure in genomic studies (Lucas et al., 2006). Such a sparse factor model implies that only those genes with non-zero loadings on those factors are relevant, and higher values indicate more significant gene-factor relationship.

3.3 Sparse regression model of Bayesian factor analysis

Our statistical framework utilizes high-dimensional sparse factor model, and is extended to incorporate gene expression, CNVs and other high-throughput genomic data. The underlying hypothesis is that the gene signatures of expression variation can be represented by the estimated factors. Furthermore, given the potential contribution of chromosomal aneuploidy and CNVs to the altered mRNA expression of relevant genes during oncogenesis, we could use the factor model to test for the association between gene expression signatures and CNVs. The model assumes that the input data are from the same organism. Suppose the data structure is given as $\mathbf{X} = [\mathbf{x}_1, \ldots, \mathbf{x}_n]$ with dimension $n \times p_x$, where n denotes the sample size, p_x the number of genes, and $\mathbf{x}_i$ the fluorescence level from probes of gene expression measurements. The CNV data is represented by $\mathbf{Y} = [\mathbf{y}_1, \ldots, \mathbf{y}_n]$ with similar strucutre. Therefore, the linear regression model for sample i can be expressed as

$$\mathbf{x}_i = \mathbf{B}_h \mathbf{h}_i + \mathbf{B}\mathbf{F}_i + \epsilon_i \quad (1)$$

$$\mathbf{y}_i = \mathbf{A}_h \mathbf{h}_i + \mathbf{A}\mathbf{G}_i + \zeta_i \quad (2)$$

with the following components:

- $\mathbf{B}$ is the $p_x \times k$ factor loadings matrix for sample $\mathbf{x}_i$, with elements $\beta_{g,j}$ for $g = 1, \ldots, p_x$ and $j = 1, \ldots, k$.
- $\mathbf{F}_i = [\mathbf{f}_i^C; \mathbf{f}_i^{(r)}]^T$. $\mathbf{f}_i$ is a k-dimension vector of factor scores, where $\mathbf{f}_i^{(r)}$, the r-th factor for sample i, are specific to data $\mathbf{x}_i$, and $\mathbf{f}_i^C$ consists of the factors ***common*** between both data.
- $\mathbf{B}_h$ is the $p_x \times r$ regression matrix for dataset $\mathbf{x}_i$, with elements $b_{g,j}$ for $g = 1, \ldots, p_x$ and $j = 1, \ldots, r$.
- $\mathbf{h}_i = \left[h_{1,i}, \ldots, h_{q,i}\right]^T$ is the q design factors of sample i.
- $\epsilon_i = \left[\epsilon_{1,i}, \ldots, \epsilon_{p_x,i}\right]^T$ is the idiosyncratic noise vector with dimension p_x.

The priors for each parameters are defined as follows:

$$\beta_{g,j} \sim (1-\rho_j)\delta_0(\beta_{g,j}) + \rho_j \mathcal{N}(\beta_{g,j}; 0, \tau_j) \quad (3)$$

$$\rho_j \sim Beta(\rho_j; s_0, l_0); \tau_j \sim Gamma(\tau_j^{-1}; \frac{a_\tau}{2}, \frac{b_\tau}{2}) \quad (4)$$

$$b_{g,j} \sim (1-\pi_j)\delta_0(b_{g,j}) + \pi_j \mathcal{N}(b_{g,j}; \mu_{0,j}, \sigma_0^2) \quad (5)$$

$$\pi_j \sim Beta(\pi_j; t_0, v_0) \quad (6)$$

$$\mathbf{f}_i^{(r)} \sim \mathcal{N}(\mathbf{f}_i^{(r)}; \mathbf{0}, \mathbf{I}) \qquad \mathbf{f}_i^C \sim \mathcal{N}(\mathbf{f}_i^C; \mathbf{g}_i^C, \Sigma) \quad (7)$$

$$\epsilon_i^{(r)} \sim \mathcal{N}(\epsilon_i^{(r)}; \mathbf{0}, \mathbf{\Phi}); \mathbf{\Phi} = \text{diag}(\phi_1, \ldots, \phi_{p_x}); \phi_g \sim Gamma(\phi_g; \frac{a_{\phi_x}}{2}, \frac{b_{\phi_x}}{2}) \quad (8)$$

The parameters and prior structures are similar for copy number data $\mathbf{y}_i$.

Prior Choices

• $\beta_{g,j}$: The regression coefficient. Here we consider the long-standing problem of variable selection in a multivariate linear regression model. That is, in gene expression analysis the number of gene features is huge (usually larger than 20,000) compared with the number of samples available. A direct way is to use regression model on the high-dimensional genomic data and impose sparseness on the coefficients. In this way, most of the coefficients will be shrunk towards zero. Bayesian spike and slab approaches (George & McCulloch, 1993; Ishwaran & Rao, 2005; Mitchell & Beauchamp, 1988) have been proposed to address the variable selection problem. As indicated in 3, it sets up a two-component mixture distribution with the spike part centered at zero and the slab part distributed diffusely without informed prior knowledge.

• ρ_j: This parameter controls the prior probability of a coefficient being non-zero. We assume coefficients that are promising have posterior latent variables $\hat{\rho}_j = 1$ (the slab). The opposite occurs when $\hat{\rho}_j = 0$ with a delta function $\delta_0(\cdot)$ indicating the point-mass at zero (the spike). Here we use beta priors, defining the probability ρ_j distributed on the interval (0,1). The hyperparameters s_0 and l_0 determine the domain of the beta distribution. Small values of ρ_j reflect high prior skepticism about the coefficients, while large ρ_j means the knowledge of more theoretical importance of the variables and more skeptical about the sampling of the data.

• τ_j: the variance for the slab part of the mixture prior for $\beta_{g,j}$. This gamma distribution is the conjugate prior for the precision of the normal distribution $\mathcal{N}(\beta_{g,j}; 0, \tau_j)$. In addition, it allows the Markov chain to identify and adjust the appropriate sample space for updating coefficients. Different combinations of ρ_j and τ_j prior choices are usually required to obtain desirable mixing and shrinkage in $\beta_{g,j}$.

• $\mathbf{f}_i$: Unknown latent factors for sample i. For factors unique for each data, we use a diffuse, conjugate prior distribution such that $f_{j,i} \sim \mathcal{N}(0,1)$, in order to alleviate issues with identifiability of $\mathbf{f}_i$ and $\boldsymbol{\beta}$ due to scaling. On the other hand, since high-throughput data can vary in size by orders of magnitude, e.g. CGH data is approximately ten times larger than gene expression. Thus one data set may dominate the factor model given a large size discrepancy. Therefore, rather than utilizing the uninformative prior, we link individual factors from each data using $\mathbf{f}_i^C \sim \mathcal{N}(\mathbf{g}_i^C, \Sigma)$ based on the hypothesis that gene expression is directly influenced by CNVs. This will prevent difference in data size from overwhelming the information available on associations between them. In addition, the systematic error between two data sets will be considered by estimation of the covariance matrix Σ.

Updated Distributions

• $p(\beta_{g,j}|-)$:

For factor j, let $x^*_{g,j} = x_{g,j} - \sum_{j=1}^{r} b_{g,j}h_{j,i} - \sum_{l\neq j}^{k} \beta_{g,l}f_{l,i}$, so that $x^*_{g,j} \sim \mathcal{N}(\beta_{g,j}f_{j,i}, \phi_g)$. In order to be mathematically identifiable for $\mathbf{B}$, we assume the regression coefficients a lower triangular matrix with positive diagonal elements (Carvalho & West, 2006). This gives the following posterior updates where $g \neq j$:

$$\begin{aligned} p(\beta_{g,j}|-) &\propto \prod_{i=1}^{n} p(x^*_{g,j}|\beta_{g,j} f_{j,i}, \phi_g) p(\beta_{g,j}) \\ &= \prod_{i=1}^{n} \mathcal{N}(x^*_{g,j}; \beta_{g,j} f_{j,i}, \phi_g)((1-\rho_j)\delta_0(\beta_{g,j}) + \rho_j \mathcal{N}(\beta_{g,j}; 0, \tau_j)) \\ &= (1-\hat{\rho}_j)\delta_0(\beta_{g,j}) + \hat{\rho}_j \mathcal{N}(\beta_{g,j}; \mu_{g,j}, \Omega_{g,j}) \end{aligned}$$

where $\Omega_{g,j} = (\tau_j^{-1} + \sum_{j=1}^{k} f_{j,i}^2/\phi_g)^{-1}, \mu_{g,j} = \Omega_{g,j}(\sum_{i=1}^{n} x^*_{g,i} f_{j,i})\phi_g^{-1}$ and $\beta_{g,j} \neq 0$ with probability

$$\hat{\rho}_j = \frac{\rho_j}{\rho_j + (1-\rho_j)\frac{\mathcal{N}(0;0,\tau_j)}{\mathcal{N}(0;\mu_{g,j},\Omega_{g,j})}}$$

For the constrained diagonal elements of **B**, the posterior conditional distribution is given as

$$p(\beta_{j,j}|-) \sim \mathcal{N}(\mu_{j,j}, \Omega_{j,j})\mathbf{I}(\beta_{j,j} > 0)$$

with similar forms of $\mu_{j,j}$ and $\Omega_{j,j}$.

- $p(\rho_j|-)$:

$$\begin{aligned} p(\rho_j|-) &\propto \prod_{j=1}^{k} p(\beta_{g,j}|\rho_j)p(\rho_j) = (1-\rho_j)^{p_x - j - S_j}\rho_j^{S_j} Beta(\rho_j; s_0, l_0) \\ &\sim Beta(s_0 + S_j, l_0 + p_x - j - S_j) \end{aligned}$$

with $S_j = \sum_{g=j}^{p_x} \mathbf{I}(\beta_{g,j} \neq 0)$.

$$\begin{aligned} p(\tau_j|-) &\propto \prod_{g=1}^{p_x} p(\beta_{g,j}|\rho_j, \tau_j)p(\tau_j) = \prod_{g=1}^{p_x} \mathcal{N}(\beta_{g,j}; 0, \tau_j) Ga(\tau_j^{-1}; \frac{a_\tau}{2}, \frac{b_\tau}{2}) \\ &\sim InvGamma(\tau_j; \frac{a_\tau + \omega_j}{2}, \frac{b_\tau + \sum_{g=1}^{p_x} \beta_{g,j}^2}{2}) \end{aligned}$$

with $\omega_j = \sum_{g=j}^{p_x} \mathbf{I}(\beta_{g,j} \neq 0)$.

- $p(\mathbf{f}_i|-), p(\mathbf{g}_i|-)$:

Let $\mathbf{F} = [\mathbf{f}_1, \ldots, \mathbf{f}_n]$. The posterior distribution of **F** can be updated as:

$$\begin{aligned} p(\mathbf{F}|-) &\propto p(\mathbf{X}|\mathbf{F}, \mathbf{B}, \mathbf{\Phi})p(\mathbf{F}) = \prod_{i=1}^{n} p(\mathbf{x}_i|\mathbf{f}_i, \mathbf{B}, \mathbf{\Phi})p(\mathbf{f}_i) \\ &= \prod_{i=1}^{n} \mathcal{N}(\mathbf{x}_i - \mathbf{B}_h \mathbf{H}_i; \mathbf{B}\mathbf{f}_i, \mathbf{\Phi}) \mathcal{N}(\mathbf{f}_i; \mathbf{g}_i, \Sigma) \\ &\propto \prod_{i=1}^{n} \mathcal{N}(\mathbf{f}_i; \mathbf{E1}_i, \mathbf{V1}_i) \end{aligned}$$

where $\mathbf{V1}_i = (\Sigma^{-1} + \mathbf{B}'\mathbf{\Phi}^{-1}\mathbf{B})^{-1}$, $\mathbf{E1}_i = \mathbf{V1}_i(\mathbf{B}'\mathbf{\Phi}^{-1}(\mathbf{x}_i - \mathbf{B}_h\mathbf{H_i}) + \mathbf{G}_i\Sigma^{-1})$.

Similarly $p(\mathbf{g}_i|-)$ takes the form

$$p(\mathbf{G}|-) \propto \prod_{i=1}^{n} \mathcal{N}(\mathbf{g}_i; \mathbf{E2}_i, \mathbf{V2}_i)$$

where $\mathbf{V2}_i = (\mathbf{I} + \mathbf{A}'\mathbf{\Psi}^{-1}\mathbf{A})^{-1}$, $\mathbf{E2}_i = \mathbf{V2}_i(\mathbf{A}'\mathbf{\Psi}^{-1}(\mathbf{y}_i - \mathbf{A}_h\mathbf{H_i}))$. $\mathbf{\Psi}$ is the covariance matrix of $\mathbf{y}_i$.

- $p(\phi_g|-)$:

$$\begin{aligned} p(\phi_g|-) &\propto \prod_{i=1}^{n} p(x_{g,i}|\beta_g f_i, \phi_g)p(\phi_g) \\ &= \prod_{i=1}^{n} \mathcal{N}(x_{g,i} - \sum_{j=1}^{r} b_{g,j}h_{j,i}; \beta_g f_i, \phi_g)Ga(\phi_g{}^{-1}; \frac{a_{\phi_x}}{2}, \frac{b_{\phi_x}}{2}) \\ &\sim InvGamma(\phi_g; \frac{a_{\phi_x} + n}{2}, \frac{b_{\phi_x} + \sum_{i=1}^{n}(x_{g,i} - b_g h_i - \beta_g f_i)^2}{2}) \end{aligned}$$

3.4 Example: joint analysis of ovarian cancer gene expression and CNVs

We applied our joint factor model on ovarian cancer gene expression and CNV data from TCGA project. This study is aimed to detect correlations between them, which will lead to the identification of pivotal genomic determinants of cancer phenotypes. We adopted 74 ovarian cancer individuals and 1 disease-free patient's data. In order to capture genes with differential expression patterns and their association with the CNVs in the narrowed chromosomal regions, we established a filtering criteria: 1) select Affymetrix HT_HG-U133A probes with sample mean above 8, and standard deviation above 0.6; take out probes without matched gene symbols. It results in a gene expression data set downsized from 22277 to 921 probes; 2) apply the basic Bayesian factor model 1, i.e., the one that only analyzes one data set, and generate signature expression factors; 3) remove CNV segments (Agilent Human Genome CGH 244A probes) not showing significant correlation (p-value < 0.01 after Bonferroni correction) with the gene expression factors. It reduced the CNV data dimension from 227613 to 7278. Therefore, we fitted our joint factor model 1 and 2 to the shrunk data.

We obtained 11 factors in the two data sets, i.e., $\mathbf{F}_{11*75}$ and $\mathbf{G}_{11*75}$, and selected the most strongly associated pair using Pearson correlation. It turns out that the largest factor loadings in the corresponding CNV factor come mostly from the long arm of chromosome 8 (figure 1A), that the factor correlates well with the paired gene expression factor (figure 1B), and that the gene expression factor correlates with individual SNP observations in the long arm of chromosome 8 (figure 1C). Based on these results, we further examined the genes loaded on this correlated CGH factor and gene expression factor. By ranking the squared factor loadings, we selected the top 16 Affymetrix probe sets (Table 1) and 178 CGH probe sets, because the variance in these probes are best explained by the corresponding factors compared with all other data. Pearson correlation between the values of mRNA expression levels and copy number variations were calculated on these heavily loaded genes. We noted that the copy number gains of EBAG9 (CGH probe position: 8q23.2, size 60 bp; mean copy number 2.63 (1-6)) and MTDH (CGH probe position: 8q22.1, size 60 bp; mean copy number 2.38

(1-6)) significantly accompanies their overexpression of mRNAs in the corresponding regions, where correlation coefficients indicate a good linearity between CNVs and gene expression with r = 0.758 for EBAG9 and r = 0.806 for MTDH. Interestingly, in the same factor, 3 CGH loci with duplicated DNAs show significant correlation with MTDH overexpression (r>0.8, p-val<0.01) and are located 0.2M upstream, 5M and 12M downstream of MTDH CGH locus, respectively; and 11 CGH loci are identified with copy number gain and 3Mb upstream of EBAG9 CGH clone (r>0.75, p-val<0.01). These findings may provide evidence for distant regulatory of transcription elements or interactions within a potential gene network.

Gene symbol	Gene
MTDH	LYRIC/3D3 (UID: 92140)
EBAG9	estrogen receptor binding site associated, antigen, 9 (UID:9166)
YWHAZ	tyrosine 3-monooxygenase (UID:7534)
LAPTM4B	lysosomal protein transmembrane 4 beta (UID:55353)
ESRP1	epithelial splicing regulatory protein 1 (UID:54845)
NBN	nibrin (UID:9048)
RAD21	RAD21 homolog (S. pombe) (UID:5885)
RNF139	ring finger protein 139 (UID:11236)
ZNF706	HSPC038 protein (UID:51123)
AZIN1	antizyme inhibitor 1 (UID:51582)
DERL1	Der1-like domain family, member 1 (UID:79139)
ENY2	enhancer of yellow 2 homolog (Drosophila) (UID:56943)
EXT1	exostoses (multiple) 1 (UID:2131)
CTSB	cathepsin B (UID:1508)
DECR1	2,4-dienoyl CoA reductase 1, mitochondrial (UID:1666)
PTDSS1	phosphatidylserine synthase 1 (UID:9791)

Table 1. Genes on chromosome 8 showing significantly differential expression in ovarian cancer. The list is ranked by the squared factor loadings.

The product of EBAG9 has been identified as an estrogen receptor binding site associated antigen 9 identical to RCAS1 (Nakashima et al., 1999). Overexpression of EBAG9/RCAS1 inhibits growth of tumor-stimulated host immune cells and induces their apoptosis (Nakashima et al., 1999). Furthermore, it has been reported that RCAS1 is expressed with high frequency in ovarian and lung cancers (Akahira et al., 2004; Iwasaki et al., 2000), and the copy numbers of the region increase in breast cancer (Rennstam et al., 2003). These lines of evidence, together with the results obtained above, imply that overexpression of EBAG9 in ovarian serous cystadenocarcinoma may be triggered by increased gene copy number, which is likely to play an important role in the immune escape of tumor cells and causing cancer progression.

In addition, MTDH, also known as AEG1, is an oncogene cooperating with Ha-ras as well as functioning as a downstream target gene of Ha-ras and may perform a central role in Ha-ras-mediated carcinogenesis (Lee et al., 2007). Overexpression of this gene has been reported in various cancers including breast, brain, prostate, melanoma and glioblastoma multiforme (Emdad et al., 2007; Kikuno et al., 2007). In particular, it has been revealed that MTDH overexpression is associated with 8q22 genomic gain in breast cancer, and has been considered as an important therapeutic target for enhancing chemotherapy efficacy and reducing metastasis risk (Hu et al., 2009). Therefore, we believe that, our results along with the

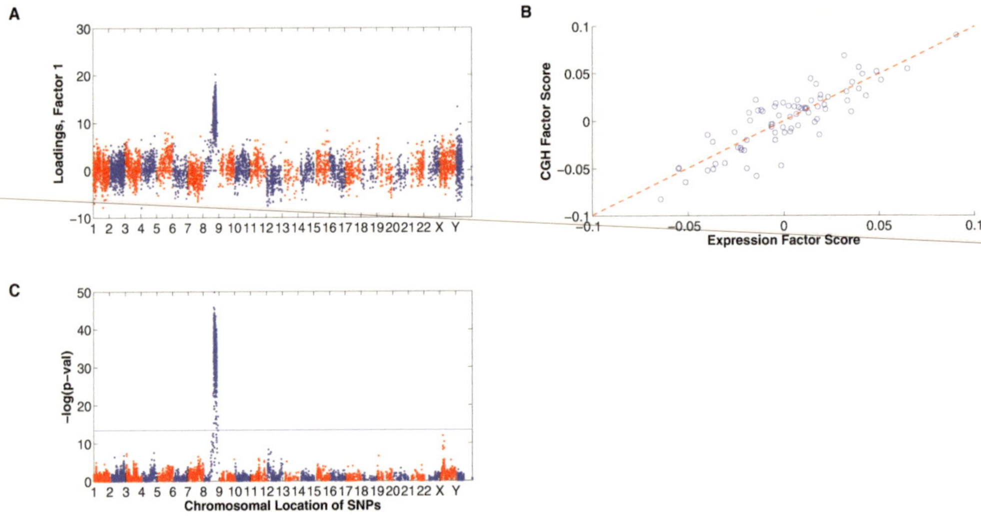

Fig. 1. Factor analytic relationship between CNV and gene expression. Panel A shows the factor loadings from the first factor of the joint factor model fit to CNV data. Panel B shows a scatterplot of significant correlation between gene expression factor and the CNV factor, of which it is linked to. Panel C shows the significance of correlation between the expression factor and each individual SNP from the high-density CGH array. The y-axis shows the -log(p-value) of the Pearson correlation between CNVs and gene expression factor. The horizontal line shows the threshold of p-value less than 0.01 after Bonferroni correction for multiple testing.

above findings suggest the copy number gain activated MTDH overexpression is a potential indicator in epithelial ovarian cancer.

Validations on the above hypotheses regarding critical genes in cancer progression and their regulation mechanisms can be carried out in several directions. A number of databases can be used to validate these hypotheses. For instance, GATHER and GOrilla are good resources to annotate gene functions; Tumorscape helps interpret copy number variations; DAVID Bioinformatics provides pathway analysis for genes identified by the model. In addition, experimental validation can be performed to quantitatively justify that the activation/inactivation of identified genes are caused by copy number variations. Moreover, we could identify drug susceptibilities of these candidates by searching against reference information from DrugBank (http://www.drugbank.ca), then using these results for experimental validation. The general approach is to grow cell lines in the presence of a particular treatment, whose genomic drivers are disrupted by the introduction of RNA inference and transfection with viral plasmids. Similar strategy can also been applied to predict potential therapies by the identification of new drug targets. Therefore, these will lead to a greater understanding of cancer progression, and allow the identification of combined therapies for individual tumors.

Tumor segmental aneuploidy association with gene expression factors has been demonstrated in a previous study (Lucas et al., 2010) that it makes significant contributions to variation in gene signature of breast cancer under the stress of lactic acidosis or hypoxia. We are interested to test if this is consistent in other tumor tissues, which will provide potential treatment choices for different cancers. We used a similar approach (Lucas et al., 2010) by projecting the breast expression factors into TCGA ovarian and glioblastoma gene expression data and identified correlated CNVs under the same interventions of lactic acidosis/hypoxia. The ability of projecting the factor model into other data sets allows the possibility of comparing new experimental data to different genomic information, such as CNVs from aCGH. The underlying assumption is that genes showing shared expression patterns in tumors of different origins can be represented by the same loadings matrix. Therefore, in order to estimate the factor scores for the new data, this translates into a well known problem of inverse regression $\mathbf{F}_y = (\mathbf{I}_k + \mathbf{B}'\mathbf{\Phi}^{-1}\mathbf{B})^{-1}\mathbf{B}'\mathbf{\Phi}^{-1}\mathbf{Y}$, where $\mathbf{B}$ is the loadings matrix and $\mathbf{\Phi}$ the diagonal matrix containing the gene by gene variance estimators in the original data, $\mathbf{Y}$ the new set of expression data and $\mathbf{F}_y$ the factor scores on the new data set. With this approach, we estimated factor scores for the TCGA data and calculated their correlations with CNVs. In our analysis, about half of the breast expression factors are also associated with copy number variations in ovarian cancer and that about a quarter are associated with CNVs in glioblastoma. For example, the CNV activated expression pattern in breast cancer (not shown) is also discovered in both ovarian cancer and glioblastoma within the same region

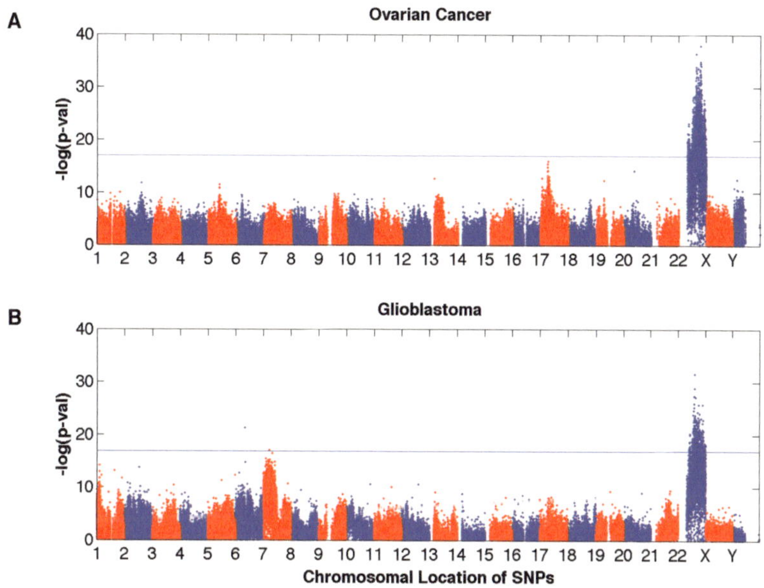

Fig. 2. Panel A and B show the the association between gene expression factor and CNVs across tumors of different origins. Each scatter plot indicates the evidence of association between the same factor that was learned on breast cancer data and copy number changes of different tumor tissues. Plot A shows correlation between the factor, projected onto ovarian cancer expression data, and ovarian CGH data. Plot B shows the same for Glioblastoma. Each point corresponds to one of the SNPs measured in the high-dimensional CGH array. The y-axis shows the -log(p-value) of the Pearson correlation between CNVs and gene expression factor. The horizontal line shows the threshold of p-value less than 0.01 after Bonferroni correction for multiple testing.

(figure 2A and 2B). Therefore, it is likely that similar CNVs might be selected under the same pressure of hypoxia/ lactic acidosis in difference cancers.

4. Conclusion

This chapter has built upon a basic understanding of a layout on the correlation between copy number variations and gene expression to deepen knowledge of key concepts and methods. By introducing and comparing a diverse range of techniques for measuring CNVs, we provide the scope of localizing cancer related genes using different platforms. By describing an appreciation of the use of several statistical methods to assist the positioning of CNV regions, we are aimed to better identify cancer driven mutations within the copy number gain/loss regions. Moreover, we have also included examples from TCGA project to show the unique features of CNV data.

The key challenge of finding candidate drivers is to distinguish it from passenger genes, which are physically located close to the driver mutations and whose variations are not causal to convey growth advantage on cancer cells. In our analysis, we focus on genes with cis-regulated CNVs, and postulate that cancer driven mutation is associated with the expression of a group of genes, and it is likely to localize in DNA amplified or deleted regions in tumors. Since DNA dosage variations may result in functional changes of affected genes and cause expression change of downstream genes. We have proposed a generic framework to jointly analyze disparate data sets, which is extendable to incorporate diverse information such as proteomics data. This will allow for more robust analysis of the relationship between mRNA expression and protein abundance. Our results not only identify candidate genes whose mRNA expression is statistically significantly correlated with their CNVs, but also successfully recover the region where similar gene expression pattern is triggered by the same genomic program across tumors of different organ systems. This approach is able to estimate the probability of each gene regulated by genomic sources and the relative importance of each source. Additionally, two genes, EBAG9 and MTDH, suggest that abnormal abundance in their DNA copy numbers may contribute to proliferation in ovarian serous cystadenocarcinoma. For these two predicted drivers, we also find many CNVs in the same region but poorly correlated with their gene expression, thus consider them no apparent effect in cancer. Copy number variation is only one of many ways that gene expression can be altered. We believe that a number of complementary approaches are needed to validate possibly driving alterations, as illustrated in the previous section. Therefore, We envision that our model is used as screening guidance to assist the identification of potential cancer drivers with possibly therapeutic importance.

Our work presents a framework toward a broad understanding of the genomic determinants of cancer. With this approach, we anticipate to generate testable biological hypothesis regarding the regulation of cellular responses, which is a tremendous advantage over any single data analyses that can be obtained from gene expression or CNVs alone. This will lead to a greater, more integrated understanding of cellular mechanism, and will allow the identification of genomic regulators as well as enhancement of anticancer drug specificity targeting those regulators. This is key to the discovery of potential combination therapies for the treatment of human cancer. Moreover, genomic patterns related to therapeutic response and clinical outcomes can be identified as biomarkers, which will improve early cancer detection, prognosis and outcome prediction as well as treatment selection. All in all, this will create a comprehensive picture of heterogeneity in tumor genomes, and offer a valuable starting point for new therapeutic approaches.

5. References

Akahira, J.-i., Aoki, M., Suzuki, T., Moriya, T., Niikura, H., Ito, K., Inoue, S., Okamura, K., Sasano, H. & Yaegashi, N. (2004). Expression of ebag9/rcasl is associated with advanced disease in human epithelial ovarian cancer, *Br J Cancer* 90(11): 2197–2202. URL: *http://dx.doi.org/10.1038/sj.bjc.6601832*

Akavia, U. D., Litvin, O., Kim, J., Sanchez-Garcia, F., Kotliar, D., Causton, H. C., Pochanard, P., Mozes, E., Garraway, L. A. & Pe'er, D. (2010). An integrated approach to uncover drivers of cancer, *Cell* 143(6): 1005 – 1017. URL: *http://www.sciencedirect.com/science/article/pii/S0092867410012936*

Albertson, D. G. (2003). Profiling breast cancer by array cgh, *Breast Cancer Research and Treatment* 78(3): 289–298. URL: *http://dx.doi.org/10.1023/A:1023025506386*

Beheshti, B., Braude, I., Marrano, P., Thorner, P., Zielenska, M. & Squire, J. (2003). Chromosomal localization of dna amplifications in neuroblastoma tumors using cdna microarray comparative genomic hybridization., *Neoplasia (New York, N.Y.)* 5(1). URL: *http://ukpmc.ac.uk/abstract/MED/12659670*

Carvalho, C. M., Chang, J., Lucas, J. E., Nevins, J. R., Wang, Q. & West, M. (2008). High-Dimensional Sparse Factor Modelling: Applications in Gene Expression Genomics, *Journal of the American Statistical Association* 103(484): 1438–1456. URL: *http://pubs.amstat.org/doi/pdf/10.1198/016214508000000086*

Carvalho, C. M. & West, M. (2006). Structure and sparsity in high-dimensional multivariate analysis, *ProQuest Dissertations and Theses* . URL: *http://search.proquest.com/docview/305329670?accountid=10598*

Cleveland, W. S. (1979). Robust locally weighted regression and smoothing scatterplots, *Journal of the American Statistical Association* 74(368): 829–836. URL: *http://www.jstor.org/stable/2286407*

Comprehensive genomic characterization defines human glioblastoma genes and core pathways (2008). *Nature* 455(7216): 1061–1068. URL: *http://dx.doi.org/10.1038/nature07385*

Du, L., Chen, M., Lucas, J. & Carin, L. (2010). Sticky hidden markov modeling of comparative genomic hybridization, *Signal Processing, IEEE Transactions on* 58(10): 5353 –5368.

Emdad, L., Sarkar, D., Su, Z.-Z., Lee, S.-G., Kang, D.-C., Bruce, J. N., Volsky, D. J. & Fisher, P. B. (2007). Astrocyte elevated gene-1: Recent insights into a novel gene involved in tumor progression, metastasis and neurodegeneration, *Pharmacology and Therapeutics* 114(2): 155 – 170. URL: *http://www.sciencedirect.com/science/article/pii/S0163725807000332*

Fridlyand, J. (2004). Hidden Markov models approach to the analysis of array CGH data, *Journal of Multivariate Analysis* 90(1): 132–153. URL: *http://dx.doi.org/10.1016/j.jmva.2004.02.008*

Garraway, L. A., Widlund, H. R., Rubin, M. A., Getz, G., Berger, A. J., Ramaswamy, S., Beroukhim, R., Milner, D. A., Granter, S. R., Du, J., Lee, C., Wagner, S. N., Li, C., Golub, T. R., Rimm, D. L., Meyerson, M. L., Fisher, D. E. & Sellers, W. R. (2005). Integrative genomic analyses identify mitf as a lineage survival oncogene amplified

in malignant melanoma, *Nature* 436(7047): 117–122.
URL: *http://dx.doi.org/10.1038/nature03664*

George, E. I. & McCulloch, R. E. (1993). Variable selection via gibbs sampling, *Journal of the American Statistical Association* 88(423): 881–889.
URL: *http://www.jstor.org/stable/2290777*

Hsu, L., Self, S. G., Grove, D., Randolph, T., Wang, K., Delrow, J. J., Loo, L. & Porter, P. (2005). Denoising array-based comparative genomic hybridization data using wavelets, *Biostatistics* 6(2): 211–226.
URL: *http://biostatistics.oxfordjournals.org/content/6/2/211.abstract*

Hu, G., Chong, R. A., Yang, Q., Wei, Y., Blanco, M. A., Li, F., Reiss, M., Au, J. L.-S., Haffty, B. G. & Kang, Y. (2009). Mtdh activation by 8q22 genomic gain promotes chemoresistance and metastasis of poor-prognosis breast cancer, *Cancer Cell* 15(1): 9 – 20.
URL: *http://www.sciencedirect.com/science/article/pii/S1535610808003796*

Hup, P., Stransky, N., Thiery, J.-P., Radvanyi, F. & Barillot, E. (2004). Analysis of array cgh data: from signal ratio to gain and loss of dna regions, *Bioinformatics* 20(18): 3413–3422.
URL: *http://bioinformatics.oxfordjournals.org/content/20/18/3413.abstract*

Integrated genomic analyses of ovarian carcinoma (2011). *Nature* 474(7353): 609–615.
URL: *http://dx.doi.org/10.1038/nature10166*

Ishwaran & Rao, J. S. (2005). Spike and slab variable selection: frequentist and bayesian strategies.

Iwasaki, T., Nakashima, M., Watanabe, T., Yamamoto, S., Inoue, Y., Yamanaka, H., Matsumura, A., Iuchi, K., Mori, T. & Okada, M. (2000). Expression and prognostic significance in lung cancer of human tumor-associated antigen rcas1, *International Journal of Cancer* 89(6): 488–493.
URL: *http://dx.doi.org/10.1002/1097-0215(20001120)89:6<488::AID-IJC4>3.0.CO;2-D*

Jonsson, G., Staaf, J., Vallon-Christersson, J., Ringner, M., Holm, K., Hegardt, C., Gunnarsson, H., Fagerholm, R., Strand, C., Agnarsson, B., Kilpivaara, O., Luts, L., Heikkila, P., Aittomaki, K., Blomqvist, C., Loman, N., Malmstrom, P., Olsson, H., Th Johannsson, O., Arason, A., Nevanlinna, H., Barkardottir, R. & Borg, A. (2010). Genomic subtypes of breast cancer identified by array-comparative genomic hybridization display distinct molecular and clinical characteristics, *Breast Cancer Research* 12(3): R42.
URL: *http://breast-cancer-research.com/content/12/3/R42*

Kiechle, M., Jacobsen, A., Schwarz-Boeger, U., Hedderich, J., Pfisterer, J. & Arnold, N. (2001). Comparative genomic hybridization detects genetic imbalances in primary ovarian carcinomas as correlated with grade of differentiation, *Cancer* 91(3): 534–540.
URL: *http://dx.doi.org/10.1002/1097-0142(20010201)91:3<534::AID-CNCR1031>3.0.CO;2-T*

Kikuno, N., Shiina, H., Urakami, S., Kawamoto, K., Hirata, H., Tanaka, Y., Place, R. F., Pookot, D., Majid, S., Igawa, M. & Dahiya, R. (2007). Knockdown of astrocyte-elevated gene-1 inhibits prostate cancer progression through upregulation of foxo3a activity, *Oncogene* 26(55): 7647–7655.
URL: *http://dx.doi.org/10.1038/sj.onc.1210572*

Lanckriet, G. R. G., De Bie, T., Cristianini, N., Jordan, M. I. & Noble, W. S. (2004). A statistical framework for genomic data fusion, *Bioinformatics* 20(16): 2626–2635.
URL: *http://bioinformatics.oxfordjournals.org/content/20/16/2626.abstract*

Lee, S.-G., Su, Z.-Z., Emdad, L., Sarkar, D., Franke, T. F. & Fisher, P. B. (2007). Astrocyte elevated gene-1 activates cell survival pathways through pi3k-akt signaling,

Oncogene 27(8): 1114–1121.
URL: *http://dx.doi.org/10.1038/sj.onc.1210713*

Lockwood, W. W., Chari, R., Chi, B. & Lam, W. L. (2005). Recent advances in array comparative genomic hybridization technologies and their applications in human genetics, *Eur J Hum Genet* 14(2): 139–148.
URL: *http://dx.doi.org/10.1038/sj.ejhg.5201531*

Lucas, J., Carvalho, C., Wang, Q., Bild, A., Nevins, J. & West, M. (2006). *Sparse Statistical Modelling in Gene Expression Genomics*, pp. 155–176.

Lucas, J., Carvalho, C. & West, M. (2009). A bayesian analysis strategy for cross-study translation of gene expression biomarkers., *Statistical applications in genetics and molecular biology* 8(1).
URL: *http://dx.doi.org/10.2202/1544-6115.1436*

Lucas, J. E., Kung, H.-N. & Chi, J.-T. A. (2010). Latent factor analysis to discover pathway-associated putative segmental aneuploidies in human cancers, *PLoS Comput Biol* 6(9): e1000920.
URL: *http://dx.doi.org/10.1371/journal.pcbi.1000920*

McKay, S. C., Unger, K., Pericleous, S., Stamp, G., Thomas, G., Hutchins, R. R. & Spalding, D. R. C. (2011). Array comparative genomic hybridization identifies novel potential therapeutic targets in cholangiocarcinoma, *HPB* 13(5): 309–319.
URL: *http://dx.doi.org/10.1111/j.1477-2574.2010.00286.x*

Mitchell, T. J. & Beauchamp, J. J. (1988). Bayesian variable selection in linear regression, *Journal of the American Statistical Association* 83(404): 1023–1032.
URL: *http://www.jstor.org/stable/2290129*

Nakashima, M., Sonoda, K. & Watanabe, T. (1999). Inhibition of cell growth and induction of apoptotic cell death by the human tumor-associated antigen rcas1, *Nat Med* 5(8): 938–942.
URL: *http://dx.doi.org/10.1038/11383*

Olshen, A. B., Venkatraman, E. S., Lucito, R. & Wigler, M. (2004). Circular binary segmentation for the analysis of arrayâĂŘbased dna copy number data, *Biostatistics* 5(4): 557–572.
URL: *http://biostatistics.oxfordjournals.org/content/5/4/557.abstract*

Parsons, D. W., Jones, S., Zhang, X., Lin, J. C.-H., Leary, R. J., Angenendt, P., Mankoo, P., Carter, H., Siu, I.-M., Gallia, G. L., Olivi, A., McLendon, R., Rasheed, B. A., Keir, S., Nikolskaya, T., Nikolsky, Y., Busam, D. A., Tekleab, H., Diaz, L. A., Hartigan, J., Smith, D. R., Strausberg, R. L., Marie, S. K. N., Shinjo, S. M. O., Yan, H., Riggins, G. J., Bigner, D. D., Karchin, R., Papadopoulos, N., Parmigiani, G., Vogelstein, B., Velculescu, V. E. & Kinzler, K. W. (2008). An integrated genomic analysis of human glioblastoma multiforme, *Science* 321(5897): 1807–1812.
URL: *http://www.sciencemag.org/content/321/5897/1807.abstract*

Pinkel, D. & Albertson, D. G. (2005). Array comparative genomic hybridization and its applications in cancer, *Nat Genet* .

Rennstam, K., Ahlstedt-Soini, M., Baldetorp, B., Bendahl, P.-O., Borg, Å., Karhu, R., Tanner, M., Tirkkonen, M. & Isola, J. (2003). Patterns of chromosomal imbalances defines subgroups of breast cancer with distinct clinical features and prognosis. a study of 305 tumors by comparative genomic hybridization, *Cancer Research* 63(24): 8861–8868.
URL: *http://cancerres.aacrjournals.org/content/63/24/8861.abstract*

Rueda, O. M. & Díaz-Uriarte, R. (2007). Flexible and accurate detection of genomic copy-number changes from acgh, *PLoS Comput Biol* 3(6): e122.
URL: *http://dx.plos.org/10.1371%2Fjournal.pcbi.0030122*

3

Sister Chromatid Cohesion and Aneuploidy

Erwan Watrin* and Claude Prigent*
Research Institute of Genetics and Development
Centre National de la Recherche Scientifique
University of Rennes I
France

1. Introduction

In all living organisms, cells arise from the division of a pre-existing cell and inherit one copy of the genome identical to that of the mother cell. Any defect in chromosome segregation can lead to aneuploidy *via* chromosome gain or loss, and consequently to genetic instability, thereby paving the way for malignant growth and cancer. Thus, the faithful distribution of one copy of each chromosome between the two daughter cells is essential to maintain genome stability. Cells have evolved elaborate control mechanisms to ensure that chromosome segregation occurs in an accurate manner. From yeast to human, replicated DNA molecules are held together from their synthesis during S-phase until their separation in mitosis. This sister chromatid cohesion is absolutely essential for faithful transmission of replicated chromosomes during mitosis (for review, see Nasmyth, 2001). Indeed, in early mitosis, cohesion between sister chromatids counteracts the pulling forces exerted by the microtubule filaments emanating from the opposite poles of the mitotic spindle, thereby allowing the proper alignment of chromosomes on the metaphase plate, and their faithful segregation during the subsequent anaphase. In the case of a defective cohesion, the sister chromatids would float around in the cellular space and, as a consequence, would fail to be equally distributed between the two future daughter cells. Cohesion between sister chromatid is not only required for the proper distribution of replicated genomes during mitosis, but is also essential in postreplicative interphase cells for the repair of DNA double-strand breaks by homologous recombination (Sjogren and Nasmyth, 2001)(for review, see Strom and Sjogren, 2007; Watrin and Peters, 2006). The homologous recombination pathway uses an identical copy of the damaged DNA fibre, typically the sister chromatid, as a template to faithfully repair the altered DNA. For the homologous recombination machinery to process chromosome breaks, the broken chromatid and the sister chromatid that is used as a template have to be positioned and maintained in close proximity. It is believed that sister chromatid cohesion provides this spatial proximity between damaged and template chromatids. Consistently, proteins that are required for sister chromatid cohesion are also required for the repair of DNA double-strand breaks in postreplicative cells (for review, see Watrin and Peters, 2006). Therefore, sister chromatid cohesion plays an essential role in restoring and maintaining the integrity of the genome upon genotoxic stress.

---

* Corresponding Author

In all eukaryotes studied so far, sister chromatid cohesion depends on a multi-subunit complex called cohesin (Losada et al., 1998; Strunnikov et al., 1993; Toth et al., 1999). This complex forms a ring-like structure, and it has been proposed that cohesin entraps replicated DNA molecules in this proteinaceous ring (Gruber et al., 2003; Haering et al., 2002). In addition to its role in sister chromatid cohesion, the cohesin complex has also been shown to be involved in other aspects of chromosome biology, which include the control of gene expression and the regulation of the DNA damage checkpoint that will not be further discussed here.

Over the last decade, we began to understand at the molecular level how cohesin functions in sister chromatid cohesion and how the cohesion apparatus is regulated during the cell cycle. In addition, accumulating evidence in human and animal models highlighted the importance of the cohesion apparatus in protecting somatic cells from aneuploidy and cancer, and germ cells from improper meiotic segregation that leads to aneuploid gametes and infertility. Here we present an overview of the current knowledge on the sister chromatid cohesion apparatus, its molecular actors and regulatory mechanisms in human. In addition we will discuss a defective cohesion as a cause for aneuploidy in somatic and germinal cells, and its involvement in human pathologies. Finally we will try to identify future directions that we need to explore to better understand the basis of aneuploidy-driven genomic instability.

2. Composition and architecture of the cohesin complex

2.1 The cohesin core complex

The cohesin core complex consists of four subunits (Figure 1). The two core subunits Smc1 and Smc3 belong to the structural maintenance of chromosome (SMC) protein family. SMC proteins fold back on themselves creating a long intramolecular anti-parallel coiled-coil that separates a "hinge" domain and a globular ATPase head which is formed by the reunion of the C- and N-terminal regions (Melby et al., 1998; Michaelis et al., 1997; Strunnikov et al., 1993). Within the cohesin complex, Smc1 and Smc3 bind tightly to each other *via* their hinge domain, and form a V-shaped heterodimer. In somatic cells, the ATPase domains of Smc1 and Smc3 are physically linked to each other by the kleisin subunit Scc1 (also called Rad21 or Mcd1). Scc1 subunit associates by its N- and C-termini to the ATPase heads of Smc3 and Smc1, respectively (Haering et al., 2002; Haering et al., 2004). The reunion of the Smc1/Smc3 heterodimer together with the Scc1 protein forms a tripartite molecular ring with an inner diameter of 40 nm (Figure 1) (Haering et al., 2002). This ring structure has been observed by electron microscopy imaging of cohesin complexes isolated from human cells as well as from *Xenopus laevis* interphase egg extract (Anderson et al., 2002). The cohesin ring is large enough to accommodate two 10-nanometer DNA fibres, and it has been proposed that cohesin maintains the cohesion between replicated chromatids by embracing them within its ring (Gruber et al., 2003; Haering et al., 2002). According to the widely accepted ring model (Figure 1), cohesin complex mediates cohesion between replicated DNA fibres simply by topological links. Alternative ring-based models have also been proposed for cohesin-mediated sister chromatid cohesion, like the "handcuff" model, where each sister chromatid of a pair would be encircled within distinct cohesin complexes that would interact with each others and may thereby physically connect sister chromatids (Zhang et al., 2008b). Also, it has been proposed that two cohesin complexes would oligomerise into a larger ring around DNA (Huang et al., 2005). Besides interacting with Smc1 and Smc3, Scc1 protein also binds to the fourth cohesin subunit called Scc3 in yeast, of which two orthologs exist in vertebrates, called stromalin antigen 1 and 2 (SA1 and SA2). Within the cohesin complex, SA1 and SA2 interact with Scc1 in a mutually exclusive manner (Losada et al., 2000, Sumara et al., 2000), implying that two cohesin core complexes, referred to as cohesin^{SA1} and cohesin^{SA2}, coexist in vertebrates somatic cells. It has recently been suggested that cohesin complexes containing SA1 or SA2 have specialised function in sister chromatid cohesion at telomeres and at centromeres, respectively (Canudas and Smith, 2009).

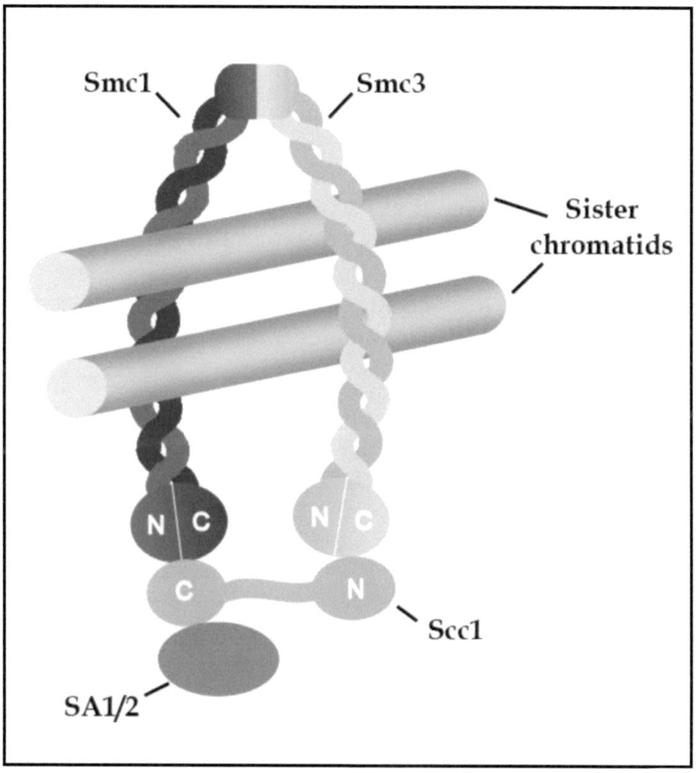

The vertebrate cohesin core complex consists of the four subunits Smc1, Smc3, Scc1 and SA1 or SA2. The association of Smc1, Smc3 and Scc1 forms a tripartite molecular ring. According to the ring model (Gruber et al., 2003; Haering et al., 2002), cohesin maintains sister chromatid cohesion by embracing the replicated chromatids within its ring. Cohesion is therefore mediated solely by physical, topological linkages.

Fig. 1. Composition and architecture of the cohesin core complex and the ring model

2.2 Cohesin associated factors

Besides the four core cohesin subunits, additional proteins have also been shown to be part of the cohesin complex. These evolutionary conserved proteins are named Pds5, Wapl and Sororin. In vertebrates, two homologs of Pds5 exist, called Pds5A and Pds5B, which are both able to associate with either cohesin^{SA1} or cohesin^{SA2} (Losada et al., 2000; Sumara et al., 2000). Therefore four distinct cohesin complexes are present in vertebrates cells. From yeast to fly, Pds5 is essential for the proper cohesion between sister chromatids (Dorsett et al., 2005;

Hartman et al., 2000; Panizza et al., 2000; Tanaka et al., 2001; Wang et al., 2002. In vertebrate cells, however, depletion of Pds5A or Pds5B does not result in strong sister chromatid cohesion defects (Losada, 2005). Quite the opposite, it has recently been shown that depletion of both Pds5A and Pds5B from *Xenopus laevis* egg extract does not impair sister chromatid cohesion, but instead, severely affects cohesin dissociation and cohesion loss from chromosome arms in mitosis (Shintomi and Hirano, 2009), suggesting that Pds5A and Pds5B function in the dissociation of cohesin complexes from chromosome arms and thereby in the resolution, i.e. the physical separation, of the sister chromatids in early mitosis (see below).

Vertebrate cohesin also binds to Wapl (Gandhi et al., 2006; Kueng et al., 2006), a protein that was first identified in *Drosophila,* where it has been involved in the establishment of heterochromatin (Verni et al., 2000). Wapl homologs also exist in yeasts (called Rad61 or Wpl1) where it also associates with the cohesin complex (Rolef Ben-Shahar et al., 2008). It has been shown in human that the interaction of Wapl with cohesin depends on the SA1/SA2 and Scc1 subunits (Kueng et al., 2006). Furthermore, Wapl interacts with Pds5 proteins (Shintomi and Hirano, 2009) through a conserved motif that consists of the triplet sequence phenylalanine-glycin-phenylalanine residues (called the FGF motif). In vertebrates, Wapl is dispensable for sister chromatid cohesion, but plays an essential role in the removal of cohesin complexes from chromosome arms during early mitosis, similarly to Pds5 proteins (see below).

Finally, a small protein called Sororin also interacts with cohesin complexes (Rankin et al., 2005; Schmitz et al., 2007). Like the core cohesin complex, Sororin has been shown to be essential for cohesion between sister chromatids in vertebrates (Rankin et al., 2005; Schmitz et al., 2007), but is dispensable for cohesin's ability to associate with chromatin (Schmitz et al., 2007). Recent work has shown that the function of Sororin in sister chromatid cohesin depends on its ability to compete with Wapl for its binding to Pds5 proteins *via* its FGF motif (Nishiyama et al., 2010), strongly suggesting that Sororin acts in cohesion by antagonising Wapl's capacity to dissociate cohesin complexes from the chromatin (see below).

2.3 Composition of cohesin in meiosis

Similar to mitosis, faithful segregation of homologous chromosomes and sister chromatids during meiosis also depends on sister chromatid cohesion and on cohesin complexes (see below). However, the composition of the cohesin complex in meiotic cells slightly differs from that of somatic cells (for review, see Petronczki et al., 2003). The subunit Scc1 is replaced by a meiosis-specific variant called Rec8, and the Smc1β isoform can substitute for the canonical Smc1 (also referred to as Smc1α). Finally, SA1 and SA2 proteins can both be replaced by the meiotic form STAG3. Therefore, meiotic cells contain different forms of cohesin complexes, specific functions of which are still largely unknown.

3. Regulating cohesin and sister chromatid cohesion

In vertebrate cells, cohesin is loaded onto chromatin from telophase to early G1 phase. During S phase, sister chromatid cohesion is established, and maintained throughout G2 phase. Finally, cohesin complexes are removed from chromosomes during mitosis to allow physical separation of sister chromatids and faithful segregation of replicated chromosomes during anaphase (Figure 2).

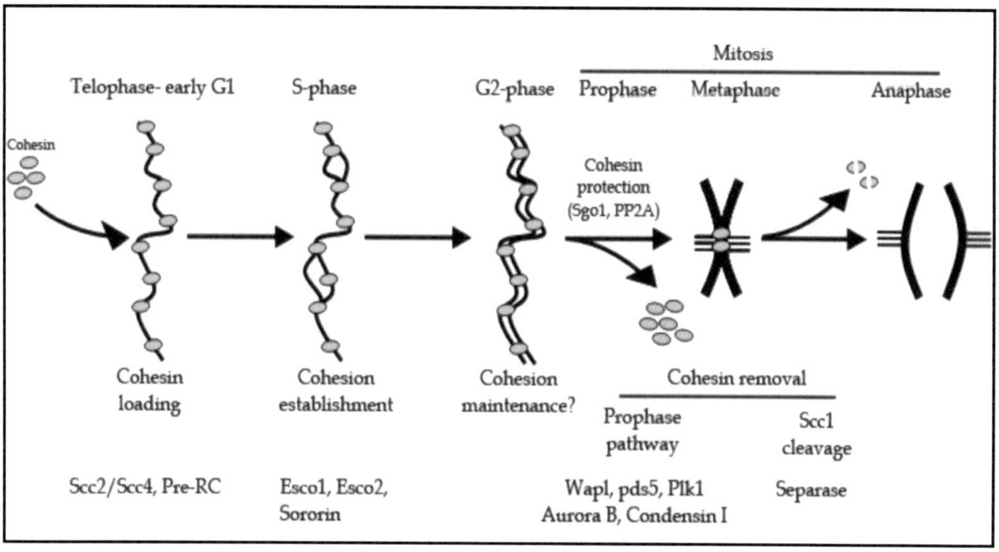

Cohesin loading onto chromatin occurs from telophase to early G1 and depends on the loading complex Scc2/Scc4. In addition, this process also requires that pre-RC complexes have assembled on chromatin. During S phase, cohesion between duplicated sister chromatids is established. This process depends on the activity of the two acetyltransferases Esco1 and Esco2. The protein sororin is also essential for cohesion establishment. Sister chromatid cohesion is maintained during G2, although it is still unclear whether cohesion maintenance requires specific factors. Cohesin is removed from chromosomes during early mitosis in a two-step manner. During prophase, cohesin complexes dissociate from chromosome arms in a process that depends on the activity of the mitotic kinases Plk1 and Aurora B, the association of condensin I with chromosomes, as well as on Wapl and Pds5 proteins. Centromeric cohesin is protected from removal by the prophase pathway by Sgo1 and PP2A. At the metaphase-to-anaphase transition, the protease separase is activated and cleaves centromeric cohesin complexes. Complete removal of cohesin from chromosomes allows segregation of sister chromatids.

Fig. 2. Regulation of sister chromatid cohesion during cell cycle in human

3.1 Loading of cohesin onto chromatin

In all eukaryotes studied so far, loading of cohesin onto chromatin depends on an additional complex formed by two proteins, called Scc2 and Scc4 (Bernard et al., 2006; Ciosk et al., 2000; Furuya et al., 1998; Gillespie and Hirano, 2004; Rollins et al., 2004; Takahashi et al., 2004; Watrin et al., 2006). Furthermore, cohesin loading onto chromatin in *Xenopus* egg extract also requires that the pre-replication complex (pre-RC) assembles on chromatin during the exit from mitosis (Gillespie and Hirano, 2004; Takahashi et al., 2004). It has also been show that the ATPase activity of the Smc1/Smc3 heterodimer is essential for cohesin to bind to chromatin (Arumugam et al., 2003; Weitzer et al., 2003). How the chromatin fibre can enter the cohesin ring has been a long-lasting question in the field. Biochemical approaches combined with genetics studies have provided insights into molecular events that govern this process, which have been reviewed elsewhere (for review, see Nasmyth and Haering, 2009; Peters et al., 2008). Therefore, we will present here only an overview of key findings. The cohesin ring must be opened to allow the entry of the DNA therein. It has been proposed that Smc1 and Smc3 transiently dissociate at the hinge domain, thereby allowing

DNA to enter into the cohesin ring (Gruber et al., 2006; Milutinovich et al., 2007). Given that in *S. cerevisiae*, the hinge domain of Smc1/Smc3 is able to interact with their ATPase heads (Mc Intyre et al., 2007), one can envision that ATP hydrolysis by Smc1/Smc3 ATPase heads triggers a conformational change of the cohesin complex, which would *in fine* result in the transient opening of the hinge and in the entry of DNA into the cohesin ring.

3.2 Establishment of sister chromatid cohesion

The establishment of cohesion between sister chromatids takes place while DNA is replicated during S phase (Uhlmann and Nasmyth, 1998) and depends on the activity of an acetyltransferase called Eco1/Ctf7 in yeast (Skibbens et al., 1999; Toth et al., 1999). Eco1 becomes dispensable once replication has been achieved, indicating that the cohesion can only be established during replication, i.e. when sister chromatids are synthesised. However, it has to be noticed that cohesion can be established *de novo* in postreplicative cells, but only upon DNA double-strand break (Kim et al., ; Strom et al., 2007; Unal et al., 2007). It has recently been shown that in yeast, Eco1 acetylates two lysine residues in the ATPase region of Smc3, and that these acetylations are essential for the establishment of sister chromatid cohesion (Rolef Ben-Shahar et al., 2008; Unal et al., 2008; Zhang et al., 2008a). In vertebrate cells, two orthologs of Eco1 exist, called Esco1 and Esco2 (Hou and Zou, 2005). Similar to the situation in yeast, Smc3 becomes acetylated during replication at two evolutionary conserved lysine residues, at position 105 and 106 (Zhang et al., 2008a). Simultaneous inactivation in human cells of Esco1 and Esco2 impairs the acetylation of Smc3 whereas depletion of either Esco1 or Esco2 has little impact, if any, on Smc3 acetylation (Nishiyama et al., 2010; Zhang et al., 2008a), indicating that these two acetyltransferases are at least partly redundant for their function in Smc3 acetylation. Interestingly, acetylation of Smc3 becomes dispensable for sister chromatid cohesion when either Wapl or Pds5 are inactivated (Feytout et al., 2011; Rowland et al., 2009; Sutani et al., 2009). This is consistent with the function of Wapl and Pds5 in destabilising sister chromatid cohesion. Recently, it has further been shown that the acetylation of Smc3 triggers a rearrangement in cohesin subunit interactions (Nishiyama et al., 2010). Indeed, Smc3 acetylation promotes binding of Sororin to cohesin, where Sororin displaces Wapl from its interaction with Pds5 proteins. The authors further showed that Sororin also contains an FGF motif that competes with that of Wapl for its binding to Pds5. Therefore the establishment of sister chromatid cohesion depends on the protein Sororin that might counteracts Wapl's ability to dissociate cohesin complexes from chromatin (Nishiyama et al., 2010). In human cultured cells, fluorescence recovery after photobleaching (FRAP) experiments have shown that the binding of cohesin complexes to chromatin is very dynamic in G1 phase cells, and that the binding of half of chromatin-bound cohesin pool becomes very stably associated with DNA in G2 phase cells (Gerlich et al., 2006). It has been proposed that this stably-bound pool of cohesin is responsible for sister chromatid cohesion (Gerlich et al., 2006). Consistent with this possibility, the inactivation of Sororin results in the reduction of the stably-bound pool of cohesin (Schmitz et al., 2007). Conversely, inactivating Wapl induces an increase in the stable pool of chromatin-bound cohesin (Kueng et al., 2006).

Altogether, these data are in favour of a model, in which the acetylation of Smc3 during replication triggers the recruitment of Sororin, the consequent displacement of the cohesion-destabilising protein Wapl, ultimately leading to the creation of a cohesive state of cohesin complexes and to the establishment of sister chromatid cohesion.

3.3 Removal of cohesin from chromosomes during mitosis

Cohesion between sister chromatid is maintained during G2 until mitosis, when it must be dissolved to allow the physical separation of the two sets of replicated chromosomes. Unlike in yeasts, vertebrate cohesin is removed from chromosomes in a two-step manner from the onset of mitosis until the metaphase-to-anaphase transition (Figure 2).

3.3.1 The prophase pathway

In vertebrates, the bulk of cohesin complexes (~ 90 - 95 %) is removed from the chromosome arms during prophase and prometaphase (Sumara et al., 2000; Waizenegger et al., 2000), whereas some cohesin complexes remain bound to chromosomes at centromeric regions (Waizenegger et al., 2000). This first wave of cohesin removal from chromosomes is referred to as the prophase pathway, which depends on several factors that include the mitotic kinases Aurora B (Dai et al., 2006; Losada et al., 2002) and Plk1 (Lenart et al., 2007; Losada et al., 2002; Sumara et al., 2002) and the proteins Wapl (Gandhi et al., 2006; Kueng et al., 2006) and Pds5 (Shintomi and Hirano, 2009). Plk1 is thought to promote cohesin release from chromatin by phosphorylating the SA2 subunit (Losada et al., 2002; Sumara et al., 2002). Consistent with this possibility, the expression of a mutated version of SA2 that can no longer be phosphorylated in mitosis triggers a persistent binding of cohesin complexes on chromosome arms in prometaphase (Hauf et al., 2005). This strongly suggests that Plk1 participates in the dissociation of cohesin from the chromosomes by directly phosphorylating the SA2 subunit. In addition, it has also been shown that the cohesin-related complex Condensin I is required for cohesin removal from chromosome arms (Hirota et al., 2004), although the role of Condensin I in the prophase pathway remains unclear.

Central actors to the removal of cohesin by the prophase pathway are Wapl and Pds5 proteins (Gandhi et al., 2006; Kueng et al., 2006; Shintomi and Hirano, 2009). Consistently, inactivation of either Wapl or Pds5 results in the persistence of cohesin complexes along the chromosome arms, which leads to unresolved sister chromatids in prometaphase (Gandhi et al., 2006; Kueng et al., 2006; Shintomi and Hirano, 2009). Recently, it was shown that sororin, which promotes sister chromatid cohesion by counteracting cohesin-destabilising activity of Wapl (see above), is phosphorylated in mitosis (Nishiyama et al., 2010). Sororin phosphorylation correlates with the loss of its ability to displace Wapl from Pds5 *in vitro*. Therefore, it has been proposed that the mitotic phosphorylation of Sororin inactivates its ability to displace Wapl from binding to Pds5, which in turn leads to the association of Wapl to Pds5 and the dissociation of cohesin complexes from chromosomes (Nishiyama et al., 2010).

Whereas most of cohesin complexes are removed from the chromosome arms during prophase, the cohesin complexes located at centromeric regions are protected from the prophase pathway. This protection of centromeric cohesion is essential to maintain sister chromatid cohesion until anaphase onset, and allows the proper bipolar attachment of mitotic chromosomes on the metaphase plate. At this stage of mitosis, sister chromatids are held together only at centromeres, giving rise to the classical X-shaped mitotic chromosomes. Cohesin protection at centromeres depends on a protein called Shugoshin (guardian spirit in Japanese) also known as Sgo1 (Kitajima et al., 2004; McGuinness et al.,

2005; Salic et al., 2004). Sgo1 interacts with the protein phosphatase PP2A and both proteins are enriched at centromeres in early mitosis. It is believed that Sgo1 recruits PP2A to the centromeres, where PP2A dephosphorylates the cohesin subunit SA2, thereby counteracting the dissociation activity of the kinase Plk1 (Kitajima et al., 2006). The inhibition of the kinase Aurora B has been shown to trigger abnormal localisation of Sgo1 along chromosome arms (Dai et al., 2006). This indicates that Aurora B is required for the proper enrichment of Sgo1 at centromeres, and might account for its role in the prophase pathway. Finally other factors have also been shown to be important for the protection of cohesin complexes at centromeres, including the mitotic kinases Haspin (Dai et al., 2006) and Bub1 (Tang et al., 2004). Recently, it has been shown that Bub1 kinase is required for the phosphorylation of the centromeric histone H2A at threonine 120 (T120), for Sgo1 enrichment at centromeres and for sister chromatid cohesion (Kawashima et al., 2010), suggesting that Bub1-mediated phosphorylation of H2A-T120 recruits Sgo1 and thereby participates in the protection of centromeric cohesion. Additional experimental works will be required to substantiate this view, and, more importantly, to obtain an integrated view of the molecular actors and mechanisms involved in the protection of sister chromatid cohesion at centromeres.

3.3.2 Cleavage of cohesin by separase

During early mitosis, sister chromatids remain tightly associated at centromeric regions until all the chromosomes have been properly bi-oriented on the mitotic spindle (Waizenegger et al., 2000). As long as all chromosomes have not been correctly aligned on the metaphase plate, a surveillance mechanism, called the spindle assembly checkpoint (SAC), inhibits the activity of the anaphase promoting complex, or cyclosome, (APC/c) thereby preventing the activation of separase and the inactivation of cyclin-dependent kinase 1 (Cdk1). Once all chromosomes have been bi-oriented on the mitotic spindle, the SAC is satisfied and, consequently, the inhibition of the APC/c is relieved. Activated APC/c can then ubiquitinate the separase inhibitory protein securin as well as the Cdk1 activator cyclin B, leading to their degradation by the 26S proteasome (reviewed in Peters, 2002). Once it has been activated, separase cleaves the cohesin subunit Scc1, which triggers opening of the cohesin ring, dissociation of cohesin complexes from chromosomes, dissolution of sister chromatid cohesion and separation of the two sets of replicated chromosomes to the opposite poles of the mitotic spindle (Tomonaga et al., 2000; Uhlmann et al., 1999; Waizenegger et al., 2000). The concomitant degradation of cyclin B inactivates Cdk1, which leads to cell's exit from mitosis and to the formation of the two daughter cells.

4. Meiosis

Meiosis is a specialised form of cell division that produces gametes, which contain either the maternal or the parental copy of each chromosome. Nonetheless, meiosis shares common features with mitosis as well as specific mechanisms. Meiosis involves a single S phase followed by two successive rounds of chromosome segregation without intervening DNA replication, and produces haploid germinal cells. Similar to mitosis, replication of DNA prior meiotic division gives rise to replicated sister chromatids that are linked to each other along their entire length by meiotic cohesin complexes (Figure 3). During prophase I, homologous paternal and maternal chromosomes become attached to each other through a mechanism called homolog pairing or synapsis. This pairing depends on a large protein complex called the synaptonemal complex. These homologs pairs (also called tetrads or bivalents) undergo exchanges of DNA segments between paternal and maternal non-sister chromatids by homologous recombination, which give rise to crossover. Once homologous recombination has occurred in late prophase I, the synaptonemal complex is dissolved. Therefore, homologous chromosomes are held together solely by cohesion between sister chromatids distal to the site of recombination. At metaphase I, bivalents are aligned on the meiotic microtubule spindle in a monopolar fashion, that is, with the two kinetochores of each sister chromatid pair facing toward the same spindle pole. At the metaphase I-to-anaphase I transition, the meiotic cohesin subunit Rec8 located on the arms of chromosomes is cleaved by separase, allowing the segregation of homologous chromosomes to opposite poles during anaphase I. Thus, the meiosis I gives rise to two cells that only contains either the maternal or the paternal copy of each chromosome, eventually recombined. Due to this peculiarity, meiosis I is also referred to as the reductional division. Central to meiosis is the protection of Rec8 cleavage from separase at centromeric regions by a mechanism that is conserved throughout evolution and that depends on Shugoshin. Unlike in budding yeast and in fruit fly where only one shugoshin protein is found, two shugoshin-like proteins exist in other eukaryotes, and are called Sgo1 and Sgo2. In all eukaryotes cohesin is protected from cleavage by separase in meiosis I, whereas it is protected from non-proteolytic removal in mitosis (Katis et al., 2004; Kitajima et al., 2004; Kitajima et al., 2006; Rabitsch et al., 2004; Riedel et al., 2006). Recent data indicate that Shugoshin-PP2A complex protects Rec8 from cleavage by separase by counteracting its phosphorylation, thereby rendering Rec8 a poor substrate for separase (Katis et al., 2010). In mouse oocyte, although both Sgo1 and Sgo2 are

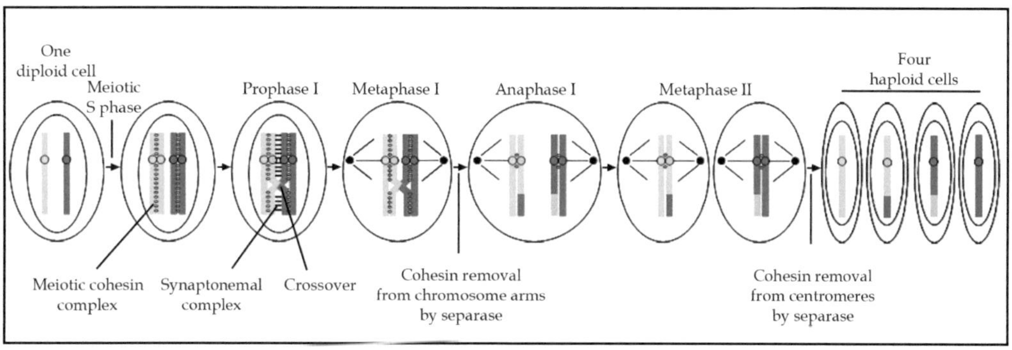

After completion of the meiotic S phase, sister chromatids are held together by meiotic cohesin complexes along their entire length. During prophase I, homologous chromosomes pair and remain associated to each other by the synaptonemal complex, and homologous recombination occurs and results in crossover. Once the synaptonemal complex has been dissolved late in prophase I, homologues remain associated only by cohesin located at distal position from the site of recombination. At metaphase I, homologues are bi-oriented on the first meiotic spindle, with both kinetochores from the same pair of sister chromatids facing the same spindle pole. Active separase cleaves Rec8 from chromosome arms, while cohesin complexes present at centromeres are protected by Shugoshin from cleavage by separase, thereby allowing proper bipolar attachment of sister chromatids on the microtubule spindle at metaphase II. Centromeric Rec8 is then cleaved by separase, allowing sister chromatid segregation. Once meiosis has been completed, four haploid cells are formed.

Fig. 3. Overview of meiosis

present in meiotic cells, Sgo2 appears to be the main protector of Rec8 cleavage (Lee et al., 2008; Llano et al., 2008). During meiosis II, also referred to as equational division, sister chromatids align on the second meiotic spindle in a bipolar manner, similar to the situation in mitosis. Once all chromosomes have been properly bi-oriented, separase cleaves centromeric Rec8 and sister chromatids are segregated between the two future haploid cells. How the function of Sgo2 in protecting Rec8 from its cleavage by separase is alleviated is still unknown. Once meiosis has been completed, four haploid cells are formed. It has to be noted that during spermatogenesis, four gametes arise from one meiotic division, whereas during oogenesis meiotic divisions are asymmetric and produce only one gamete. Furthermore, vertebrate oocytes are arrested at the metaphase stage of the second meiotic division and the completion of oocyte meiosis is triggered by fertilisation that induces the metaphase II-to-anaphase II transition.

5. Defective cohesion and aneuploidy

The sister chromatid cohesion is absolutely essential for the accurate distribution of the replicated genomes during mitosis and meiosis, and therefore, for the faithful transmission of genetic information from one generation of cells or organisms to the next. As a consequence, cohesion defects in somatic cells would lead to unequal distribution of chromosomes that leads to genomic instability and would thereby participate in the appearance of cancers. Similarly, during gametogenesis, defects in cohesion could lead to aneuploid gametes and infertility.

5.1 Mitosis

For more than a century, it is well known that genome instability and chromosomal aberrations are associated with cancer. Already in the early 20th century Theodor Boveri proposed that chromosomal instability contributes to cancer development. However, the causal link between aneuploidy and carcinogenesis has remained difficult to be experimentally addressed. Recently, it has been reported that, in yeast cells, aneuploidy induces an increase in DNA recombination and a decrease in DNA damage repair efficiency (Sheltzer et al., 2011), which are two frequent forms of genomic instability that are found in cancer cells. This clearly demonstrates that aneuploidy *per se* is able to induce chromosomal instability. Thus, defective sister chromatid cohesion can result in chromosome missegregation (Figure 4) that leads to aneuploidy and chromosomal instability, which *in fine* promotes tumourigenesis. Consistent with the association between an altered sister chromatid cohesion apparatus and tumourigenesis, both mutations and abnormal expression of genes encoding cohesin subunits have been found in various human cancers (for review see Mannini and Musio, 2011; (Xu et al., 2011). For instance, the core cohesin subunits Scc1 and Smc3 are overexpressed in breast and prostate cancers, and in colon carcinomas, respectively. Also, separase is found overexpressed in a variety of cancers including breast cancers (70 %) and osteosarcomas (for review see Mannini and Musio). More importantly, somatic mutations of Smc1α, Smc3 and STAG3 genes have been found in colorectal cancers (4 , 1 and 1 of 130, respectively) (Barber et al., 2008) and mutation of Scc1, SA2, STAG3 were found in lung carcinomas (1 , 1 and 1 of 12, respectively) (Xu et al., 2011) and references therein). Furthermore, genes encoding proteins involved in the regulation of cohesin are also found mutated in different types of cancer. In particular, Scc2 gene was

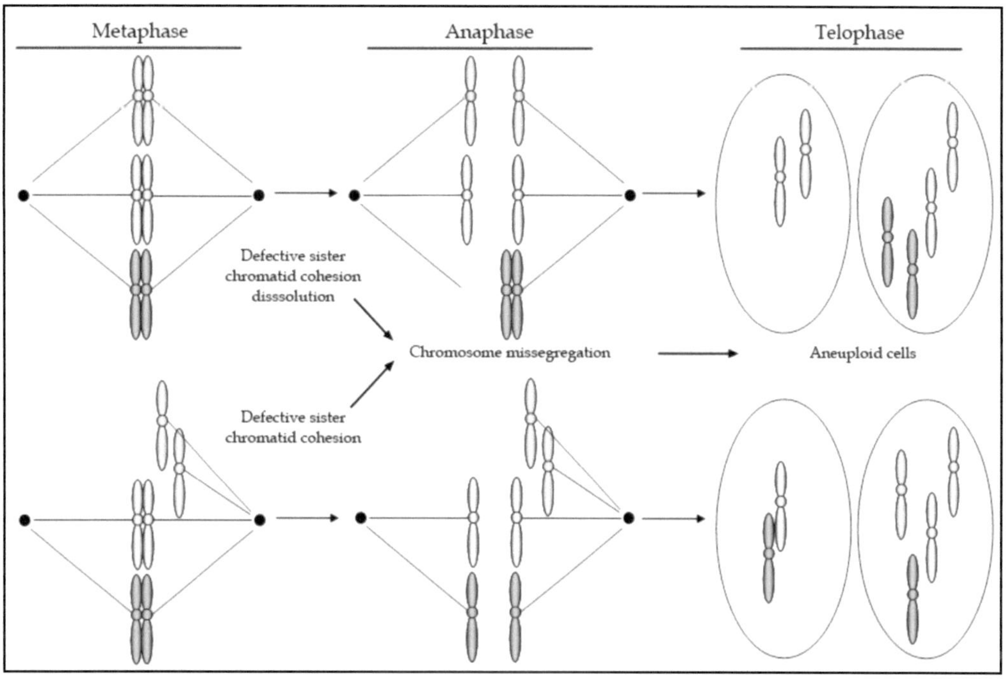

Schematic representation of chromosome missegregation as a cause of aneuploidy in somatic cells. During early mitosis, the spindle microtubule forces align condensed chromosomes on the metaphase plate. At the anaphase, one copy of each chromosome is pulled to one spindle pole. If the cohesin release from chromosomes is altered, sister chromatids would fail to separate and the two sister chromatids would be inherited by one daughter cell. Similarly, the deficient sister chromatid cohesion would lead in the premature separation of sister chromatids. Separated sisters would fail to align on the metaphase plate, which could eventually lead to their co-segregation into one daughter cell.

Fig. 4. Misregulation of sister chromatid cohesion leads to aneuploidy

shown to carry mutations in breast (1 of 48), lung (2 of 11) and kidney (1 of 101) carcinomas as well as in colorectal cancers (4 of 130), whereas mutations in separase gene were identified in kidney (1 of 101) and lung (1 of 12) carcinomas (Xu et al., 2011). Altogether, these observations underline the strong association that exists between altered sister chromatid cohesion apparatus and cancers. The direct implication of cohesin mutations in aneuploidy and chromosomal instability has been directly addressed recently (Solomon et al., 2011). The authors used single-nucleotide polymorphism analysis to characterise chromosomal rearrangements in human glioblastoma cell lines and thereby identified a genomic deletion of the X chromosome that contains the cohesin subunit SA2 gene. Accordingly, no expression of SA2 could be observed in these cell lines. Absence of functional SA2 protein expression was extended to others genomic rearrangement (frame-shift insertions and deletions, mutations of splicing regulatory elements) in other cancer cell lines (Solomon et al., 2011). Then, the authors addressed whether SA2 gene mutations induce genomic instability and aneuploidy by correcting endogenous locus using gene targeting in glioblastoma cell lines. Non-corrected cell lines exhibited premature separation of sister chromatids similar to the phenotype observed when cohesin is inactivated. Quite remarkably, the correction of SA2 was sufficient to rescue the loss-of-cohesion phenotype in this cancer cell line, demonstrating that SA2 mutation were the cause of the observed defective cohesion. Furthermore, the authors showed that the correction of SA2 not only rescues sister chromatid cohesion, but also reduces the number of defective mitotic divisions and the chromosome missegregation at anaphase. Finally, restoring SA2 expression also triggered a reduction in the variability in chromosome numbers between independent cells, indicative of an increase in genome stability. Altogether these works demonstrate that alteration of sister chromatid cohesion apparatus leads to missegregation of chromosomes and to aneuploidy and chromosome instability. This indicates that the function of the cohesin complex in maintaining the sister chromatid cohesion acts as an important barrier against tumorigenesis. Whether other known functions of cohesin, *i.e.* in the DNA damage response or in gene expression, also participate in carcinogenesis still needs to be uncovered.

5.2 Meiosis

The proper segregation of chromosomes during meiosis is of crucial importance in all living organisms, as aneuploidy leads to embryonic death and severe disorders, such as infertility and Down syndrome. Recent efforts from the scientific community have highlighted the importance of cohesin in preventing aneuploidy during meiosis in mammals. In human, oocytes wait up to several decades until they finally resume the first meiotic division, and it is well established that oocyte aneuploidy increases with age. Accordingly, age-related aneuploidy in oocyte correlates with a dramatic increase of trisomic pregnancy. Aneuploidy commonly arises from segregation errors during oocyte meiosis I, and relates to the long arrest of oocytes in preceding stages of meiosis. In these oocytes, the cohesion between chromosomes must be maintained for an extraordinary long period of time (up to ~ fifty years in human), and depends on cohesin complexes. Recent studies in mouse have suggested that the loss of sister chromatid cohesion is a leading cause of aneuploidy in oocyte, and is due to a progressive deterioration of cohesin itself. Indeed, these studies have reported that the meiotic cohesin subunit Rec8 (Chiang et al., 2010; Lister et al., 2010) and the protein Sgo2 that protects centromeric cohesin in meiosis I (Lister et al., 2010) decrease on meiotic chromosomes with age. The degradation of cohesin correlates with an increased distance between sister kinetochores and with the loss of sister chromatid cohesion (Chiang et al., 2010; Lister et al., 2010). Altogether, these data indicate that cohesin is essential to maintain sister chromatid cohesion in arrested oocytes, and highlight the importance of the cohesin function in preventing aneuploidy and infertility in mammalian oocytes. Determining how cohesin gets degraded, if and how it can be prevented would be of great interest in the future.

6. Conclusion

The sister chromatid cohesion apparatus protects somatic and germinal cells from unequal chromosome segregation and aneuploidy. Recent advances in the field have pointed to the misregulation of cohesion factors, mainly cohesin, as a cause for aneuploidy-based human disorders from cancer to trisomies and infertility. In the future, we will have to decipher the molecular mechanisms of both normal and defective sister chromatid cohesion, as well as its links with human pathologies, including cancers. Furthermore, it will be interesting to address whether one could take advantage of our knowledge on the molecular function of cohesin to develop new approaches to treat cancer cells. Finally, it is of great importance to determine if, and to which extent, the other known functions of cohesin and its associated factors, namely regulation of gene expression and the DNA damage response, also participate in tumourigenesis.

7. Further reading

In this chapter, we aimed at presenting the basic current knowledge about the sister chromatid cohesion apparatus, its role and regulation in the segregation of replicated chromosomes during mitosis and meiosis, and how cohesion defects lead to aneuploidy. For those colleagues who wish to learn more about particular aspects of cohesin in chromosome biology, there are some dedicated reviews that we shall recommend: cohesin mechanistic and its regulation (Nasmyth and Haering, 2009; Onn et al., 2008; Peters et al., 2008), cohesin in gene regulation (Dorsett, 2007; Wendt and Peters, 2009), DNA damage response (Strom and Sjogren, 2007; Watrin and Peters, 2006), meiosis and gametogenesis (Jessberger, 2003; Petronczki et al., 2003), aneuploidy and cancer (Barbero, 2011; Nicholson and Cimini, 2011).

8. Acknowledgment

We are grateful to Jacek Kubiak for his comments on the manuscript. Work in Claude Prigent 's lab is funded by the Centre National de la Recherche Scientifique (CNRS), the University of Rennes I, and by grants from the Agence Nationale pour la Recherche, the Association pour la Recherche contre le Cancer and the Ligue Nationale contre le Cancer.

9. References

Anderson, D.E., Losada, A., Erickson, H.P. and Hirano, T. (2002) Condensin and cohesin display different arm conformations with characteristic hinge angles. *J Cell Biol*, 156, 419-424.

Arumugam, P., Gruber, S., Tanaka, K., Haering, C.H., Mechtler, K. and Nasmyth, K. (2003) ATP hydrolysis is required for cohesin's association with chromosomes. *Curr Biol*, 13, 1941-1953.

Barber, T.D., McManus, K., Yuen, K.W., Reis, M., Parmigiani, G., Shen, D., Barrett, I., Nouhi, Y., Spencer, F., Markowitz, S., Velculescu, V.E., Kinzler, K.W., Vogelstein, B., Lengauer, C. and Hieter, P. (2008) Chromatid cohesion defects may underlie chromosome instability in human colorectal cancers. *Proc Natl Acad Sci U S A*, 105, 3443-3448.

Barbero, J.L. (2011) Sister chromatid cohesion control and aneuploidy. *Cytogenet Genome Res*, 133, 223-233.

Bernard, P., Drogat, J., Maure, J.F., Dheur, S., Vaur, S., Genier, S. and Javerzat, J.P. (2006) A screen for cohesion mutants uncovers Ssl3, the fission yeast counterpart of the cohesin loading factor Scc4. *Curr Biol.*, 16, 875-881.

Canudas, S. and Smith, S. (2009) Differential regulation of telomere and centromere cohesion by the Scc3 homologues SA1 and SA2, respectively, in human cells. *J Cell Biol*, 187, 165-173.

Chiang, T., Duncan, F.E., Schindler, K., Schultz, R.M. and Lampson, M.A. (2010) Evidence that weakened centromere cohesion is a leading cause of age-related aneuploidy in oocytes. *Curr Biol*, 20, 1522-1528.

Ciosk, R., Shirayama, M., Shevchenko, A., Tanaka, T., Toth, A. and Nasmyth, K. (2000) Cohesin's binding to chromosomes depends on a separate complex consisting of Scc2 and Scc4 proteins. *Mol Cell*, 5, 243-254.

Dai, J., Sullivan, B.A. and Higgins, J.M. (2006) Regulation of mitotic chromosome cohesion by Haspin and Aurora B. *Dev Cell*, 11, 741-750.

Dorsett, D. (2007) Roles of the sister chromatid cohesion apparatus in gene expression, development, and human syndromes. *Chromosoma.*, 116, 1-13. Epub 2006 Jul 2004.

Dorsett, D., Eissenberg, J.C., Misulovin, Z., Martens, A., Redding, B. and McKim, K. (2005) Effects of sister chromatid cohesion proteins on cut gene expression during wing development in Drosophila. *Development*, 5, 5.

Feytout, A., Vaur, S., Genier, S., Vazquez, S. and Javerzat, J.P. (2011) Psm3 acetylation on conserved lysine residues is dispensable for viability in fission yeast but contributes to Eso1-mediated sister chromatid cohesion by antagonizing Wpl1. *Mol Cell Biol*, 31, 1771-1786.

Furuya, K., Takahashi, K. and Yanagida, M. (1998) Faithful anaphase is ensured by Mis4, a sister chromatid cohesion molecule required in S phase and not destroyed in G1 phase. *Genes Dev*, 12, 3408-3418.

Gandhi, R., Gillespie, P.J. and Hirano, T. (2006) Human Wapl is a cohesin-binding protein that promotes sister-chromatid resolution in mitotic prophase. *Curr Biol.*, 16, 2406-2417. Epub 2006 Nov 2416.

Gerlich, D., Koch, B., Dupeux, F., Peters, J.M. and Ellenberg, J. (2006) Live-cell imaging reveals a stable cohesin-chromatin interaction after but not before DNA replication. *Curr Biol*, 16, 1571-1578.

Gillespie, P.J. and Hirano, T. (2004) Scc2 couples replication licensing to sister chromatid cohesion in Xenopus egg extracts. *Curr Biol*, 14, 1598-1603.

Gruber, S., Arumugam, P., Katou, Y., Kuglitsch, D., Helmhart, W., Shirahige, K. and Nasmyth, K. (2006) Evidence that loading of cohesin onto chromosomes involves opening of its SMC hinge. *Cell*, 127, 523-537.

Gruber, S., Haering, C.H. and Nasmyth, K. (2003) Chromosomal cohesin forms a ring. *Cell*, 112, 765-777.

Haering, C.H., Lowe, J., Hochwagen, A. and Nasmyth, K. (2002) Molecular architecture of SMC proteins and the yeast cohesin complex. *Mol Cell*, 9, 773-788.

Haering, C.H., Schoffnegger, D., Nishino, T., Helmhart, W., Nasmyth, K. and Lowe, J. (2004) Structure and stability of cohesin's Smc1-kleisin interaction. *Mol Cell.*, 15, 951-964.

Hartman, T., Stead, K., Koshland, D. and Guacci, V. (2000) Pds5p is an essential chromosomal protein required for both sister chromatid cohesion and condensation in Saccharomyces cerevisiae. *J Cell Biol*, 151, 613-626.

Hauf, S., Roitinger, E., Koch, B., Dittrich, C.M., Mechtler, K. and Peters, J.M. (2005) Dissociation of cohesin from chromosome arms and loss of arm cohesion during early mitosis depends on phosphorylation of SA2. *PLoS Biol*, 3, e69. Epub 2005 Mar 2001.

Hirota, T., Gerlich, D., Koch, B., Ellenberg, J. and Peters, J.M. (2004) Distinct functions of condensin I and II in mitotic chromosome assembly. *J Cell Sci*, 117, 6435-6445. Epub 2004 Nov 6430.

Hou, F. and Zou, H. (2005) Two human orthologues of Eco1/Ctf7 acetyltransferases are both required for proper sister-chromatid cohesion. *Mol Biol Cell.*, 16, 3908-3918. Epub 2005 Jun 3915.

Huang, C.E., Milutinovich, M. and Koshland, D. (2005) Rings, bracelet or snaps: fashionable alternatives for Smc complexes. *Philos Trans R Soc Lond B Biol Sci*, 360, 537-542.

Jessberger, R. (2003) SMC proteins at the crossroads of diverse chromosomal processes. *IUBMB Life*, 55, 643-652.

Katis, V.L., Galova, M., Rabitsch, K.P., Gregan, J. and Nasmyth, K. (2004) Maintenance of cohesin at centromeres after meiosis I in budding yeast requires a kinetochore-associated protein related to MEI-S332. *Curr Biol*, 14, 560-572.

Katis, V.L., Lipp, J.J., Imre, R., Bogdanova, A., Okaz, E., Habermann, B., Mechtler, K., Nasmyth, K. and Zachariae, W. (2010) Rec8 phosphorylation by casein kinase 1 and Cdc7-Dbf4 kinase regulates cohesin cleavage by separase during meiosis. *Dev Cell*, 18, 397-409.

Kawashima, S.A., Yamagishi, Y., Honda, T., Ishiguro, K. and Watanabe, Y. (2010) Phosphorylation of H2A by Bub1 prevents chromosomal instability through localizing shugoshin. *Science*, 327, 172-177.

Kim, B.J., Li, Y., Zhang, J., Xi, Y., Li, Y., Yang, T., Jung, T., Jung, S.Y., Pan, X., Chen, R., Li, W., Wang, Y. and Qin, J. (2010) Genome-wide reinforcement of cohesin binding at pre-existing cohesin sites in response to ionizing radiation in human cells. *J Biol Chem*, 285, 22784-22792.

Kitajima, T.S., Kawashima, S.A. and Watanabe, Y. (2004) The conserved kinetochore protein shugoshin protects centromeric cohesion during meiosis. *Nature*, 427, 510-517. Epub 2004 Jan 2018.

Kitajima, T.S., Sakuno, T., Ishiguro, K., Iemura, S., Natsume, T., Kawashima, S.A. and Watanabe, Y. (2006) Shugoshin collaborates with protein phosphatase 2A to protect cohesin. *Nature*, 441, 46-52.

Kueng, S., Hegemann, B., Peters, B.H., Lipp, J.J., Schleiffer, A., Mechtler, K. and Peters, J.M. (2006) Wapl controls the dynamic association of cohesin with chromatin. *Cell.*, 127, 955-967. Epub 2006 Nov 2016.

Lee, J., Kitajima, T.S., Tanno, Y., Yoshida, K., Morita, T., Miyano, T., Miyake, M. and Watanabe, Y. (2008) Unified mode of centromeric protection by shugoshin in mammalian oocytes and somatic cells. *Nat Cell Biol*, 10, 42-52.

Lenart, P., Petronczki, M., Steegmaier, M., Di Fiore, B., Lipp, J.J., Hoffmann, M., Rettig, W.J., Kraut, N. and Peters, J.M. (2007) The small-molecule inhibitor BI 2536 reveals novel insights into mitotic roles of polo-like kinase 1. *Curr Biol.*, 17, 304-315. Epub 2007 Feb 2008.

Lister, L.M., Kouznetsova, A., Hyslop, L.A., Kalleas, D., Pace, S.L., Barel, J.C., Nathan, A., Floros, V., Adelfalk, C., Watanabe, Y., Jessberger, R., Kirkwood, T.B., Hoog, C. and Herbert, M. (2010) Age-related meiotic segregation errors in mammalian oocytes are preceded by depletion of cohesin and Sgo2. *Curr Biol*, 20, 1511-1521.

Llano, E., Gomez, R., Gutierrez-Caballero, C., Herran, Y., Sanchez-Martin, M., Vazquez-Quinones, L., Hernandez, T., de Alava, E., Cuadrado, A., Barbero, J.L., Suja, J.A. and Pendas, A.M. (2008) Shugoshin-2 is essential for the completion of meiosis but not for mitotic cell division in mice. *Genes Dev*, 22, 2400-2413.

Losada, A., Hirano, M. and Hirano, T. (1998) Identification of Xenopus SMC protein complexes required for sister chromatid cohesion. *Genes Dev*, 12, 1986-1997.

Losada, A., Hirano, M. and Hirano, T. (2002) Cohesin release is required for sister chromatid resolution, but not for condensin-mediated compaction, at the onset of mitosis. *Genes Dev*, 16, 3004-3016.

Losada, A., Yokochi, T., Kobayashi, R. and Hirano, T. (2000) Identification and Characterization of SA/Scc3p Subunits in the Xenopus and Human Cohesin Complexes. *J Cell Biol*, 150, 405-416.

Mc Intyre, J., Muller, E.G., Weitzer, S., Snydsman, B.E., Davis, T.N. and Uhlmann, F. (2007) In vivo analysis of cohesin architecture using FRET in the budding yeast Saccharomyces cerevisiae. *Embo J*, 26, 3783-3793.

McGuinness, B.E., Hirota, T., Kudo, N.R., Peters, J.M. and Nasmyth, K. (2005) Shugoshin prevents dissociation of cohesin from centromeres during mitosis in vertebrate cells. *PLoS Biol*, 3, e86. Epub 2005 Mar 2001.

Melby, T.E., Ciampaglio, C.N., Briscoe, G. and Erickson, H.P. (1998) The symmetrical structure of structural maintenance of chromosomes (SMC) and MukB proteins: long, antiparallel coiled coils, folded at a flexible hinge. *J Cell Biol*, 142, 1595-1604.

Michaelis, C., Ciosk, R. and Nasmyth, K. (1997) Cohesins: chromosomal proteins that prevent premature separation of sister chromatids. *Cell*, 91, 35-45.

Milutinovich, M., Unal, E., Ward, C., Skibbens, R.V. and Koshland, D. (2007) A multi-step pathway for the establishment of sister chromatid cohesion. *PLoS Genet.*, 3, e12. Epub 2006 Dec 2008.

Nasmyth, K. (2001) Disseminating the genome: joining, resolving, and separating sister chromatids during mitosis and meiosis. *Annu Rev Genet*, 35, 673-745.

Nasmyth, K. and Haering, C.H. (2009) Cohesin: its roles and mechanisms. *Annu Rev Genet*, 43, 525-558.

Nicholson, J.M. and Cimini, D. (2011) How mitotic errors contribute to karyotypic diversity in cancer. *Adv Cancer Res*, 112, 43-75.

Nishiyama, T., Ladurner, R., Schmitz, J., Kreidl, E., Schleiffer, A., Bhaskara, V., Bando, M., Shirahige, K., Hyman, A.A., Mechtler, K. and Peters, J.M. (2010) Sororin mediates sister chromatid cohesion by antagonizing Wapl. *Cell*, 143, 737-749.

Onn, I., Heidinger-Pauli, J.M., Guacci, V., Unal, E. and Koshland, D.E. (2008) Sister chromatid cohesion: a simple concept with a complex reality. *Annu Rev Cell Dev Biol*, 24, 105-129.

Panizza, S., Tanaka, T., Hochwagen, A., Eisenhaber, F. and Nasmyth, K. (2000) Pds5 cooperates with cohesin in maintaining sister chromatid cohesion. *Curr Biol*, 10, 1557-1564.

Peters, J.M. (2002) The anaphase-promoting complex: proteolysis in mitosis and beyond. *Mol Cell*, 9, 931-943.

Peters, J.M., Tedeschi, A. and Schmitz, J. (2008) The cohesin complex and its roles in chromosome biology. *Genes Dev*, 22, 3089-3114.

Petronczki, M., Siomos, M.F. and Nasmyth, K. (2003) Un menage a quatre: the molecular biology of chromosome segregation in meiosis. *Cell*, 112, 423-440.

Rabitsch, K.P., Gregan, J., Schleiffer, A., Javerzat, J.P., Eisenhaber, F. and Nasmyth, K. (2004) Two fission yeast homologs of Drosophila Mei-S332 are required for chromosome segregation during meiosis I and II. *Curr Biol*, 14, 287-301.

Rankin, S., Ayad, N.G. and Kirschner, M.W. (2005) Sororin, a substrate of the anaphase-promoting complex, is required for sister chromatid cohesion in vertebrates. *Mol Cell*, 18, 185-200.

Riedel, C.G., Katis, V.L., Katou, Y., Mori, S., Itoh, T., Helmhart, W., Galova, M., Petronczki, M., Gregan, J., Cetin, B., Mudrak, I., Ogris, E., Mechtler, K., Pelletier, L., Buchholz, F., Shirahige, K. and Nasmyth, K. (2006) Protein phosphatase 2A protects centromeric sister chromatid cohesion during meiosis I. *Nature*, 441, 53-61.

Rolef Ben-Shahar, T., Heeger, S., Lehane, C., East, P., Flynn, H., Skehel, M. and Uhlmann, F. (2008) Eco1-dependent cohesin acetylation during establishment of sister chromatid cohesion. *Science*, 321, 563-566.

Rollins, R.A., Korom, M., Aulner, N., Martens, A. and Dorsett, D. (2004) Drosophila nipped-B protein supports sister chromatid cohesion and opposes the stromalin/Scc3 cohesion factor to facilitate long-range activation of the cut gene. *Mol Cell Biol*, 24, 3100-3111.

Rowland, B.D., Roig, M.B., Nishino, T., Kurze, A., Uluocak, P., Mishra, A., Beckouet, F., Underwood, P., Metson, J., Imre, R., Mechtler, K., Katis, V.L. and Nasmyth, K. (2009) Building sister chromatid cohesion: smc3 acetylation counteracts an antiestablishment activity. *Mol Cell*, 33, 763-774.

Salic, A., Waters, J.C. and Mitchison, T.J. (2004) Vertebrate shugoshin links sister centromere cohesion and kinetochore microtubule stability in mitosis. *Cell*, 118, 567-578.

Schmitz, J., Watrin, E., Lenart, P., Mechtler, K. and Peters, J.M. (2007) Sororin is required for stable binding of cohesin to chromatin and for sister chromatid cohesion in interphase. *Curr Biol*, 17, 630-636.

Sheltzer, J.M., Blank, H.M., Pfau, S.J., Tange, Y., George, B.M., Humpton, T.J., Brito, I.L., Hiraoka, Y., Niwa, O. and Amon, A. (2011) Aneuploidy drives genomic instability in yeast. *Science*, 333, 1026-1030.

Shintomi, K. and Hirano, T. (2009) Releasing cohesin from chromosome arms in early mitosis: opposing actions of Wapl-Pds5 and Sgo1. *Genes Dev*, 23, 2224-2236.

Sjogren, C. and Nasmyth, K. (2001) Sister chromatid cohesion is required for postreplicative double-strand break repair in Saccharomyces cerevisiae. *Curr Biol*, 11, 991-995.

Skibbens, R.V., Corson, L.B., Koshland, D. and Hieter, P. (1999) Ctf7p is essential for sister chromatid cohesion and links mitotic chromosome structure to the DNA replication machinery. *Genes Dev*, 13, 307-319.

Solomon, D.A., Kim, T., Diaz-Martinez, L.A., Fair, J., Elkahloun, A.G., Harris, B.T., Toretsky, J.A., Rosenberg, S.A., Shukla, N., Ladanyi, M., Samuels, Y., James, C.D., Yu, H., Kim, J.S. and Waldman, T. (2011) Mutational inactivation of STAG2 causes aneuploidy in human cancer. *Science*, 333, 1039-1043.

Strom, L., Karlsson, C., Lindroos, H.B., Wedahl, S., Katou, Y., Shirahige, K. and Sjogren, C. (2007) Postreplicative formation of cohesion is required for repair and induced by a single DNA break. *Science.*, 317, 242-245.

Strom, L. and Sjogren, C. (2007) Chromosome segregation and double-strand break repair - a complex connection. *Curr Opin Cell Biol.*, 19, 344-349. Epub 2007 Apr 2026.

Strunnikov, A.V., Larionov, V.L. and Koshland, D. (1993) SMC1: an essential yeast gene encoding a putative head-rod-tail protein is required for nuclear division and defines a new ubiquitous protein family. *J Cell Biol*, 123, 1635-1648.

Sumara, I., Vorlaufer, E., Gieffers, C., Peters, B.H. and Peters, J.M. (2000) Characterization of vertebrate cohesin complexes and their regulation in prophase. *J Cell Biol*, 151, 749-762.

Sumara, I., Vorlaufer, E., Stukenberg, P.T., Kelm, O., Redemann, N., Nigg, E.A. and Peters, J.M. (2002) The dissociation of cohesin from chromosomes in prophase is regulated by Polo-like kinase. *Mol Cell*, 9, 515-525.

Sutani, T., Kawaguchi, T., Kanno, R., Itoh, T. and Shirahige, K. (2009) Budding yeast Wpl1(Rad61)-Pds5 complex counteracts sister chromatid cohesion-establishing reaction. *Curr Biol*, 19, 492-497.

Takahashi, T.S., Yiu, P., Chou, M.F., Gygi, S. and Walter, J.C. (2004) Recruitment of Xenopus Scc2 and cohesin to chromatin requires the pre-replication complex. *Nat Cell Biol*, 6, 991-996. Epub 2004 Sep 2026.

Tanaka, K., Hao, Z., Kai, M. and Okayama, H. (2001) Establishment and maintenance of sister chromatid cohesion in fission yeast by a unique mechanism. *Embo J*, 20, 5779-5790.

Tang, Z., Sun, Y., Harley, S.E., Zou, H. and Yu, H. (2004) Human Bub1 protects centromeric sister-chromatid cohesion through Shugoshin during mitosis. *Proc Natl Acad Sci U S A*, 101, 18012-18017. Epub 12004 Dec 18016.

Tomonaga, T., Nagao, K., Kawasaki, Y., Furuya, K., Murakami, A., Morishita, J., Yuasa, T., Sutani, T., Kearsey, S.E., Uhlmann, F., Nasmyth, K. and Yanagida, M. (2000) Characterization of fission yeast cohesin: essential anaphase proteolysis of Rad21 phosphorylated in the S phase. *Genes Dev*, 14, 2757-2770.

Toth, A., Ciosk, R., Uhlmann, F., Galova, M., Schleiffer, A. and Nasmyth, K. (1999) Yeast cohesin complex requires a conserved protein, Eco1p(Ctf7), to establish cohesion between sister chromatids during DNA replication. *Genes Dev*, 13, 320-333.

Uhlmann, F., Lottspeich, F. and Nasmyth, K. (1999) Sister-chromatid separation at anaphase onset is promoted by cleavage of the cohesin subunit Scc1. *Nature*, 400, 37-42.

Uhlmann, F. and Nasmyth, K. (1998) Cohesion between sister chromatids must be established during DNA replication. *Curr Biol*, 8, 1095-1101.

Unal, E., Heidinger-Pauli, J.M., Kim, W., Guacci, V., Onn, I., Gygi, S.P. and Koshland, D.E. (2008) A molecular determinant for the establishment of sister chromatid cohesion. *Science*, 321, 566-569.

Unal, E., Heidinger-Pauli, J.M. and Koshland, D. (2007) DNA double-strand breaks trigger genome-wide sister-chromatid cohesion through Eco1 (Ctf7). *Science.*, 317, 245-248.

Verni, F., Gandhi, R., Goldberg, M.L. and Gatti, M. (2000) Genetic and molecular analysis of wings apart-like (wapl), a gene controlling heterochromatin organization in Drosophila melanogaster. *Genetics*, 154, 1693-1710.

Waizenegger, I.C., Hauf, S., Meinke, A. and Peters, J.M. (2000) Two distinct pathways remove mammalian cohesin from chromosome arms in prophase and from centromeres in anaphase. *Cell*, 103, 399-410.

Wang, S.W., Read, R.L. and Norbury, C.J. (2002) Fission yeast Pds5 is required for accurate chromosome segregation and for survival after DNA damage or metaphase arrest. *J Cell Sci*, 115, 587-598.

Watrin, E. and Peters, J.M. (2006) Cohesin and DNA damage repair. *Exp Cell Res.*, 312, 2687-2693. Epub 2006 Jun 2622.

Watrin, E., Schleiffer, A., Tanaka, K., Eisenhaber, F., Nasmyth, K. and Peters, J.M. (2006) Human scc4 is required for cohesin binding to chromatin, sister-chromatid cohesion, and mitotic progression. *Curr Biol.*, 16, 863-874.

Weitzer, S., Lehane, C. and Uhlmann, F. (2003) A model for ATP hydrolysis-dependent binding of cohesin to DNA. *Curr Biol*, 13, 1930-1940.

Wendt, K.S. and Peters, J.M. (2009) How cohesin and CTCF cooperate in regulating gene expression. *Chromosome Res*, 17, 201-214.

Xu, H., Tomaszewski, J.M. and McKay, M.J. (2011) Can corruption of chromosome cohesion create a conduit to cancer? *Nat Rev Cancer*, 11, 199-210.

Zhang, J., Shi, X., Li, Y., Kim, B.J., Jia, J., Huang, Z., Yang, T., Fu, X., Jung, S.Y., Wang, Y., Zhang, P., Kim, S.T., Pan, X. and Qin, J. (2008a) Acetylation of Smc3 by Eco1 is required for S phase sister chromatid cohesion in both human and yeast. *Mol Cell*, 31, 143-151.

Zhang, N., Kuznetsov, S.G., Sharan, S.K., Li, K., Rao, P.H. and Pati, D. (2008b) A handcuff model for the cohesin complex. *J Cell Biol*, 183, 1019-1031.

4

Mouse Models for Chromosomal Instability

Floris Foijer
European Institute for the Biology of Aging (ERIBA)
University Medical Center Groningen, Groningen
The Netherlands

1. Introduction

Chromosomal instability

Cancer is the result of several genetic alterations that overrule a cell's protection mechanisms against unscheduled proliferation (Hanahan & Weinberg, 2000). As the vast majority of human tumours show chromosomal instability (CIN), CIN is believed to be an important driver and facilitator of oncogenic transformation. CIN can result in structural abnormalities such as focal deletions, amplifications or translocations (structural CIN). Alternatively, CIN causes numerical abnormalities (*i.e.* aneuploidy) with cells showing high rates of losses and gains of whole chromosomes leading to dramatic karyotypic variability between cells. Whereas alterations to single or small groups of oncogenes/ tumour suppressor genes can explain the malignant effect of structural CIN, the cancerous effect of numerical CIN is mostly attributed to the loss of heterozygosity (LOH) of tumour suppressor genes (Jallepalli & Lengauer, 2001, Kops et al., 2005). Structural and numerical CIN often coincide in tumours and numerical CIN can in fact provoke structural CIN as well (Janssen et al., 2011). Although CIN appears to be a potent driver of genomic reorganization, it comes at cost for cells. For instance, numerical CIN in tissue culture cells kills cells within six generations (Kops et al., 2004). Furthermore, in depth analysis of aneuploid yeast strains and mouse embryonic fibroblasts (MEFs) carrying an extra chromosome revealed that aneuploidy slows cell proliferation down and deregulates the metabolic homeostasis (Torres et al., 2007, Williams et al., 2008). However, as the majority of human tumours are aneuploid, cancer cells must have found a way to circumvent the detrimental consequences of CIN. This chapter reviews several mechanisms that can drive numerical CIN and discusses several of the mouse models that were engineered to mimic these conditions with the aim to study the *in vivo* consequences of numerical CIN.

2. Origins of whole chromosome instability

Kinetochores and centromeric proteins

Correct chromosome distribution critically depends on correct attachment of chromosomes to a bipolar mitotic spindle. Defects in the machinery regulating the formation of a proper bipolar spindle have been associated with human cancer and aneuploidy (Fukasawa, 2005, Kops et al., 2005, Yuen et al., 2005). Kinetochores are macromolecular protein structures that link the centromeric DNA to the mitotic spindle. The inner kinetochore plate is the DNA interacting domain and is comprised of several structural proteins such as the centromeric proteins (CENP). Some of these CENP genes (*e.g. CENPA, CENPF* and *CENPH*) frequently show altered expression in human cancer, underscoring the importance of a precisely balanced protein composition of the kinetochore (Yuen et al., 2005).

The mitotic spindle checkpoint

To ensure the accurate segregation of chromosomes, cells initiate segregation only after the correct attachment of all chromosomes to microtubules of the mitotic spindle. The spindle checkpoint (SAC) operates at the outer kinetochore plate by monitoring the attachment of the kinetochore to the microtubules. Improperly attached kinetochores recruit a family of SAC proteins (Mad1, Mad2, Bub1, BubR1, Bub3, Mps1, Rod and ZW10) (Musacchio & Salmon, 2007). Additionally, CENPE, a motor protein, is recruited to unattached kinetochores, where it is implicated in regulating microtubule attachment (Kops et al., 2005). Even a single unattached kinetochore is sufficient to trigger a robust spindle checkpoint response that prevents premature anaphase onset and thus missegregation of chromosomes (Rieder et al., 1995, Rieder et al., 1994). This robust response is achieved by CDC20 sequestering by the SAC proteins, the specificity factor required for anaphase promoting complex/cyclosome (APC/C) activity. Activation of the APC/C, an E3 ubiquitin ligase, is essential for anaphase progression, as it is responsible for the degradation of several mitotic proteins including Securin and Cyclin B1. Securin degradation leads to activation of Separase, which cleaves Cohesin that glues sister chromatids together. Cyclin B1 degradation results in the inactivation of CDK1 and thereby allows mitotic exit (Karess, 2005, Kops et al., 2005, Musacchio & Salmon, 2007). Thus, precise regulation of APC/C activity by the SAC allows for timely and accurate progression of mitosis preventing numerical CIN.

Tension versus attachment

Kinetochore-microtubule attachment by itself is not sufficient to satisfy the spindle checkpoint. To achieve proper segregation, it is also essential that one kinetochore of a pair is attached to microtubules from one spindle pole and the other kinetochore to the opposite pole (Biggins & Walczak, 2003). This correct geometry of attachment generates tension between the sister chromatids, which is another prerequisite for mitotic progression. Aurora B is implicated in sensing this tension and correcting erroneous attachments (Andrews et al., 2003). In the absence of tension, for instance when both sister chromatid kinetochores are connected to the same centrosome, Aurora B kinase activity remains uninhibited. This results in the release of improper microtubule attachments and allows reattachment of the kinetochores with microtubules emanating from the opposite pole (Andrews et al., 2003, Liu et al., 2009, Musacchio & Salmon, 2007). While details of error correction mechanisms are just emerging, drugs targeting this pathway (*e.g.* Aurora inhibitors) are already in clinical trials for cancer (Jackson et al., 2007).

Centrosomes

Centrosomes are essential for bipolar spindle formation during mitosis, as they are the major microtubule organizing centres of the cell. The presence of two centrosomes is therefore critical for accurate chromosome segregation into two daughter cells. Centrosome number is tightly controlled: centrosomes are duplicated during S-phase and segregated into the two daughter cells during mitosis (see for detailed review: (Doxsey et al., 2005, Fukasawa, 2005, Nigg, 2007, Tsou & Stearns, 2006)). Defects in these control mechanisms can lead to abnormal centrosome numbers and are thus another cause of numerical CIN. In agreement with this, most tumours exhibit abnormal centrosome numbers (Nigg, 2006, Pihan et al., 1998). It was originally hypothesized that abnormal centrosome numbers would provoke CIN through multipolar mitoses. Although careful tracking revealed that such divisions occasionally do take place, the resulting daughter cells all died in the next cell cycle. It's therefore unlikely that cells undergoing multipolar divisions contribute to a developing tumour. Instead, in a large proportion of the cells supranumeral centrosomes clustered to form one 'supercentrosome' allowing 'normal' bivalent divisions to take place. Such divisions frequently coincided with lagging chromosomes in the next mitosis, presumably the result of merotelic attachments caused by abnormal centrosomal structure (Ganem et al., 2009). Therefore, lagging chromosomes might very well be the driving force behind numerical CIN associated with supranumeral centrosomes.

3. Mouse models for whole chromosome instability

To test whether numerical CIN is an early event in tumourigenesis and thereby infer whether it can be causative of cancer, several proteins playing a role in accurate segregation were disrupted in mice. The results of these studies are discussed below and collectively underscore the importance of the spindle checkpoint in the different aspects of tumourigenesis.

Loss of centromeric (CENP) genes frequently causes embryonic lethality

CENPA, B and C reside at the inner plate of the kinetochore and bridge between the centromeric DNA and the kinetochore-docking microtubules emanating from the centrosomes. Several of these genes have been knocked out in mice to determine their role in the prevention of aneuploidy. Whereas homozygous CENPB loss resulted in no overt phenotypes other than slightly lower testis and body weights (Hudson et al., 1998, Kapoor et al., 1998, Perez-Castro et al., 1998), disruption of CENPA or CENPC led to embryonic lethality in early stages of embryogenesis (E3.5-E6.5). The early embryos show micronuclei, a lowered mitotic index (indicative of mitotic delay), and enlarged nuclei (suggestive of tetraploid cells). Heterozygous mice develop normally and are fertile, although animals were not tested for cancer predisposition using carcinogens or in combination with other predisposing mutations (Howman et al., 2000, Kalitsis et al., 1998). Animal longevity and spontaneous cancer predisposition are currently being tested [Andy Choo, personal communication].

Spindle checkpoint inactivation interferes with mammalian development

The first mouse model for germline SAC inactivation was the Mad2 knockout. Homozygous Mad2 loss results in embryonic lethality at approximately day E6.5 (Dobles et al., 2000). Similar to the Mad2 knockout, BubR1, Bub1, Mad1, Bub3, Rae1 and CENPE inactivation are also incompatible with mammalian development beyond day E6.5-E8.5. In all cases, massive apoptosis of the inner cell mass (ICM) was observed, presumably a consequence of numerous missegregation events in these highly proliferative cells (Baker et al., 2004, Baker et al., 2006, Iwanaga et al., 2007, Jeganathan et al., 2007, Kalitsis et al., 2000, Putkey et al., 2002, Q. Wang et al., 2004, Weaver et al., 2007). Inactivation of the APC/C activating factors

Cdc20 or Cdh1 provoke embryonic lethality as well, but later in gestation with embryos developing up to E12.5 (Garcia-Higuera et al., 2008, Li et al., 2009).

The chromosomal passenger proteins Incenp, Survivin and Aurora B are part of the chromosomal passenger complex. This complex is essential for forming a bipolar spindle by measuring tension during metaphase and is involved in later events in cytokinesis as well (Lens et al., 2006). Knockouts for Survivin or Incenp revealed that ablation of either protein causes embryonic lethality before day E8.5, similar as observed for CENP proteins and SAC protein knockouts (Cutts et al., 1999, Uren et al., 2000).

Does reduced expression of CIN protective genes result in spontaneous tumour formation?

Several cancers show decreased expression of spindle checkpoint proteins, indicating that a partially compromised checkpoint can be the underlying cause for tumour aneuploidy (Weaver & Cleveland, 2006). As homozygous inactivation of SAC components aborts embryonic development well before mid-gestation, heterozygous mice (Mad1, Mad2, BubR1, Bub1, Bub3, Rae1, Cdc20, Cdh1 and Cenp-E) were used to study the *in vivo* consequences of a partially defective spindle checkpoint. In all cases, heterozygotes are born at a Mendelian ratio and none show clear developmental defects, except for a mild hematopoietic defect in BubR1 heterozygotes (Babu et al., 2003, Baker et al., 2006, Garcia-Higuera et al., 2008, Iwanaga et al., 2007, Jeganathan et al., 2007, Kalitsis et al., 2005, Li et al., 2009, Michel et al., 2001, Q. Wang et al., 2004, Weaver et al., 2007). However, despite normal development, Mad2, Mad1 and CENPE heterozygotes develop cancers in a substantial number of the animals (20-30%), albeit relatively late (at 18-20 months of age). Lung tumours are predominant, and CENPE heterozygotes develop hematopoietic malignancies as well (Iwanaga et al., 2007, Michel et al., 2001, Weaver et al., 2007), indicating that Mad1, Mad2 and CENPE function as haplo-insufficient tumour suppressors in the mouse by suppressing CIN. Heterozygousity for the SAC-downstream-targets Cdh1 or Cdc20 predisposes for late tumours as well: up to 50% of the Cdc20 hypomorphic mice develop tumours, mostly in the hematopoietic compartment, whereas Chd1 heterozygotes mainly develop solid tumours in the mammary gland, lungs, liver and testes (Garcia-Higuera et al., 2008, Li et al., 2009). Heterozygous BubR1, Bub1, Bub3 and Rae1, and even Bub3; Rae1 double heterozygotes do not develop any malignancies, suggesting that in those models aneuploidy is not sufficient for tumours to arise (Baker et al., 2004, Baker et al., 2006, Jeganathan et al., 2007, Q. Wang et al., 2004). Finally, similar to SAC knockout heterozygotes, Survivin$^{+/-}$ and Incenp$^{+/-}$ mice are indistinguishable from their wildtype littermates. Whether these animals are cancer-predisposed is currently not known [Andy Choo, personal communication].

In another approach, a hypomorphic allele for Bub1 was created, reducing protein levels down to 20% of wildtype levels. These mice develop several malignancies within 18-20 months of age, mainly lymphomas, lung and liver tumours (Jeganathan et al., 2007). Using the same approach, a hypomorphic allele for BubR1 was engineered (reducing BubR1 protein levels by 90%). Surprisingly, although these mice develop massive aneuploidy in several tissues, they are not cancer-predisposed, suggesting that aneuploidy does not cause cancer *per se* (Baker et al., 2004).

BubR1 hypomorphs develop another phenotype though: they age prematurely, as evidenced by decreased subcutaneous fat and spinal kyphosis (spinal deformation or hump) and muscle atrophy. The median lifespan of these animals is six months and none of them age over 15 months (Baker et al., 2004), which might obscure a late-in-life cancer phenotype. Bub3; Rae1 double heterozygotes develop a similar phenotype, albeit less severe as these animals survive up to 27 months (Jeganathan et al., 2007). Interestingly, BubR1 levels seem to decline in aging wildtype tissue, which suggests a role for this gene and possibly aneuploidy in natural aging as well (Baker et al., 2004). However, why the premature aging phenotype affects these two knockouts and not other aneuploidy-related mouse models is currently unknown.

Phenotypes of the various mouse models are summarized in Table 1. Taken together, the results show that SAC defects have a profound effect on development and cancer predisposition. Additionally, mouse models targeting the SAC have revealed a potential role for aneuploidy in aging.

Aneuploidy as a collaborating factor in tumorigenesis

Even though mouse models clearly indicate that numerical CIN can contribute to *tumour initiation*, the actual tumour phenotypes of these mouse models are relatively weak, with tumours arising sporadically and relatively late in life. Why is this effect so weak despite the high incidence of aneuploidy in human cancer? One explanation is that the current mouse models rely on partial inactivation of the spindle checkpoint, since complete inactivation is incompatible with embryonic development. Another possible explanation for the weak phenotypes is that aneuploidy requires predisposing mutations in order to be tumorigenic and therefore plays a more important role in *tumour progression*. To test the latter hypothesis, several of the described models were exposed to carcinogenic drugs or combined with other mouse models carrying predisposing mutations in established tumour suppressor genes.

Indeed, tumour phenotypes are exacerbated by carcinogenic insults. For instance, whereas Bub1, Bub3, Rae1 and Bub3; Rae1 double heterozygous mice are not clearly cancer predisposed, DMBA treatment (a known carcinogen) provokes more tumours in all four knockouts than in wildtype mice (Baker et al., 2006, Jeganathan et al., 2007). This is also true for DMBA-treated BubR1 hypomorphs (Baker et al., 2004). Furthermore, BubR1 heterozygotes are more susceptible to the formation of intestinal tumours in response to treatment with the colon carcinogen azoxymethane (Dai et al., 2004). Finally, 40% of Mad1 heterozygous mice treated with Vinicristine (a microtubule-depolymerizing agent) develop tumours whereas control-treated mice do not develop any (Iwanaga et al., 2007). Similarly, numerical CIN synergizes with predisposing mutations. For instance, decreased levels of Bub1 accelerate tumorigenesis in a $p53^{+/-}$ or $Apc^{+/Min}$ background. In this setting, numerical CIN acts by facilitating LOH of the remaining wildtype allele of the tumour suppressor gene (Baker et al., 2009).

Aneuploidy as a tumour suppressor?

Although decreased levels of Bub1 have a profound effect on tumour initiation in p53- of Apc-mutated backgrounds, this synergy is not observed in Rb or Pten heterozygous mice. Paradoxically, Bub1 hypomorphism acts tumour suppressive in $Pten^{+/-}$ mice, with $Pten^{+/-}$; Bub1 hypomorphs developing fewer hyperplastic prostate lesions than $Pten^{+/-}$ mice expressing wildtype Bub1 levels (Baker et al., 2009). Similarly CENPE heterozygousity delays tumourigenesis in a $p19^{Arf}$-deficient background. Whereas normally $p19^{Arf-/-}$ animals develop lymphomas and sarcomas with an average latency of 6-7 months (Kamijo et al.,

1997), tumour latency is delayed to 12 months in CENPE$^{+/-}$ mice. Furthermore, despite a predisposition for hematopoietic malignancies, the number of spontaneous liver tumours in CENPE$^{+/-}$ mice is reduced 3-fold and liver tumour sizes are remarkably smaller. Finally, CENPE heterozygousity also delays DMBA-induced tumours (Weaver et al., 2007). These observations suggest that aneuploidy can delay tumourigenesis as well and that the response to aneuploidy might very well be tissue specific.

Overexpression of genes with a role in chromosome segregation

Diminished Mad2 expression, mutations and even gene loss do occur in cancer, but are infrequent (Percy et al., 2000, X. Wang et al., 2002, X. Wang et al., 2000). More often Mad2 expression is elevated (Alizadeh et al., 2000, Hernando et al., 2004, van 't Veer et al., 2002). This upregulation is likely the result of increased E2F activity in cancers, as the RB (retinoblastoma) - E2F pathway is altered in more than 80% of human tumours (Malumbres & Barbacid, 2001) and the E2F transcription factor family is an important modulator of Mad2 transcription (Hernando et al., 2004). Furthermore, deregulation of the RB pathway has been associated with CIN (Lentini et al., 2006, Lentini et al., 2002, Schaeffer et al., 2004), and elevated Mad2 levels can provide an explanation for this. Indeed, reducing Mad2 protein levels to wildtype levels in Rb deficient cells reduces the number of aneuploid cells. Conversely, overexpression of either E2F or Mad2 in wildtype cells increases aneuploidy (Hernando et al., 2004). These results strongly suggest that unscheduled activation of E2F contributes to aneuploidy through elevated Mad2 expression. To test if this is true *in vivo*, an inducible Mad2 overexpression mouse model was engineered. These mice display a wide spectrum of tumours (lung adenomas, lymphomas, hepatocellular carcinomas and fibrosarcomas) with a similar latency (~20 months), but higher frequency (~50% at 20 months) than Mad2 heterozygous mice (Sotillo et al., 2007). These results seem somewhat counterintuitive: why would increasing levels of checkpoint protein lead to cancer? Perhaps, delayed degradation of both Securin and Cyclin B1 during mitosis causes defects in mitotic exit and thus explains the observed chromosomal aberrations and subsequent tumourigenesis. Even though this data indicates a clear role for Mad2 overexpression in tumorigenesis, several other mechanisms might contribute to the CIN phenotype of cells with aberrant E2F activity. For instance, Rb inactivation in mouse embryonic fibroblasts also reduces cohesion between sister chromatids, leading to premature chromosome segregation and CIN (Coschi et al., 2010, Manning et al., 2010, van Harn et al., 2010). Furthermore, inducible overexpression of Hec1, another Rb-interacting protein residing at the kinetochore, provokes aneuploid cancers 15-18 months following induction (Diaz-Rodriguez et al., 2008) similar to Mad2 overexpressing mice. Therefore, even though overexpression of Mad2 has a clear cancer phenotype, it is unlikely that Mad2 is the only downstream target of the RB pathway involved in the maintenance of a euploid genome.

Other mouse models for numerical CIN

Not all aneuploidy is the result of spindle checkpoint failure; other mitotic defects can also perturb chromosome segregation and thus cause aneuploidy. Lzts1 was discovered as a gene that is frequently lost in breast, lung, gastric, esophageal, prostate, and bladder cancers. Lzts1 impairs Cyclin B1 activation late in mitosis, resulting in lowered Cyclin B1-Cdk1 activity in mitosis and premature mitotic exit, similar to Mad2 overexpression. Indeed, Lzts1-deficient mice develop a wide spectrum of tumours within 19 months of age with a high penetrance. Lzts1 loss also facilitates carcinogen-induced tumourigenesis, as NMBA treatment resulted in a tumour incidence of 100% in both Lzts1-deficient and heterozygous animals, whereas only 15% of the treated control animals develop tumours. Therefore, premature mitotic exit through decreased Cyclin B1 levels might be an important driver of (numerical) CIN and cancer (Vecchione et al., 2007).

Entry into mitosis is guarded by a prophase checkpoint that can be activated by chromosomal damage or disruption of microtubules (Mikhailov et al., 2002, Pines & Rieder, 2001). Chfr is a potential E3 ubiquitin ligase that functions early in prophase (Matsusaka & Pines, 2004), presumably by controlling expression levels of mitotic proteins such as Aurora A. Unlike SAC components, homozygous deletion of Chfr in the mouse is dispensable for normal development. However, half of the Chfr-deficient animals develop tumours (lymphomas, lung, liver and intestinal tumours) within 20 months of age and furthermore the knockouts show accelerated tumour development upon carcinogenic insults (DMBA). (Yu et al., 2005). Both phenotypes (Lzts1, Chfr) are very similar to those of the cancer-predisposed SAC-compromised heterozygotes, emphasizing the importance of accurately regulated mitotic kinase activity (Cyclin B1-Cdk1, Aurora A) in preserving normal chromosomal numbers and suppression of cancer.

Micronuclei formation is another indication of chromosomal instability. An elegant genetic screen for genes that facilitate micronucleus formation in erythrocytes identified a point mutation in Mcm4 (Chaos3). Mcm4 is part of the Mcm2-7 replication licensing complex and therefore a crucial part of the DNA replication machinery. Mcm4 mutant mice showed decreased expression of several Mcm proteins and primary cells from this mouse also showed increased sensitivity for the replication inhibitor aphidicolin in line with a defect in DNA replication (Shima et al., 2007). However, as this mutation was identified as a mutation that provokes micronuclei formation, this model suggests that defects in DNA replication can cause numerical chromosomal abnormalities as well.

The Adenomatous polyposis coli (APC) gene is a tumour suppressor gene that is often mutated in human colorectal cancers (note that this gene is unrelated to the anaphase promoting complex APC/C). In addition to APC's well-known role in regulating/dampening β-catenin's transcriptional activity and cell proliferation, multiple lines of evidence indicate that mutated APC contributes to chromosome missegregation and numerical CIN. For instance, cell culture studies have shown that APC localizes to kinetochores and microtubule ends. Perturbing APC function by mutation, overexpression or depletion causes aneuploidy (Draviam et al., 2006, Green et al., 2005, Tighe et al., 2004). In addition, mice expressing truncated APC mutant protein display multiple intestinal tumours with aberrant mitosis and polyploidy, indicating a strong link between the loss of APC's mitotic function and tumourigenesis (Caldwell et al., 2007, Dikovskaya et al., 2007, Oshima et al., 1995, Su et al., 1992). Interestingly, this phenotype can be substantially aggravated by concomitant heterozygous BubR1 loss (Rao et al., 2005). Finally, transcriptome analysis of APC-mutated cells revealed that the mutation resulted in the increase of BubR1 and Mad2 expression, which is also observed in adenomas and colorectal carcinomas (Dikovskaya et al., 2007). Together, these findings illustrate an important link between deregulation of APC and the proteins that control mitosis in the progression from early adenomas to aggressive carcinomas.

Lessons learnt from Mouse Embryonic Fibroblasts

MEFs isolated from several of these mouse models have been invaluable in estimating the levels of aneuploidy occurring *in vivo*. However, as complete ablation of spindle checkpoint genes resulted in embryonic lethality before day E8.5 and MEFs are typically isolated at E15.5-14.5, it has been difficult to generate MEFs from the homozygous knockouts. Therefore heterozygous MEFs were analyzed for the extent of aneuploidy (Table I). All heterozygous MEFs show significantly elevated numbers of aneuploid cells compared to wildtype control MEFs, ranging from 10% aneuploidy in the Mad1$^{+/-}$ MEFs to 50% in the Mad2 heterozygotes and Mad2 overexpressing cells. Note that wildtype MEFs typically show less than 10% aneuploid cells (Iwanaga et al., 2007, Michel et al., 2001, Sotillo et al., 2007). In addition, BubR1 hypomorphic and Bub3; Rae1 heterozygous MEFs exhibit premature senescence and increased protein levels of senescence-associated p19^{Arf}, p21^{Cip1} and p16^{Ink4a} (Baker et al., 2004, Baker et al., 2006) in agreement with the observed premature aging phenotype.

Even though all SAC-compromised MEFs show aneuploidy to a greater or lesser extent, the level of aneuploidy in MEFs does not fully correlate with cancer incidence (Table I). However, aneuploidy analyses might lead to different results depending on the passage number of the MEFs. For instance, detailed analysis of Cenp-E heterozygous MEFs revealed that up to 70% of the cells are aneuploid at high passage numbers whereas only 20% are aneuploid in early passages (Weaver et al., 2007). Furthermore, culturing MEFs *in vitro* might not be the best representation for every cell type *in vivo*. Therefore, even though MEF studies are useful to estimate CIN rates *in vitro, in vivo* assessment of aneuploidy will be crucial to link the extent of aneuploidy to cell fate.

4. Conclusions

Aneuploidy as a primary cause for cancer?

Since the first notion of a possible link between chromosomal abnormalities and malignant transformation by Theodore Boveri (Boveri, 1902, Boveri, 1914), we have learned a great deal about the causes and consequences of chromosome missegregation. Mouse models have provided crucial insight into how the SAC and mitotic machinery protect against CIN en cancer. The mouse models discussed in this chapter are far from complete especially as structural CIN and numerical CIN appear to be intertwined (Janssen et al., 2011). Therefore, mutations in genes protecting against structural CIN (Brca2, Mcm4, p53bp1, etc) might very well lead to aneuploidy too, even though these models were not the focus of the current chapter.

Complete inactivation of genes involved in chromosome segregation appears to be uncommon in human cancer. Why then is the vast majority of human cancers aneuploid? Transcriptome analysis of numerous cancers has revealed that overexpression of spindle checkpoint genes is more frequent than reduced expression (Oncomine database (Rhodes et al., 2004)). However, in many cases SAC gene products show mutations or truncations (Cahill et al., 1998, Kim et al., 2005, Olesen et al., 2001, Percy et al., 2000, Scintu et al., 2007, Tsukasaki et al., 2001). Possibly, mutated SAC proteins can act in a dominant-negative fashion, and therefore attenuate spindle checkpoint function. Careful biochemical analysis of such mutant gene products for their effect on the SAC status in combination with new mouse models for these cancer-associated mutations should clarify this issue.

Mouse models for systemic SAC inactivation unequivocally show that removing the spindle checkpoint is not tolerated during embryonic development, when cells are dividing at maximum speed, and results in massive aneuploidy and apoptosis. This agrees fully with the observation that SAC inactivation is not tolerated in cancer cell lines (Kops et al., 2004). However, p53 inactivation in Mad2 deficient MEFs (derived from Mad2$^{-/-}$; p53$^{-/-}$embryonic stem cell lines) partly rescues this lethality, as these cell lines show better survival than Mad2$^{-/-}$ MEFs, even though both cell lines become highly aneuploid (Burds et al., 2005). Therefore, p53 inactivation might synergize with SAC inactivation in malignant transformation by (partly) rescuing SAC-deficiency-induced cell death. Indeed, p53 heterozygosity appears to collaborate with Bub1 hypomorphism in transformation.

Partial inactivation of spindle checkpoint genes does not interfere with normal development (Table 1) and the average life span of these mice is unaltered. While some heterozygotes succumb to tumours at 18-20 months, others age without any cancer phenotype. The Bub3; Rae1 double heterozygotes show signs of premature aging (but not cancer), but do not succumb to the consequences of this phenotype earlier than their wildtype littermates (Baker et al., 2006). All together, the current mouse models for CIN argue that aneuploidy can provoke cancer. It remains unclear why some models are more prone to cancers than other, despite the fact that heterozygous MEFs from all mouse models show substantial aneuploidy, where tested. The only effect on life span is observed in BubR1 hypomorphic mice, which die a few months earlier due to premature aging (Baker et al., 2004). Premature aging coincides with increased numbers of senescent cells *in vivo* and furthermore, MEFs showed increased levels of the senescence-associated p16^{Ink4a}, p19^{Arf} and p21^{Cip1} proteins. Remarkably, *in vivo* clearance of p16^{Ink4A} positive (*i.e.* senescent) cells can delay several of the premature aging sings in BubR1 hypomorphic mice (Baker et al., 2011), suggesting that senescence and aging , in addition to cancer, are important consequences of (numerical) CIN *in vivo*.

Premature senescence might also explain why Cenp-E$^{+/-}$ mice are less susceptible to tumours in a p19^{Arf} negative background or when tumours were induced chemically (Weaver et al., 2007). For instance, loss of p19^{Arf}, an activator of p53 activity, might lead to aberrant DNA damage signalling resulting in genomic instability. Similarly, challenging animals with carcinogenic compounds will induce CIN. Together with Cenp-E heterozygosity, the cumulative aneuploidy might rise to levels that ultimately result in senescence, instead of increased proliferation and cancer. These findings emphasize once more the importance of studying the relationship between senescence, aneuploidy and cancer.

Future directions

What are the next steps that will bring us closer to a therapy that specifically targets aneuploid cancers? We have now learnt that dramatic numerical CIN (e.g. by SAC inactivation) kills cells *in vitro* and interferes with development *in vivo*. We also now know that aneuploidy deregulates cell metabolism and restricts cell proliferation at the cellular level. Partial SAC inactivation appears to predispose for cancer in some models and to provoke a progeria/senescence phenotype in others. However, even though the vast majority of human tumours are aneuploid, few mutations in the SAC cascade have been identified, even though many human cancer cell lines display an abnormal response to anti-cancer drugs that normally activate the SAC, such as Paclitaxel.

Now that several conventional knockout mouse models have been analyzed in depth, we need to address more specific questions on the role that aneuploidy plays in cancer, for instance:

- Is full SAC inactivation tolerated in adult tissues and if so, does it require additional mutations such as p53 inactivation?
- What are the consequences of aneuploidy *in vivo* and do these resemble the consequences as found in aneuploid MEFs or yeast strains (Torres et al., 2007, Williams et al., 2008)?
- Which genes collaborate with expansion of aneuploid cell progeny?
- What determines the cellular response to aneuploidy (proliferation/senescence)?
- Can we specifically kill aneuploid cells, leaving euploid cells untouched?

To answer these questions more sophisticated mouse models are required. For instance, to answer the first question, conditional mouse models are needed. In such models the knockout allele can be deleted in tissues of choice leaving other tissues unaffected. Using this approach embryonic lethality can be circumvented in many cases. In addition, such models allow for comparing the differential responses to aneuploidy from tissue to tissue for each conditional knockout.

In addition, highly aneuploid tumour panels are required to extract the molecular consequences to aneuploidy in transformed cells. For instance, by comparing the molecular responses in different aneuploid tumour types (different knockouts, different tissues), common responses to aneuploidy can be extracted. Understanding this response is of vital importance before even starting to develop drugs that specifically kill aneuploid cells. These tumour cohorts can also be used to screen for additional mutations that occurred during tumour development. By extracting common mutations occurring in aneuploid tumours arising in different tissues and models, recurring pathways can be identified that aneuploid cells rely on to survive. With the recent advances in high throughput sequencing technology such endeavours are becoming more and more feasible.

Does this mean that we are still far away from the first therapies that target aneuploid cells? Maybe not. A recent study has identified a few promising compounds that specifically target aneuploid cell lines making use of the deregulated metabolism of these cells (Tang et al., 2011). Such drugs can be tested in an *in vivo* setting using conditional mouse models for CIN.

Finally, we need a nifty model to visualize aneuploid cells and their response in the *in vivo* setting. One possible approach is to engineer a mouse model in which a single chromosome can be tracked, for instance a transgenic mouse strain expressing a fluorescent artificial transcription factor. By tracking aneuploidy as it arises in early tumour lesions or in aging tissues the direct consequences, but also the more long term effects of aneuploidy can be monitored in an *in vivo* setting. Such a model will provide unique insight into a developing tumour or otherwise affected tissue, but, even more important, can also be used to visualize the clearance of aneuploid cell progeny in response to newly developed drugs.

Spindle checkpoint genes	Phenotypes +/- animals							
Genes	*-/-*	*+/-*	*Cancer prone?*	*Chemical induced cancer?*	*Other Phenotypes*	*Aneuploidy in tissue?*	*% Aneuploid MEFs*	*Reference*
Bub1	Embryonic lethal (E6.5)	Viable, no overt developmental defects	No	DMBA-induced	No	ND	ND	(Jeganathan et al., 2007)
Bub1 hypo-morph	NA	NA	50% have developed tumours by 20 months (lymphomas, lung and liver tumours)	ND	No	ND	15% (segregation defects)	(Jeganathan et al., 2007)
Bub3	Embryonic lethal (E6.5)	Viable, no overt developmental defects	No	DMBA-induced	No	10% (splenocytes)	20%	(Babu et al., 2003, Baker et al., 2006, Kalitsis et al., 2000, Kalitsis et al., 2005)
Bub3; Rae1	ND	Viable, no overt developmental defects	No	DMBA-induced	Premature aging	40% (splenocytes)	40%	(Babu et al., 2003, Baker et al., 2006)
BubR1	Embryonic lethal (E6.5)	Viable, no overt developmental defects	No	DMBA-induced	Hematopoietic defect	Polyploidy in megakaryocytes	15%	(Baker et al., 2004, Q. Wang et al., 2004)
BubR1 hypo-morph	NA	NA	No	DMBA-induced and azoxymethane induced	Premature aging	30% (splenocytes)	35%	(Baker et al., 2004)
$Cdc20^{AAA}$ mutant (does not bind to Mad2)	Embryonic lethal (E12.5)	Viable, no overt developmental defects	50% of the mice developed tumours by 24 months	ND	No	35% ($Cdc20^{AAA/+}$, splenocytes)	28% of $Cdc20^{AAA/+}$ and 52% of $Cdc20^{AAA/AAA}$	(Li et al., 2009)
Cdh1	Embryonic lethal (E10.5)	Viable, no overt developmental defects	17% of the females develop mammary tumours	Tumour suppression upon TPA/DMBA treatment	No	ND	Increased, not further quantified	(Garcia-Higuera et al., 2008)
CENPE	Embryonic lethal (< E7.5)	Viable, no overt developmental defects	20% develop tumours by 19-21 months of age (both lung and spleen)	Tumour suppression upon DMBA treatment	Tumour suppression in a $p19^{Arf-/-}$ background	40% (splenocytes)	20% (up to 70% at high passage)	(Weaver et al., 2003, Weaver et al., 2007)
Mad1	Embryonic lethal	Viable, no overt developmental defects	20% develop tumours within 18-20 months, (lung)	Vinicristine-induced	No	ND	10%	(Iwanaga et al., 2007)

Mad2	Embryonic lethal (E6.5)	Viable, no overt developmental defects	30% develop tumours at 18 months (lung)	ND	No	ND	55%	(Dobles et al., 2000, Michel et al., 2001)
Mad2 over-expression	NA	NA	50% develop tumours by 20 months (lymphomas, lung and liver)	DMBA-induced	No	Aneuploid tumours (not quantified)	50%	(Sotillo et al., 2007)
Rae1	Embryonic lethal (E6.5)	Viable, without developmental defects	No	DMBA-induced	No	10% (splenocytes)	20%	(Babu et al., 2003, Baker et al., 2006)
Structural centromeric proteins				**Phenotypes +/- animals**				
	-/-	*+/-*	*Cancer prone?*	*Chemical induced cancer?*	*Other Phenotypes*	*Aneuploidy in embryos or tissues?*	*% Aneuploid MEFs*	*Reference*
CENPA	Embryonic lethal (E6.5)	Viable, without developmental defects	ND	ND	NA	Chromosome missegregation in E6.5-/- embryos	NA	(Howman et al., 2000)
CENPB	Viable, no phenotype	Viable, no phenotype	ND	ND	Lower body and testis weight	ND	ND	(Hudson et al., 1998, Kapoor et al., 1998, Perez-Castro et al., 1998)
CENPC	Embryonic lethal (E3.5)	Viable, without developmental defects	ND	ND	NA	Aberrant mitosis and micronuclei in early embryos	NA	(Kalitsis et al., 1998)
Hec1 overexpression	NA	NA	13% develop lung tumours and 25% develop liver tumours 15-18 months after induction	ND	No	ND	25%	(Diaz-Rodriguez et al., 2008)
Chromosomal passenger genes/ mitotic spindle binding proteins				**Phenotypes +/- animals**				
	-/-	*+/-*	*Cancer prone?*	*Chemical induced cancer?*	*Other Phenotypes*	*Aneuploidy in embryos/ tissues?*	*% Aneuploid MEFs*	*Reference*
APC/MIN	Embryonic lethal (<E8.5)	Viable	Develop tumours within 3 months (intestine)	ND	Anaemia, presumably due to intestinal bleeding	Aneuploidy and abnormal mitosis in crypt cells	Increased, not quantified	(Caldwell et al., 2007, Oshima et al., 1995, Rao et al., 2005, Su et al., 1992)

Incenp	Embryonic lethal (E3.5-8E.5)	Viable, no overt development al defects	ND	ND	NA	Abnormal nuclear morphology hyperdiploid content in E3.5 embryos	NA	(Uren et al., 2000)
Survivin	Embryonic lethal (E6.5)	Viable, no overt development al defects	ND	ND	NA	Giant nuclei in early embryos	NA	(Uren et al., 2000)
Genes otherwise involved in mitosis	**Phenotypes -/- animals***							
	-/-	+/-	*Cancer prone?*	*Chemical induced cancer?*	*Other Phenotypes*	*Aneuploidy in tissue?*	*Aneuploidy in MEFs?*	*Reference*
Ltzs1	Viable, no development al defects	Viable, no develop-mental defects	All the -/- and 60% of the +/- mice develop tumours at 8-24 months (lymphomas, mammary, liver and liver)	NMBA-induced	No	ND	25% (lagging chromoso mes)	(Vecchione et al., 2007)
$Mcm4^{Chaos3}$	$Mcm4^{Chaos3/-}$ embryonic lethal E14.5	Viable, no development al defects	$Mcm4^{Chaos3/+}$ develop mammary tumours within a year	ND	Classic minichromoso me loss phenotype in blood	ND	ND	(Shima et al., 2007)
Chfr	Viable, no development al defects	Viable, no develop-mental defects	50% of the -/- animals develop tumours within 20 months	DMBA-induced	No	ND	25%	(Yu et al., 2005)

*in case of Mcm4 mice -/- refers to $Mcm4^{Chaos3/+}$ mice

Table 1.

5. References

A.A. Alizadeh, M.B. Eisen, R.E. Davis, C. Ma, I.S. Lossos, A. Rosenwald, J.C. Boldrick, H. Sabet, T. Tran, X. Yu, J.I. Powell, L. Yang, G.E. Marti, T. Moore, J. Hudson, Jr., L. Lu, D.B. Lewis, R. Tibshirani, G. Sherlock, W.C. Chan, T.C. Greiner, D.D. Weisenburger, J.O. Armitage, R. Warnke, R. Levy, W. Wilson, M.R. Grever, J.C. Byrd, D. Botstein, P.O. Brown, L.M. Staudt, (2000), Distinct types of diffuse large B-cell lymphoma identified by gene expression profiling, *Nature* 403, 6769. 503-511.

P.D. Andrews, E. Knatko, W.J. Moore, J.R. Swedlow, (2003), Mitotic mechanics: the auroras come into view, *Current opinion in cell biology* 15, 6. 672-683.

J.R. Babu, K.B. Jeganathan, D.J. Baker, X. Wu, N. Kang-Decker, J.M. van Deursen, (2003), Rae1 is an essential mitotic checkpoint regulator that cooperates with

Bub3 to prevent chromosome missegregation, *The Journal of cell biology* 160, 3. 341-353.

D.J. Baker, K.B. Jeganathan, J.D. Cameron, M. Thompson, S. Juneja, A. Kopecka, R. Kumar, R.B. Jenkins, P.C. de Groen, P. Roche, J.M. van Deursen, (2004), BubR1 insufficiency causes early onset of aging-associated phenotypes and infertility in mice, *Nature genetics* 36, 7. 744-749.

D.J. Baker, K.B. Jeganathan, L. Malureanu, C. Perez-Terzic, A. Terzic, J.M. van Deursen, (2006), Early aging-associated phenotypes in Bub3/Rae1 haploinsufficient mice, *The Journal of cell biology* 172, 4. 529-540.

D.J. Baker, F. Jin, K.B. Jeganathan, J.M. van Deursen, (2009), Whole chromosome instability caused by Bub1 insufficiency drives tumorigenesis through tumor suppressor gene loss of heterozygosity, *Cancer cell* 16, 6. 475-486.

D.J. Baker, T. Wijshake, T. Tchkonia, N.K. LeBrasseur, B.G. Childs, B. van de Sluis, J.L. Kirkland, J.M. van Deursen, (2011), Clearance of p16Ink4a-positive senescent cells delays ageing-associated disorders, *Nature* 479, 7372. 232-236.

S. Biggins, C.E. Walczak, (2003), Captivating capture: how microtubules attach to kinetochores, *Curr Biol* 13, 11. R449-460.

T. Boveri, (1902), Uber mehrpolige Mitosen als Mittel zur Analyse des Zellkerns (Multipolar mitoses as means of the analysis of the nucleus), *Vehr. d. phys. med. Ges. zu Wurzburg* NF35, 67-90.

T. Boveri, (1914), Zur frage der Entsehung maligner Tumoren (The origin of malignant tumors),

A.A. Burds, A.S. Lutum, P.K. Sorger, (2005), Generating chromosome instability through the simultaneous deletion of Mad2 and p53, *Proceedings of the National Academy of Sciences of the United States of America* 102, 32. 11296-11301.

D.P. Cahill, C. Lengauer, J. Yu, G.J. Riggins, J.K. Willson, S.D. Markowitz, K.W. Kinzler, B. Vogelstein, (1998), Mutations of mitotic checkpoint genes in human cancers, *Nature* 392, 6673. 300-303.

C.M. Caldwell, R.A. Green, K.B. Kaplan, (2007), APC mutations lead to cytokinetic failures in vitro and tetraploid genotypes in Min mice, *The Journal of cell biology* 178, 7. 1109-1120.

C.H. Coschi, A.L. Martens, K. Ritchie, S.M. Francis, S. Chakrabarti, N.G. Berube, F.A. Dick, (2010), Mitotic chromosome condensation mediated by the retinoblastoma protein is tumor-suppressive, *Genes & development* 24, 13. 1351-1363.

S.M. Cutts, K.J. Fowler, B.T. Kile, L.L. Hii, R.A. O'Dowd, D.F. Hudson, R. Saffery, P. Kalitsis, E. Earle, K.H. Choo, (1999), Defective chromosome segregation, microtubule bundling and nuclear bridging in inner centromere protein gene (Incenp)-disrupted mice, *Human molecular genetics* 8, 7. 1145-1155.

W. Dai, Q. Wang, T. Liu, M. Swamy, Y. Fang, S. Xie, R. Mahmood, Y.M. Yang, M. Xu, C.V. Rao, (2004), Slippage of mitotic arrest and enhanced tumor development in mice with BubR1 haploinsufficiency, *Cancer research* 64, 2. 440-445.

E. Diaz-Rodriguez, R. Sotillo, J.M. Schvartzman, R. Benezra, (2008), Hec1 overexpression hyperactivates the mitotic checkpoint and induces tumor formation in vivo, *Proceedings of the National Academy of Sciences of the United States of America* 105, 43. 16719-16724.

D. Dikovskaya, D. Schiffmann, I.P. Newton, A. Oakley, K. Kroboth, O. Sansom, T.J. Jamieson, V. Meniel, A. Clarke, I.S. Nathke, (2007), Loss of APC induces polyploidy as a result of a combination of defects in mitosis and apoptosis, *The Journal of cell biology* 176, 2. 183-195.

M. Dobles, V. Liberal, M.L. Scott, R. Benezra, P.K. Sorger, (2000), Chromosome missegregation and apoptosis in mice lacking the mitotic checkpoint protein Mad2, *Cell* 101, 6. 635-645.

S. Doxsey, W. Zimmerman, K. Mikule, (2005), Centrosome control of the cell cycle, *Trends in cell biology* 15, 6. 303-311.

V.M. Draviam, I. Shapiro, B. Aldridge, P.K. Sorger, (2006), Misorientation and reduced stretching of aligned sister kinetochores promote chromosome missegregation in EB1- or APC-depleted cells, *The EMBO journal* 25, 12. 2814-2827.

K. Fukasawa, (2005), Centrosome amplification, chromosome instability and cancer development, *Cancer letters* 230, 1. 6-19.

N.J. Ganem, S.A. Godinho, D. Pellman, (2009), A mechanism linking extra centrosomes to chromosomal instability, *Nature* 460, 7252. 278-282.

I. Garcia-Higuera, E. Manchado, P. Dubus, M. Canamero, J. Mendez, S. Moreno, M. Malumbres, (2008), Genomic stability and tumour suppression by the APC/C cofactor Cdh1, *Nature cell biology* 10, 7. 802-811.

R.A. Green, R. Wollman, K.B. Kaplan, (2005), APC and EB1 function together in mitosis to regulate spindle dynamics and chromosome alignment, *Molecular biology of the cell* 16, 10. 4609-4622.

D. Hanahan, R.A. Weinberg, (2000), The hallmarks of cancer, *Cell* 100, 1. 57-70.

E. Hernando, Z. Nahle, G. Juan, E. Diaz-Rodriguez, M. Alaminos, M. Hemann, L. Michel, V. Mittal, W. Gerald, R. Benezra, S.W. Lowe, C. Cordon-Cardo, (2004), Rb inactivation promotes genomic instability by uncoupling cell cycle progression from mitotic control, *Nature* 430, 7001. 797-802.

E.V. Howman, K.J. Fowler, A.J. Newson, S. Redward, A.C. MacDonald, P. Kalitsis, K.H. Choo, (2000), Early disruption of centromeric chromatin organization in centromere protein A (Cenpa) null mice, *Proceedings of the National Academy of Sciences of the United States of America* 97, 3. 1148-1153.

D.F. Hudson, K.J. Fowler, E. Earle, R. Saffery, P. Kalitsis, H. Trowell, J. Hill, N.G. Wreford, D.M. de Kretser, M.R. Cancilla, E. Howman, L. Hii, S.M. Cutts, D.V. Irvine, K.H. Choo, (1998), Centromere protein B null mice are mitotically and meiotically normal but have lower body and testis weights, *The Journal of cell biology* 141, 2. 309-319.

Y. Iwanaga, Y.H. Chi, A. Miyazato, S. Sheleg, K. Haller, J.M. Peloponese, Jr., Y. Li, J.M. Ward, R. Benezra, K.T. Jeang, (2007), Heterozygous deletion of mitotic arrest-deficient protein 1 (MAD1) increases the incidence of tumors in mice, *Cancer research* 67, 1. 160-166.

J.R. Jackson, D.R. Patrick, M.M. Dar, P.S. Huang, (2007), Targeted anti-mitotic therapies: can we improve on tubulin agents?, *Nat Rev Cancer* 7, 2. 107-117.

P.V. Jallepalli, C. Lengauer, (2001), Chromosome segregation and cancer: cutting through the mystery, *Nat Rev Cancer* 1, 2. 109-117.

A. Janssen, M. van der Burg, K. Szuhai, G.J. Kops, R.H. Medema, (2011), Chromosome segregation errors as a cause of DNA damage and structural chromosome aberrations, *Science (New York, N.Y* 333, 6051. 1895-1898.

K. Jeganathan, L. Malureanu, D.J. Baker, S.C. Abraham, J.M. van Deursen, (2007), Bub1 mediates cell death in response to chromosome missegregation and acts to suppress spontaneous tumorigenesis, *The Journal of cell biology* 179, 2. 255-267.

P. Kalitsis, E. Earle, K.J. Fowler, K.H. Choo, (2000), Bub3 gene disruption in mice reveals essential mitotic spindle checkpoint function during early embryogenesis, *Genes & development* 14, 18. 2277-2282.

P. Kalitsis, K.J. Fowler, E. Earle, J. Hill, K.H. Choo, (1998), Targeted disruption of mouse centromere protein C gene leads to mitotic disarray and early embryo death, *Proceedings of the National Academy of Sciences of the United States of America* 95, 3. 1136-1141.

P. Kalitsis, K.J. Fowler, B. Griffiths, E. Earle, C.W. Chow, K. Jamsen, K.H. Choo, (2005), Increased chromosome instability but not cancer predisposition in haploinsufficient Bub3 mice, *Genes, chromosomes & cancer* 44, 1. 29-36.

T. Kamijo, F. Zindy, M.F. Roussel, D.E. Quelle, J.R. Downing, R.A. Ashmun, G. Grosveld, C.J. Sherr, (1997), Tumor suppression at the mouse INK4a locus mediated by the alternative reading frame product p19ARF, *Cell* 91, 5. 649-659.

M. Kapoor, R. Montes de Oca Luna, G. Liu, G. Lozano, C. Cummings, M. Mancini, I. Ouspenski, B.R. Brinkley, G.S. May, (1998), The cenpB gene is not essential in mice, *Chromosoma* 107, 8. 570-576.

R. Karess, (2005), Rod-Zw10-Zwilch: a key player in the spindle checkpoint, *Trends in cell biology* 15, 7. 386-392.

H.S. Kim, K.H. Park, S.A. Kim, J. Wen, S.W. Park, B. Park, C.W. Gham, W.J. Hyung, S.H. Noh, H.K. Kim, S.Y. Song, (2005), Frequent mutations of human Mad2, but not Bub1, in gastric cancers cause defective mitotic spindle checkpoint, *Mutation research* 578, 1-2. 187-201.

G.J. Kops, D.R. Foltz, D.W. Cleveland, (2004), Lethality to human cancer cells through massive chromosome loss by inhibition of the mitotic checkpoint, *Proceedings of the National Academy of Sciences of the United States of America* 101, 23. 8699-8704.

G.J. Kops, B.A. Weaver, D.W. Cleveland, (2005), On the road to cancer: aneuploidy and the mitotic checkpoint, *Nat Rev Cancer* 5, 10. 773-785.

S.M. Lens, G. Vader, R.H. Medema, (2006), The case for Survivin as mitotic regulator, *Current opinion in cell biology* 18, 6. 616-622.

L. Lentini, F. Iovino, A. Amato, A. Di Leonardo, (2006), Centrosome amplification induced by hydroxyurea leads to aneuploidy in pRB deficient human and mouse fibroblasts, *Cancer letters* 238, 1. 153-160.

L. Lentini, L. Pipitone, A. Di Leonardo, (2002), Functional inactivation of pRB results in aneuploid mammalian cells after release from a mitotic block, *Neoplasia (New York, N.Y* 4, 5. 380-387.

M. Li, X. Fang, Z. Wei, J.P. York, P. Zhang, (2009), Loss of spindle assembly checkpoint-mediated inhibition of Cdc20 promotes tumorigenesis in mice, *The Journal of cell biology* 185, 6. 983-994.

D. Liu, G. Vader, M.J. Vromans, M.A. Lampson, S.M. Lens, (2009), Sensing chromosome bi-orientation by spatial separation of aurora B kinase from kinetochore substrates, *Science (New York, N.Y* 323, 5919. 1350-1353.

M. Malumbres, M. Barbacid, (2001), To cycle or not to cycle: a critical decision in cancer, *Nat Rev Cancer* 1, 3. 222-231.

A.L. Manning, M.S. Longworth, N.J. Dyson, (2010), Loss of pRB causes centromere dysfunction and chromosomal instability, *Genes & development* 24, 13. 1364-1376.

T. Matsusaka, J. Pines, (2004), Chfr acts with the p38 stress kinases to block entry to mitosis in mammalian cells, *The Journal of cell biology* 166, 4. 507-516.

L.S. Michel, V. Liberal, A. Chatterjee, R. Kirchwegger, B. Pasche, W. Gerald, M. Dobles, P.K. Sorger, V.V. Murty, R. Benezra, (2001), MAD2 haplo-insufficiency causes premature anaphase and chromosome instability in mammalian cells, *Nature* 409, 6818. 355-359.

A. Mikhailov, R.W. Cole, C.L. Rieder, (2002), DNA damage during mitosis in human cells delays the metaphase/anaphase transition via the spindle-assembly checkpoint, *Curr Biol* 12, 21. 1797-1806.

A. Musacchio, E.D. Salmon, (2007), The spindle-assembly checkpoint in space and time, *Nature reviews* 8, 5. 379-393.

E.A. Nigg, (2007), Centrosome duplication: of rules and licenses, *Trends in cell biology* 17, 5. 215-221.

E.A. Nigg, (2006), Origins and consequences of centrosome aberrations in human cancers, *International journal of cancer* 119, 12. 2717-2723.

S.H. Olesen, T. Thykjaer, T.F. Orntoft, (2001), Mitotic checkpoint genes hBUB1, hBUB1B, hBUB3 and TTK in human bladder cancer, screening for mutations and loss of heterozygosity, *Carcinogenesis* 22, 5. 813-815.

M. Oshima, H. Oshima, K. Kitagawa, M. Kobayashi, C. Itakura, M. Taketo, (1995), Loss of Apc heterozygosity and abnormal tissue building in nascent intestinal polyps in mice carrying a truncated Apc gene, *Proceedings of the National Academy of Sciences of the United States of America* 92, 10. 4482-4486.

M.J. Percy, K.A. Myrie, C.K. Neeley, J.N. Azim, S.P. Ethier, E.M. Petty, (2000), Expression and mutational analyses of the human MAD2L1 gene in breast cancer cells, *Genes, chromosomes & cancer* 29, 4. 356-362.

A.V. Perez-Castro, F.L. Shamanski, J.J. Meneses, T.L. Lovato, K.G. Vogel, R.K. Moyzis, R. Pedersen, (1998), Centromeric protein B null mice are viable with no apparent abnormalities, *Developmental biology* 201, 2. 135-143.

G.A. Pihan, A. Purohit, J. Wallace, H. Knecht, B. Woda, P. Quesenberry, S.J. Doxsey, (1998), Centrosome defects and genetic instability in malignant tumors, *Cancer research* 58, 17. 3974-3985.

J. Pines, C.L. Rieder, (2001), Re-staging mitosis: a contemporary view of mitotic progression, *Nature cell biology* 3, 1. E3-6.

F.R. Putkey, T. Cramer, M.K. Morphew, A.D. Silk, R.S. Johnson, J.R. McIntosh, D.W. Cleveland, (2002), Unstable kinetochore-microtubule capture and chromosomal instability following deletion of CENP-E, *Developmental cell* 3, 3. 351-365.

C.V. Rao, Y.M. Yang, M.V. Swamy, T. Liu, Y. Fang, R. Mahmood, M. Jhanwar-Uniyal, W. Dai, (2005), Colonic tumorigenesis in BubR1+/-ApcMin/+ compound mutant mice is linked to premature separation of sister chromatids and enhanced genomic instability, *Proceedings of the National Academy of Sciences of the United States of America* 102, 12. 4365-4370.

D.R. Rhodes, J. Yu, K. Shanker, N. Deshpande, R. Varambally, D. Ghosh, T. Barrette, A. Pandey, A.M. Chinnaiyan, (2004), ONCOMINE: a cancer microarray database and integrated data-mining platform, *Neoplasia (New York, N.Y* 6, 1. 1-6.

C.L. Rieder, R.W. Cole, A. Khodjakov, G. Sluder, (1995), The checkpoint delaying anaphase in response to chromosome monoorientation is mediated by an inhibitory signal produced by unattached kinetochores, *The Journal of cell biology* 130, 4. 941-948.

C.L. Rieder, A. Schultz, R. Cole, G. Sluder, (1994), Anaphase onset in vertebrate somatic cells is controlled by a checkpoint that monitors sister kinetochore attachment to the spindle, *The Journal of cell biology* 127, 5. 1301-1310.

A.J. Schaeffer, M. Nguyen, A. Liem, D. Lee, C. Montagna, P.F. Lambert, T. Ried, M.J. Difilippantonio, (2004), E6 and E7 oncoproteins induce distinct patterns of chromosomal aneuploidy in skin tumors from transgenic mice, *Cancer research* 64, 2. 538-546.

M. Scintu, R. Vitale, M. Prencipe, A.P. Gallo, L. Bonghi, V.M. Valori, E. Maiello, M. Rinaldi, E. Signori, C. Rabitti, M. Carella, B. Dallapiccola, V. Altomare, V.M. Fazio, P. Parrella, (2007), Genomic instability and increased expression of BUB1B and MAD2L1 genes in ductal breast carcinoma, *Cancer letters* 254, 2. 298-307.

N. Shima, A. Alcaraz, I. Liachko, T.R. Buske, C.A. Andrews, R.J. Munroe, S.A. Hartford, B.K. Tye, J.C. Schimenti, (2007), A viable allele of Mcm4 causes chromosome instability and mammary adenocarcinomas in mice, *Nature genetics* 39, 1. 93-98.

R. Sotillo, E. Hernando, E. Diaz-Rodriguez, J. Teruya-Feldstein, C. Cordon-Cardo, S.W. Lowe, R. Benezra, (2007), Mad2 overexpression promotes aneuploidy and tumorigenesis in mice, *Cancer cell* 11, 1. 9-23.

L.K. Su, K.W. Kinzler, B. Vogelstein, A.C. Preisinger, A.R. Moser, C. Luongo, K.A. Gould, W.F. Dove, (1992), Multiple intestinal neoplasia caused by a mutation in the murine homolog of the APC gene, *Science (New York, N.Y* 256, 5057. 668-670.

Y.C. Tang, B.R. Williams, J.J. Siegel, A. Amon, (2011), Identification of aneuploidy-selective antiproliferation compounds, *Cell* 144, 4. 499-512.

A. Tighe, V.L. Johnson, S.S. Taylor, (2004), Truncating APC mutations have dominant effects on proliferation, spindle checkpoint control, survival and chromosome stability, *Journal of cell science* 117, Pt 26. 6339-6353.

E.M. Torres, T. Sokolsky, C.M. Tucker, L.Y. Chan, M. Boselli, M.J. Dunham, A. Amon, (2007), Effects of aneuploidy on cellular physiology and cell division in haploid yeast, *Science (New York, N.Y* 317, 5840. 916-924.

M.F. Tsou, T. Stearns, (2006), Controlling centrosome number: licenses and blocks, *Current opinion in cell biology* 18, 1. 74-78.

K. Tsukasaki, C.W. Miller, E. Greenspun, S. Eshaghian, H. Kawabata, T. Fujimoto, M. Tomonaga, C. Sawyers, J.W. Said, H.P. Koeffler, (2001), Mutations in the mitotic check point gene, MAD1L1, in human cancers, *Oncogene* 20, 25. 3301-3305.

A.G. Uren, L. Wong, M. Pakusch, K.J. Fowler, F.J. Burrows, D.L. Vaux, K.H. Choo, (2000), Survivin and the inner centromere protein INCENP show similar cell-cycle localization and gene knockout phenotype, *Curr Biol* 10, 21. 1319-1328.

L.J. van 't Veer, H. Dai, M.J. van de Vijver, Y.D. He, A.A. Hart, M. Mao, H.L. Peterse, K. van der Kooy, M.J. Marton, A.T. Witteveen, G.J. Schreiber, R.M. Kerkhoven, C. Roberts, P.S. Linsley, R. Bernards, S.H. Friend, (2002), Gene expression profiling predicts clinical outcome of breast cancer, *Nature* 415, 6871. 530-536.

T. van Harn, F. Foijer, M. van Vugt, R. Banerjee, F. Yang, A. Oostra, H. Joenje, H. te Riele, (2010), Loss of Rb proteins causes genomic instability in the absence of mitogenic signaling, *Genes & development* 24, 13. 1377-1388.

A. Vecchione, G. Baldassarre, H. Ishii, M.S. Nicoloso, B. Belletti, F. Petrocca, N. Zanesi, L.Y. Fong, S. Battista, D. Guarnieri, R. Baffa, H. Alder, J.L. Farber, P.J. Donovan, C.M. Croce, (2007), Fez1/Lzts1 absence impairs Cdk1/Cdc25C interaction during mitosis and predisposes mice to cancer development, *Cancer cell* 11, 3. 275-289.

Q. Wang, T. Liu, Y. Fang, S. Xie, X. Huang, R. Mahmood, G. Ramaswamy, K.M. Sakamoto, Z. Darzynkiewicz, M. Xu, W. Dai, (2004), BUBR1 deficiency results in abnormal megakaryopoiesis, *Blood* 103, 4. 1278-1285.

X. Wang, D.Y. Jin, R.W. Ng, H. Feng, Y.C. Wong, A.L. Cheung, S.W. Tsao, (2002), Significance of MAD2 expression to mitotic checkpoint control in ovarian cancer cells, *Cancer research* 62, 6. 1662-1668.

X. Wang, D.Y. Jin, Y.C. Wong, A.L. Cheung, A.C. Chun, A.K. Lo, Y. Liu, S.W. Tsao, (2000), Correlation of defective mitotic checkpoint with aberrantly reduced expression of MAD2 protein in nasopharyngeal carcinoma cells, *Carcinogenesis* 21, 12. 2293-2297.

B.A. Weaver, Z.Q. Bonday, F.R. Putkey, G.J. Kops, A.D. Silk, D.W. Cleveland, (2003), Centromere-associated protein-E is essential for the mammalian mitotic checkpoint to prevent aneuploidy due to single chromosome loss, *The Journal of cell biology* 162, 4. 551-563.

B.A. Weaver, D.W. Cleveland, (2006), Does aneuploidy cause cancer?, *Current opinion in cell biology* 18, 6. 658-667.

B.A. Weaver, A.D. Silk, C. Montagna, P. Verdier-Pinard, D.W. Cleveland, (2007), Aneuploidy acts both oncogenically and as a tumor suppressor, *Cancer cell* 11, 1. 25-36.

B.R. Williams, V.R. Prabhu, K.E. Hunter, C.M. Glazier, C.A. Whittaker, D.E. Housman, A. Amon, (2008), Aneuploidy affects proliferation and spontaneous immortalization in mammalian cells, *Science (New York, N.Y* 322, 5902. 703-709.

X. Yu, K. Minter-Dykhouse, L. Malureanu, W.M. Zhao, D. Zhang, C.J. Merkle, I.M. Ward, H. Saya, G. Fang, J. van Deursen, J. Chen, (2005), Chfr is required for tumor suppression and Aurora A regulation, *Nature genetics* 37, 4. 401-406.

K.W. Yuen, B. Montpetit, P. Hieter, (2005), The kinetochore and cancer: what's the connection?, *Current opinion in cell biology* 17, 6. 576-582.

Section 2

The Impact of Aneuploidy on Human Health

5

Aneuploidy and Epithelial Cancers: The Impact of Aneuploidy on the Genesis, Progression and Prognosis of Colorectal and Breast Carcinomas

Jens K. Habermann[1], Gert Auer[2], Madhvi Upender[3], Timo Gemoll[1], Hans-Peter Bruch[1], Hans Jörnvall[2], Uwe J. Roblick[1] and Thomas Ried[3]

[1]*University of Lübeck*
[2]*Karolinska Institute*
[3]*National Cancer Institute*
[1]*Germany*
[2]*Sweden*
[3]*USA*

1. Introduction

Aneuploidy is a defining feature of epithelial cancers with an impact on the genesis, progression and prognosis of these malignancies. Essentially all sporadic, mismatch repair proficient colorectal carcinomas are defined by a non-random distribution of genomic imbalances. Regarding breast cancer, however, aneuploid and near diploid cases show almost similar frequencies. Independent of the tumor entity, increased levels of aneuploidy result in a worse clinical outcome. For breast and colorectal carcinomas, aneuploidy has been reported as an independent prognostic factor with an impact comparable to that of the tumor stage. Unfortunately, the translation of this knowledge into the clinic was slow. Prognostication in breast cancer is augmented by gene expression profiles of poor or good prognosis. Interestingly, there is growing evidence that prognostic gene expression signatures simply reflect the degree of genomic instability. This is not surprising since gross nuclear aneuploidy is reflected in a strikingly recurrent and tumor entity specific distribution of chromosomal imbalances. Chromosomal imbalances, in turn, do significantly modulate resident gene expression levels. Furthermore, aneuploidy also affects protein expression. Proteomics has therefore become a powerful tool to unravel potential new targets for diagnostics, prognostication and therapeutic stratification. There is also increasing evidence that aneuploidy precedes invasive disease and can already be detected in premalignant lesions such as colon adenomas and/or ulcerative colitis. It is therefore reasonable to assume that aneuploidy plays a crucial role during carcinogenesis, an interpretation consistent with its direct influence on disease outcome. This has triggered considerable efforts to elucidate how aneuploidy develops and what its impact is on the genetic equilibrium of cells at the molecular level.

2. Nuclear DNA content, genomic instability and chromosomal aneuploidy

In 1914, Theodor Boveri proposed that the loss or gain of "inhibiting" or "promoting" chromosomes, respectively, might cause uncontrolled cell proliferation (Boveri 1914; Ried 2009). This hypothesis could only be validated after technical progress allowed a more detailed analysis of the human genome and after the correct number of human chromosomes was established to be 46 (Tjio and Levan 1956). Each chromosome consists of two chromatids that are joined at the centromere. The centromeric region is important for the attachment of kinetochores that are responsible for the segregation of the chromatids during mitotic cell division, a central feature for maintaining genomic stability (Kops, Weaver, and Cleveland 2005). Chromosomes can be classified by their centromere position, size and banding pattern (Strachan and Read 1999). Telomeres are located at the ends of chromosomes to protect the integrity of the chromosomal DNA. They harbour proteins that protect the ends of chromosomes from, e.g., recombination, nuclease attacks, and end-to-end fusions. The DNA polymerase *telomerase* is responsible for the maintenance of the telomere length that physiologically becomes shorter with each cell division. Telomerase reactivation has been identified as an important mechanism for malignant transformation (Shay and Wright 2002). Both abnormalities of centromere and telomere function can lead to aneuploidy.

2.1 Clonal expansion and proliferation

Boveri's hypothesis that chromosomal aberrations might cause uncontrolled cell proliferation was first supported by the detection of the Philadelphia chromosome in 1960. The Philadelphia chromosome shows a translocation, t(9;22), characteristic for chronic myelogenous leukemia (Rowley 1973). This translocation causes synthesis of a fusion protein with increased tyrosine kinase activity (p210) that increases cell proliferation. Translocations belong to those mutations that affect the chromosomal structure. Inversions, deletions and duplications are also referred to as structural aberrations. Such cancer promoting chromosomal aberrations can affect different genes, causing either a gain of function (proto-oncogenes) or a loss of function (tumor suppressor genes). Whereas mutations in oncogenes are mainly dominant, mutations in tumor suppressor genes are typically recessive and follow Knudson's two-hit model: The first mutation "hits" one allele of a tumor suppressor gene. The presence of the remaining wild-type allele preserves the tumor inhibiting function. The second "hit" mutates the remaining wild-type allele, which results in the complete loss of gene function (Knudson 1979). In addition to structural chromosomal aberrations, we also observe alterations of chromosome number, i.e., aneuploidy (Giaretti et al. 2004). While one reason for the emergence of structural chromosomal aberrations are deficiencies in the repair of DNA double strand breaks (Sinicrope, Rego, Foster, et al. 2006), there is mounting evidence that numeric chromosome imbalances are caused by chromatid segregation errors during mitotic cell division (D'Amours and Jackson 2002; Jallepalli and Lengauer 2001; Loeb and Loeb 2000; Vessey, Norbury, and Hickson 1999). Loss of bub1, for instance, a gene involved in the mitotic checkpoint, increases chromosome segregation errors (Cahill et al. 1998). Alternatively, overexpression of cyclin E, a cell cycle regulator results in centrosome amplification (Nigg 1996), and has been observed in a variety of malignancies causing chromosome instability and aneuploidy (Spruck, Won, and Reed 1999; Donnellan and Chetty 1999). The completion of the cell and DNA replication cycle requires the coordination of a variety of macromolecular syntheses, assemblies and movements. These complex processes are normally tightly controlled by regulatory pathways or checkpoints in order to maintain genomic stability. However, cancer cells often exhibit mutations that allow bypassing those regulatory mechanisms leading to aberrant growth and clonal expansion. Gain-of-function of growth factor receptors, often through an increase in copy number, is also frequently observed in tumors (Scharf and Braulke 2003).

2.2 Cell cycle regulation

Cell cycle regulators, namely cyclin-dependent kinases (cdks) and their regulatory subunits (cyclins), are driving forces of the cell cycle and act at different cellular checkpoints. In 1951, Howard and Pelc divided the cell cycle into four phases (GAP1, synthetic phase, GAP2, and mitosis) (Howard and Pelc 1951). Later on, abbreviations were used that described the preceding phase as G1, the synthetic phase as S phase, the phase before cell division as G2, and the mitosis phase as M phase (Zetterberg, Larsson, and Wiman 1995). Since the genetic material is duplicated in the S phase and divided in the M phase, the transition of a cell into these two phases is crucial and regulated by the *G1/S checkpoint* and the *G2/M DNA damage checkpoint*. The cascade of interacting cyclins and cdks during the cell cycle can be briefly summarized as follows: The activation of cdk4 and cdk6 by cyclin D leads the cell from the middle of G1 to the G1/S checkpoint. Active cyclin E/cdk2 complexes then trigger the transition from G1 to S phase. The cyclin A/cdk2 complex promotes the cell cycle progress from the G1/S checkpoint into G2 (Sherr 1993). Cyclin A can therefore serve as a proliferation marker for committed cells that will pass through the S and G2 phase (Zindy et al. 1992). Cyclin A also binds cdk1 from the end of S to the beginning of the M phase. Its function has not been conclusively elucidated but aberrant expression of cyclin A/cdk1 complexes has been associated with tumorigenesis (Liao et al. 2004). In addition, cyclin A overexpression itself significantly reflects poor prognosis of carcinoma patients (Handa et al. 1999). For the transition from G2 into M phase, cyclin B activates cdk1. In addition to the cell cycle regulation by cdks and their cyclins, other regulatory factors have been described such as the transcription factor TP53 which is responsible for leading the cell into G1 and G2 arrest (Vousden 2002). Another checkpoint has been described for the M phase which has been subdivided into five phases that harbour specific stages of the mitotic cell division: prophase, prometaphase, metaphase, anaphase, and telophase. The appropriate transition from prometaphase and metaphase to anaphase is highly important to guarantee genomic stability. The cellular mechanism that could be used to delay prometaphase or metaphase in response to spindle defects or impaired chromosome segregation has been termed the spindle integrity checkpoint (Allshire 1997).

3. Aneuploidy and epithelial malignancies

Aneuploidy is a characteristic genetic alteration of the cancer genome (Duesberg et al. 1998; Lengauer, Kinzler, and Vogelstein 1998; Ried et al. 1999). When the first quantitative measurements of the DNA content were applied to cancer cells, aneuploidy was defined as a variation in the nuclear DNA content of cancer cells within a tumor (Caspersson 1979). In addition to nuclear aneuploidy, an increased resolution of cytogenetic techniques such as chromosome banding, comparative genomic hybridization (CGH), spectral karyotyping

(SKY), and multicolor fluorescence *in situ* hybridization allowed the detection of specific non-random imbalances, heretofore referred to as chromosomal aneuploidy (Caspersson et al. 1970; Kallioniemi et al. 1992; Schrock et al. 1996; Speicher, Gwyn Ballard, and Ward 1996). Indeed, despite genetic instability in cancer genomes, cancer cell populations as a whole display a surprisingly conserved, malignancy-specific pattern of genomic imbalances (Ried et al. 1999; Knuutila et al. 1998; Forozan et al. 1997). Interestingly, chromosomal aneuploidy can be the first detectable genetic aberration found during human tumorigenesis, *e.g.*, in pre-invasive dysplastic lesions (Hittelman 2001; Hopman et al. 1988; Heselmeyer et al. 1996; Solinas-Toldo et al. 1996). This suggests both an initial requirement for the acquisition of specific chromosomal aneuploidy and a requirement for the maintenance of these imbalances despite genomic and chromosomal instability. This would be consistent with continuous selective pressure to retain a specific pattern of chromosomal copy number changes in the majority of tumor cells (Bomme et al. 1994; Ried et al. 1999; Nowak et al. 2002; Desper et al. 2000). Chromosomal aneuploidy is also the earliest detectable genomic aberration in cell culture model systems in which cells are exposed to carcinogens or subject to spontaneous transformation (Barrett et al. 1985; Padilla-Nash et al. 2011). The conservation of these specific patterns of chromosomal aneuploidy indicates a fundamental biological role in tumorigenesis.

3.1 Aneuploidy and colorectal cancer

3.1.1 Chromosomal aneuploidy in sporadic colorectal cancer (SCC)

Malignant transformation of the colorectum is defined by the sequential acquisition of genetic alterations, both at gene-specific and on chromosomal levels (Fearon and Vogelstein 1990). Many of these aberrations can be visualized as specific chromosomal gains and losses resulting in a conserved and malignancy-specific pattern of genomic imbalances (Ried et al. 1996). One of the earliest acquired genetic abnormalities during colorectal tumorigenesis are copy number gains of chromosome 7 (Bomme et al. 1994) which can already be observed in benign polyps. At later stages, e.g., in high-grade adenomas or in invasive carcinomas, additional numeric aberrations such as gains of chromosomes and chromosome arms 8q, 13, and 20q, and losses that map to 8p, 17p, and 18q become prominent (**Figure 1**). For a comprehensive summary see the "Mitelman Database of Chromosome Aberrations in Cancer" at http://cgap.nci.nih.gov/Chromosomes/Mitelman. Chromosomal aneuploidy is accompanied by specific mutations in tumor suppressor genes and oncogenes, including e.g., *APC* and *TP53* (Vogelstein and Kinzler 2004). It is therefore well accepted that both chromosomal aneuploidy and specific gene mutations, are required for tumorigenesis.

3.1.2 Chromosomal aneuploidy and ulcerative colitis-associated colorectal cancer (UCC)

Unlike sporadic colorectal tumors, UCCs do not follow the adenoma–carcinoma sequence, and their sequential acquisition of chromosomal aneuploidy and gene mutations is less well established. It was therefore questioned if the pattern of chromosomal alterations in UCC is similar to that known for sporadic carcinomas. Earlier reports suggested that genomic imbalances observed in UCC cluster on the same chromosomes as those observed in sporadic colorectal carcinomas (Kern et al. 1994; Holzmann et al. 2001; Willenbucher et al. 1997; Loeb and Loeb 1999; Aust et al. 2000).

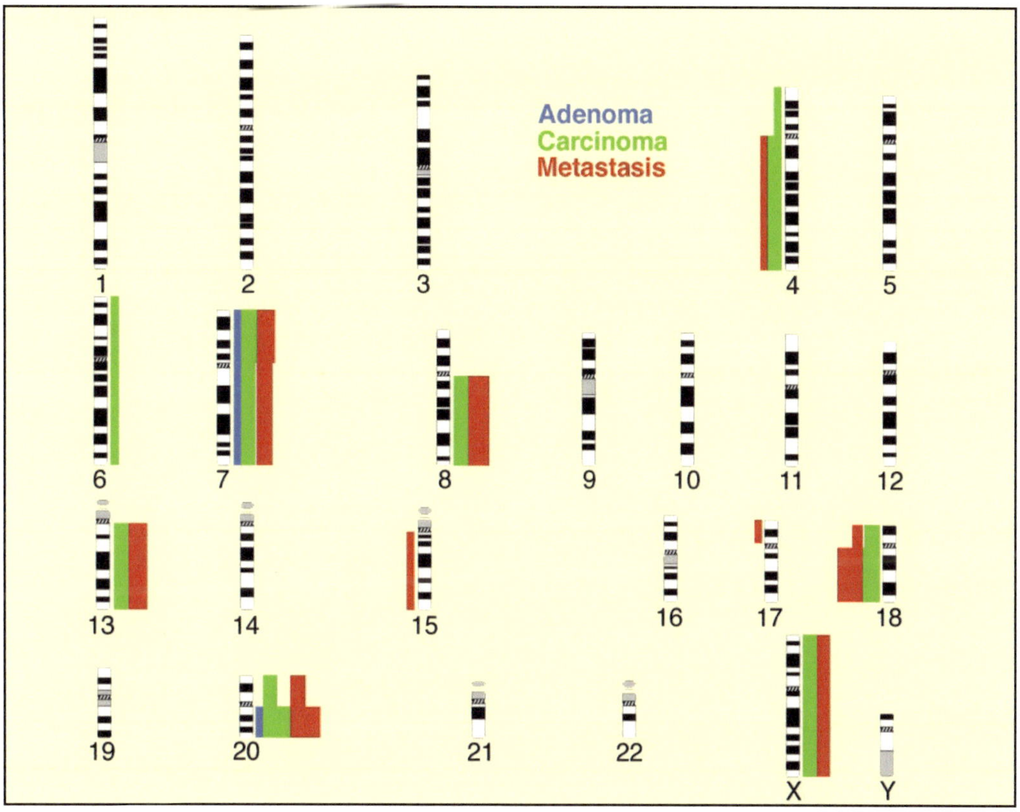

Fig. 1. Comparison of genomic imbalances in sporadic adenomas (n=14), sporadic colorectal carcinomas (n= 15), and liver metastasis of sporadic colorectal carcinomas (n=12). Bars on the left side of the chromosome ideogram denote a loss of sequence in the tumor genome, bars on the right side a gain of sequence in the tumor genome. The number of alterations per chromosome is normalized to 10 cases for each disease stage. Only ratios greater than 2 have been considered. Figure modified from (Habermann et al. 2007).

The analysis by Habermann and colleagues comprised the largest sample collection of UCCs from one clinical center and supports these findings: all 19 UCC specimens showed chromosomal imbalances by comparative genomic hybridization (CGH) (Habermann et al. 2003) that mainly cluster on the same chromosomes as described for sporadic colorectal cancer (**Figure 1**). These data clearly indicate that the tumor cell population as an entity of UCCs selects for a distribution of genomic imbalances that is similar to sporadic carcinomas. It therefore seems logic to conclude that the tissue origin of the tumor cell and not the mode of tumor induction defines the similarity between sporadic colorectal cancers and UCC. This is in striking contrast to hereditary colorectal carcinomas arising in the background of mismatch repair deficiency, where neither aneuploidy nor specific chromosomal imbalances are observed (Ghadimi et al. 2000; Schlegel et al. 1995).

3.1.3 Nuclear aneuploidy and prognosis of colorectal cancer (SCC and UCC)

The strikingly conserved pattern of chromosomal aneuploidy in sporadic and ulcerative colitis-associated colorectal carcinomas can be reflected by nuclear DNA aneuploidy. Hereby, flow and/or image cytometry are reliable tools with excellent clinical applicability also for high-throughput clinical diagnostics. Interestingly, reported frequencies of aneuploidy in UCCs vary inconsistently between 28.6% and 100% (Holzmann et al. 1998; Fozard et al. 1986). One limitation of former studies might be the overall low number of UCC cases analyzed, varying from single case studies up to 17 UCC patients (Clausen et al. 2001; Makiyama et al. 1995; Burmer, Rabinovitch, and Loeb 1991). Against this background, we had recently compiled a single center cohort comprising 31 UCCs that were assessed for the frequency of nuclear aneuploidy and its association to clinical parameters and survival and in comparison to 257 sporadic colorectal carcinomas (Gerling et al. 2010). Ploidy measurements were performed by means of image cytometry which allows the simultaneous assessment of histomorphology. Histograms were classified according to Auer (**Figure 2**) (Auer, Caspersson, and Wallgren 1980).

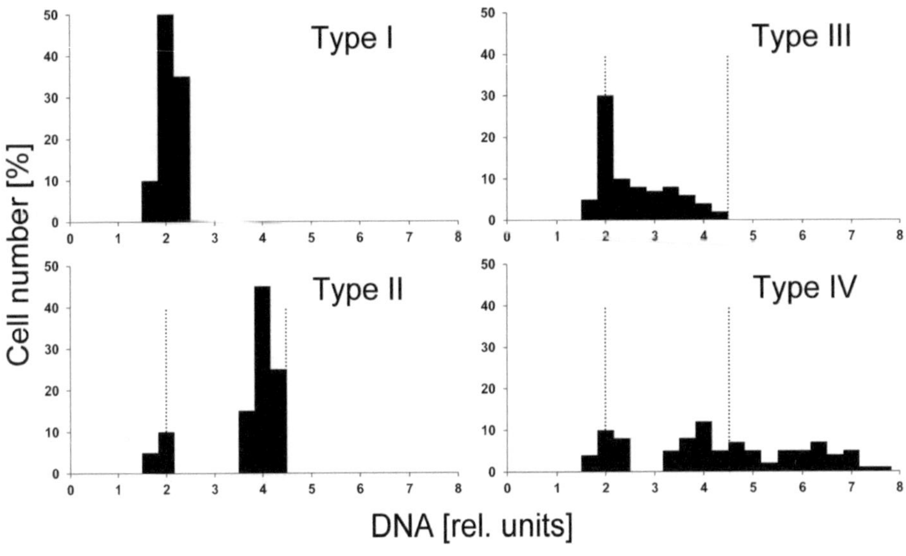

Fig. 2. DNA Histogram types according to Auer (Auer, Caspersson, and Wallgren 1980). Histograms characterized by a single peak in the diploid or near-diploid region (1.5-2.5 c) were classified as type I. The total number of cells with DNA values exceeding the diploid region (>2.5 c) was <10%. Type II histograms showed a single peak in the tetraploid region (3.5- 4.5 c) or peaks in both the diploid and tetraploid regions (>90% of the total cell population). The number of cells with DNA values between the diploid and tetraploid region and those exceeding the tetraploid region (>4.5 c) was <10%. Type III histograms represented highly proliferating near-diploid cell populations and were characterized by DNA values ranging between the diploid and the tetraploid regions. Only a few cells (<5%) showed more than 4.5 c. The DNA histograms of types I, II, and III thus characterize euploid cell populations. Type IV histograms showed increased (>5%) and/or distinctly scattered DNA values exceeding the tetraploid region (>4.5 c). These histograms reflect aneuploid populations of colon mucosa nuclei with decreased genomic stability.

Interestingly, UCCs showed aneuploidy at a significantly higher frequency than sporadic colorectal carcinomas (100% versus 74.6%; $P < 0.0006$) (Gerling et al. 2010). A logistic regression analysis assessed age, sex, UICC stage, T- and N-status, histologic tumor grading, underlying inflammation, and DNA ploidy status. Out of these features, only age and DNA ploidy status were significant parameters indicating both patients of higher age at diagnosis and patients with aneuploid malignancy have a poor survival prognosis. Additional logistic regression analysis comprising these two significant parameters only confirmed age (odds ratio [OR], 1.05; 95% CI, 1.02–1.09; $P = 0.003$) and DNA ploidy (OR, 4.07; 95% CI, 1.46 -11.36; $P = 0.007$) to be independent prognostic parameters. Among those, DNA aneuploidy with an OR of 4.07 seemed to be the strongest independent prognostic marker for R0-resected colorectal cancer patients overall. The dominance of aneuploidy as an independent prognostic factor in patients with SCC and UCC was further supported by the fact, that patients with diploid tumors at advanced stages (UICC stage III/IV) did present a survival comparable to that of patients with aneuploid tumors at early stages (**Figure 3**). The latter finding might even suggest that the presence of aneuploid tumor cell populations may influence the patient's prognosis more dominantly than tumor stage.

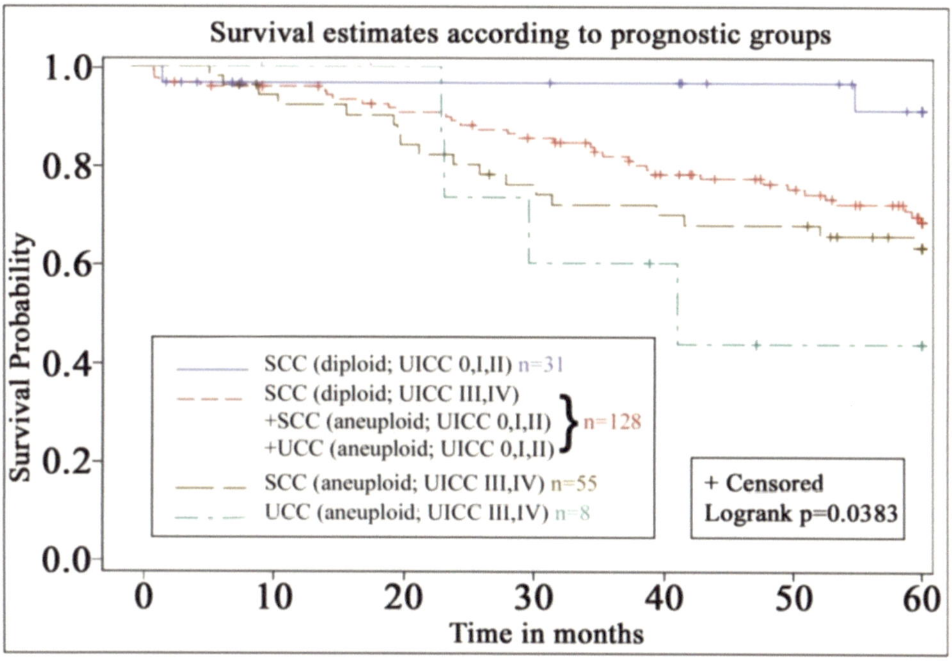

Fig. 3. Kaplan-Meier survival estimates of significant prognostic groups according to UICC stage, ploidy status, and underlying inflammatory disease. SCC, sporadic colorectal cancer; UCC, ulcerative colitis-associated colorectal cancer. Modified from (Gerling et al. 2010).

3.1.4 Nuclear aneuploidy and cancer risk assessment in ulcerative colitis and sporadic colon adenomas

The higher frequency of nuclear aneuploidy in UCCs than in sporadic colorectal cancer might indicate the dominance of genomic instability not only at the time when malignancy is overt but also for the development of malignant properties. In order to evaluate aneuploidy as a potential predictive marker in patient risk assessment, two groups were analyzed (Habermann et al. 2001): eight patients with UCC and 16 ulcerative colitis (UC) patients without malignancy but comparable risk factors according to the duration of disease, extent of inflammation and occurrence of epithelial dysplasia. A total of 683 paraffin-embedded mucosal biopsies were evaluated for inflammatory activity, grade of dysplasia and ploidy status. In all biopsies, mild or moderate inflammatory activity was present in 78% while low-grade or high-grade dysplasia was found in 5.5% overall. No difference in inflammatory activity and dysplasia between patient groups could be detected (Habermann et al. 2001). One of the most important findings of this study was the detection of highly aneuploid epithelial cell populations scattered over the colon and rectum in premalignant biopsies of all eight UCC patients. These lesions could be observed up to 11 years prior to the final cancer diagnosis (average 7.8 years). Aneuploidy was found in macro- and microscopically unsuspicious mucosa, could even be detected in regenerative epithelium, and was not related to dysplasia. DNA aneuploidy occurred more frequently in biopsies (75%) of ulcerative colitis patients with a subsequent UCC than in those without subsequent malignancy (14%, p = 0.006). All eight UCC specimens themselves also showed aneuploidy. In line with these findings, Löfberg et al. reported aneuploid biopsies in 25% of high-risk patients at least once during 10 years of observation (Lofberg et al. 1992). In other studies, aneuploidy has been repeatedly observed also in non-dysplastic mucosa of high-risk patients (Rubin et al. 1992). It seems therefore reasonable to suggest that genomic instability, represented by DNA aneuploidy, might initiate malignant transformation in colitis as an early event. However, aneuploidy may be reversible over time once cells are no longer exposed to the inducing carcinogen (Auer et al. 1982; Ono et al. 1984). Thus, nuclear aneuploidy might need to be followed by multiple cellular alterations in order to reach malignant properties.

In sporadic colorectal carcinogenesis, adenomas are considered premalignant lesions. However, individual colorectal adenomas have different propensities to progress to malignancy. We therefore explored whether these differences could be explained by chromosomal aberrations, oncogene amplifications, and/or deletions of tumor-suppressor genes. Fluorescence *in situ* hybridization (FISH) with gene specific probe sets was applied to 18 adenomas of patients without synchronous or subsequent carcinoma, 23 adenomas of carcinoma patients, and 6 matched carcinomas (Habermann et al. 2011). The probe sets included centromere probes for chromosomes 17 and 18 (CEP17 and CEP18), as well as gene-specific probes for *SMAD7* (18q21.1), *EGFR* (7p12), *NCOA3* (20q12), *TP53* (17p13.1), *MYC* (8q24.21), and *RAB20* (13q34).

First, gene copy numbers were correlated with the DNA ploidy status independent of patient groups: *EGFR* amplifications correlated with *SMAD7* deletions ($P < 0.01$) and an increased DNA stem line value ($P = 0.019$). *NCOA3* amplifications were more frequently observed in aneuploid adenomas and increasing *NCOA3* gene copy number signals correlated with higher DNA stem line values ($P = 0.023$, **Figure 4**). A deletion of *TP53* was more frequently observed in aneuploid adenoma samples ($P = 0.029$). *MYC* amplifications were more frequently observed in adenoma samples with increased DNA stem line values ($P < 0.01$) and in adenoma samples that were assessed to be aneuploid ($P = 0.029$). *RAB20* amplifications also correlated with increased DNA stem line values ($P < 0.05$).

Second, comparing adenomas with and without synchronous carcinomas showed that a higher genomic instability index of CEP18, *SMAD7*, and *EGFR* (the genomic instability index was measured by dividing the number of different signal patterns by the number of analyzed cells) could be detected in the adenoma samples of patients with carcinoma than in adenoma samples of patients without synchronous or subsequent carcinoma (P = 0.037). Furthermore, *TP53* deletions were more frequently observed in adenoma samples of patients with synchronous carcinoma (P = 0.045).

Third, evaluation of the prognostic potential for adenoma recurrence revealed that a diploid signal count for *NCOA3* was associated with a longer adenoma recurrence-free observation time (P = 0.042, **Figure 4**).

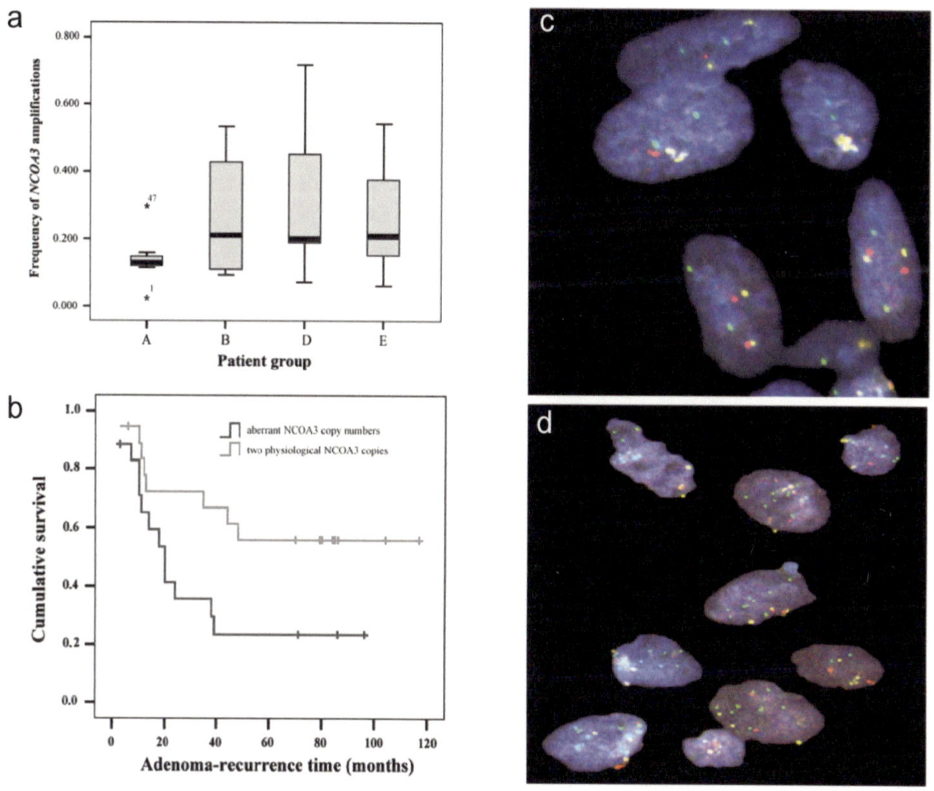

Fig. 4. (a) Frequency of *NCOA3* amplifications according to patient groups (A, patients without adenoma recurrence and without carcinoma; (B) patients with adenoma recurrence but without carcinoma; (D) patients without adenoma recurrence but with carcinoma; (E) patients with adenoma recurrence and with carcinoma). (b) Adenoma recurrence-free survival time depending on *NCOA3* copy numbers. (c) Physiological copy numbers in diploid and (d) aberrant copy numbers in aneuploid adenomas for CEP17 (yellow), *NCOA3* (green) and *TP53* (red). Modified from (Habermann et al. 2011).

Fourth, the most frequently observed alterations overall were a gain of *EGFR* (36.2%) and *RAB20* (34.2%). Although the frequency of these two aberrations was increased in the carcinoma samples (*EGFR*, 44%/*RAB20*, 41.4%), there was no difference between patients with and without malignancy. Based on the presented above results one could conclude that genomic instability in colorectal adenomas is reflected by genomic amplification of the oncogenes *EGFR, MYC, NCOA3,* and *RAB20.* These amplifications could be indicative for adenoma recurrence and for the presence of synchronous carcinomas. Detection of such amplifications using FISH could therefore contribute to the assessment of individual progression to malignancy.

4. Aneuploidy-associated gene expression

4.1 Aneuploidy-associated gene expression in colorectal cell lines

The correlation of nuclear aneuploidy with conserved patterns of chromosomal aberrations and gene specific signal enumerations with prognosis prompted us to analyze the immediate consequences of chromosomal copy number changes at the gene expression level. For this purpose, microcell-mediated chromosome transfer was used to introduce extra copies of chromosomes 3, 7, and 13 into the diploid colorectal cancer cell line DLD1 (Upender et al. 2004). The introduction of all three chromosomes individually resulted in a significant increase in average gene expression on the trisomic chromosome (all $P < 0.0001$). In order to assess whether this effect was specific for DLD1 *per se* or specific for the tissue of origin (colon), we also determined the effect of an additional copy of chromosome 3 in a mammary epithelial cell line (hTERT-HME). The introduction of an extra copy of chromosome 3 into the telomerase immortalized, karyotypically normal mammary epithelial cells resulted as well in an increase in the average gene expression of chromosome 3 genes ($P < 0.0001$, **Figure 5**). An additional analysis at the level of chromosome arms did not reveal additional changes in any of the derivative cell lines.

In addition to analysis of average, chromosome-specific gene expression levels for the introduced chromosomes, we also identified additional deregulated genes throughout the genome. The influence of the three trisomies at the individual gene expression level was examined by considering only genes with expression ratios >2.0 (up-regulated) or <0.5 (down-regulated) when compared with the parental cell line. For clone DLD1 + 7, only 18% (35 of 194) of the differentially expressed genes (DEGs) with known locus information mapped to chromosome 7 and 32 of these were up-regulated (Table 1). Regarding chromosome 13, only 6% (10 of 162) mapped to chromosome 13, of which all were up-regulated (**Table 1**). The trisomy of chromosome 3 in DLD1 revealed 12% (17 of 144) to map to this chromosome and all were up-regulated (**Table 1**). The introduction of the same trisomy 3 into the hTERT-HME cells yielded 17% (23 of 135) of the differentially expressed genes mapping to chromosome 3, of which 21were up-regulated (**Table 1**).

Strikingly, no genes were affected in common among any of the four derivative cell clones. Five percent of all genes on the array mapped to each of chromosomes 7 and 3. For chromosome 13, the percentage was 1.7%. The observed percentages of up-regulated genes located on chromosomes 7 and 3 were each >20%, and the observed percentage of up-regulated genes residing on chromosome 13 was >10%. Thus, the percentages of up-regulated genes residing on the introduced chromosomes were substantially greater than would have been expected by chance if up-regulation occurred at random. In contrast, the percentages of down-regulated genes residing on the introduced chromosomes were no more than expected by chance. Thus, the effect of a very specific increase in average

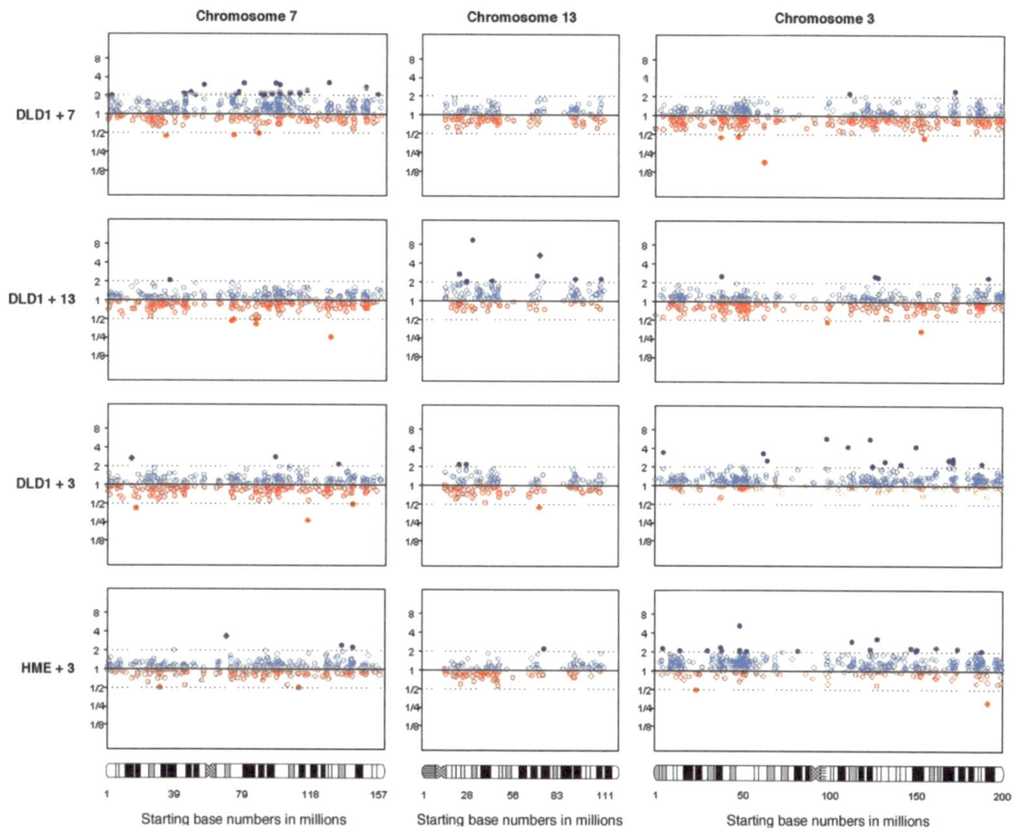

Fig. 5. Global gene expression profiles. Each scatter-plot displays all genes and their corresponding normalized expression ratio values along the length of each chromosome. Values in open light blue circles and open light orange circles represent ratio values between 0.5 and 2.0. Dark blue dots represent expression ratios > 2.0 and dark orange dots are ratios < 0.5. The X axis shows the starting base pair location of each gene (Upender et al. 2004).

	DLD1 + 7		DLD1 + 13		DLD1 + 3		HME + 3	
No. of genes two-fold altered	202		164		148		140	
No. of up-regulated genes	155		92		81		91	
Map on chromosome		32		10		17		21
Map off chromosome		117		82		64		66
Map unknown		6		0		0		4
No. of down-regulated genes	47		72		67		49	
Map on chromosome		3		0		0		2
Map off chromosome		42		70		63		46
Map unknown		2		2		4		1

NOTE. Genes up or down regulated (normalized ratio > 2.0 and < 0.5, respectively; (Upender et al. 2004).

Table 1. Summary of 2-fold altered gene lists

expression of genes on the trisomic chromosomes is further supported by an expression increase of a significant number of individual genes located on those chromosomes. Furthermore, a large number of genes located on diploid chromosomes in these derivative cell clones was also significantly increased in expression, hereby revealing a more complex global transcriptional deregulation.

The phenomenon of trisomy-associated expression alterations in the cell line model described above was further confirmed by a correlation analysis of chromosomal aberrations and gene expression changes in 16 normal mucosa specimens, 17 adenomas, 20 primary colorectal carcinomas, and 13 liver metastases (Habermann et al. 2007). In particular, we found average gene expression changes for those chromosome arms that showed copy number changes including 7p, 7q, 8p, 8q, 13q, 18p, 18q, 20p and 20q in colorectal carcinomas.

4.2 Aneuploidy-associated gene expression in breast carcinoma

Comparable to colorectal cancer, aneuploidy also has a direct impact on the prognosis of patients suffering from breast cancer. In this disease, aneuploidy serves as an indicator of poor prognosis independent from established parameters such as lymph node status and other clinical and histomorphological variables (Auer, Caspersson, and Wallgren 1980; Auer et al. 1984; Heselmeyer-Haddad et al. 2002; Ried et al. 1995). Consistent with these results, the differentiation of aneuploidy and near diploidy in genomically stable and unstable cell populations using the *Stemline Scatter Index* (SSI) has shown that patients with genomically stable tumors have a significantly better prognosis than those with unstable ones (Kronenwett et al. 2004; Kronenwett et al. 2006). To evaluate potential differences in gene expression patterns between genomically stable and unstable breast carcinomas, 48 breast carcinomas were assessed by gene expression profiling on microarrays (Habermann et al. 2009): 17 diploid tumors were genomically stable (dGS), 15 tumors assessed as aneuploid, yet genomically stable (aGS), and 16 carcinomas were classified as aneuploid and genomically unstable (aGU). No differences were observed among the three groups regarding patients' age, tumor size and number of lymph node metastases. The higher degree of genomic instability in the aGU group was also reflected in an increase in chromosomal copy number changes as measured by CGH. A detailed summary and comparison of chromosomal aberrations between the three groups is presented in **Figure 6**.

Chromosomal aberrations in the genomically stable tumors (dGS and aGS) were mainly restricted to gains of chromosome 1q and 16p and accompanied by losses on chromosome 16q. In contrast, aGU tumors showed more diverse changes including a frequent gain of the long arm of chromosome 17, the mapping position of the *ERBB2* oncogene. The similarity of the genomically stable (dGS and aGS) compared to the genomically unstable (aGU) tumors was further supported by gene expression profiles: pair-wise comparisons of the three groups showed that 38 genes were commonly differentially expressed for the comparisons *aGU versus dGS* and *aGU versus aGS*, whereas only two genes were commonly observed in the comparisons *aGU versus aGS* and *aGS versus dGS*, and three genes among *aGS versus dGS* and *aGU versus dGS*. The gene lists describing exclusive differences between all groups can be obtained from Habermann et al. (Habermann et al. 2009). In summary, both,

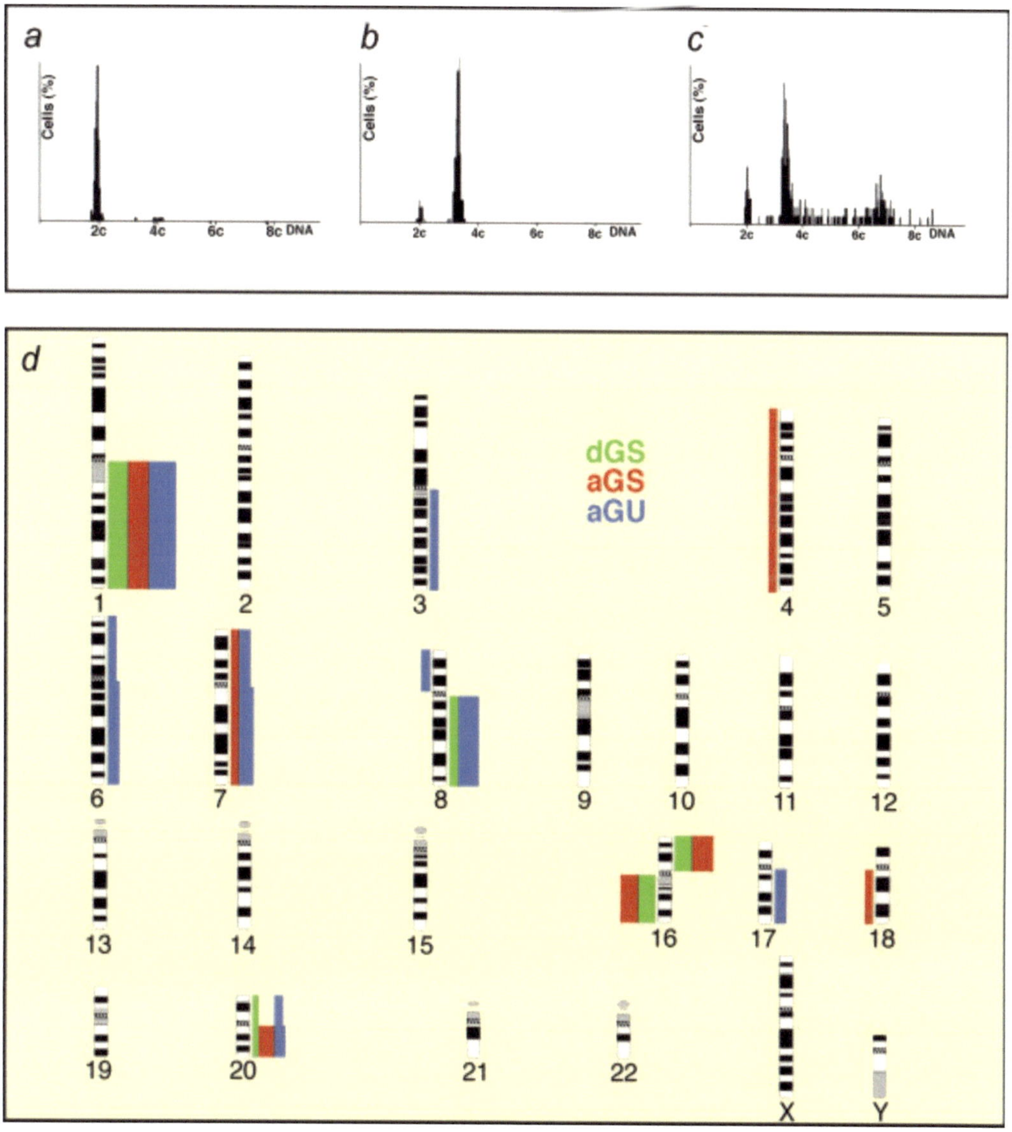

Fig. 6. Genomic instability in breast cancer: Examples of DNA histograms of (a) diploid, genomically stable tumors (dGS), (b) aneuploid, yet genomically stable tumors (aGS), and (c) aneuploid and genomically unstable (aGU) tumors. Note the profound scattering of the ploidy stemline in (c) (for details of the ploidy classification see (Kronenwett et al. 2004). (d) Summary of genomic imbalances in 15 dGS (green), 12 aGS (red), and 11 aGU (blue) breast carcinomas analyzed by comparative genomic hybridization. Bars on the left side of the chromosome ideogram denote a loss of sequence in the tumor genome, while bars on the right side designate a gain. The width of the bars indicates the relative frequency of gains and losses observed (Habermann et al. 2009).

chromosomal alterations and patterns of differentially expressed genes suggest that tumors classified as genetically unstable differed substantially from the genetically stable ones, regardless of the actual ploidy status (i.e., the position of the stemline which is at 2c in the dGS and different from 2c in the aGS).

In order to further explore the biological relevance of our gene expression differences in the genomically stable versus unstable groups, we evaluated the usefulness of our expression profiles for predicting disease outcome in previously published independent datasets. For this purpose, the classification of our samples into genomically stable and unstable carcinomas was based on a 12-gene-genome instability signature (Habermann et al. 2009). This gene set, which discerned the stable from unstable tumors, was then applied for predicting cancer outcomes in independent datasets reported by Sorlie et al. (Sorlie et al. 2003), van de Vijver et al. (van de Vijver et al. 2002), and Sotiriou et al. (Sotiriou et al. 2003). Each patient in the three validation cohorts was classified as being more similar to either the genomically stable or unstable signature, based on the correlation of this patient's gene expression pattern with the average expression profiles of the genomically stable and unstable samples in our dataset. Kaplan-Meier analyses showed that patients defined to have genomic unstable carcinomas were associated with a distinct shorter relapse-free survival and metastasis-free survival ($p < 0.04$) in the patient cohorts from Sorlie et al. (Sorlie et al. 2003), van de Vijver et al. (van de Vijver et al. 2002), and Sotiriou et al. (Sotiriou et al. 2003). Furthermore, patients presenting tumors with genomic instability had a remarkably different, shorter overall survival in Kaplan-Meier analyses ($p < 0.025$) as shown in **Figure 7**.

It was further shown, that the 12-gene signature is independent of clinicopathologic factors such as lymph node status, the NIH criteria, the St. Gallen criteria, and grading used for breast cancer prognostication (Habermann et al. 2009). Furthermore, the 12-gene genome instability signature revealed a remarkable concordance with independent classification systems for specific prognostic subtypes, i.e., luminal A and B, basal, ERBB2+, and normal-like (Sorlie et al. 2001; Sorlie et al. 2003; Perou et al. 2000; Bergamaschi et al. 2006): of the 28 genomically stable tumors in our collection, 24 were assigned to subtypes luminal A (n = 18) or normal-like (n = 6). Only four tumors were assigned to the ERBB2+ group. In contrast, all but one genomically unstable tumor (n = 16) was assigned to either the ERBB2+ group (n = 10) or the basal group (n = 5), indicating pour prognosis. Of note, most of our genomically unstable tumors showed genomic amplification of chromosome arm 17q, the mapping position of the ERBB2 oncogene (**Figure 6**).

In addition, it was explored whether other gene expression signatures for breast cancer prognosis would allow classification of the degree of genomic instability in our samples. Specifically, the 21-gene signature of the so-called Oncotype DX assay (consisting of 16 cancer-associated genes and 5 genes included for normalization purposes) (Paik et al. 2004), and the 70-gene signature of the MammaPrint ® (van de Vijver et al. 2002; van 't Veer et al. 2002) were used to predict genomic instability in our tumor collection. Twelve of the 21 genes used in the Oncotype DX test were present on our platform, whereas 21 of the 70 genes employed by MammaPrint® could be utilized in our set. Using the Oncotype DX gene set, overall prediction accuracy (measured as correct classification of unstable tumors as unstable, and stable tumors as stable) was 91%, whereas the MammaPrint® set correctly classified 84% of all cases. Therefore, these results further support a close linkage between genomic instability and poor prognosis in breast cancer.

In summary, the above data show that, firstly, differences in the degree of genomic instability were reflected in the 12-gene signature that separated our samples. Secondly, this aneuploidy-specific gene expression signature can reliably predict outcome in published datasets, and, thirdly, in turn, the gene expression signature of poor prognosis, independent of the specific platform, predicts the degree of genomic instability with convincing accuracy ($p < 0.001$).

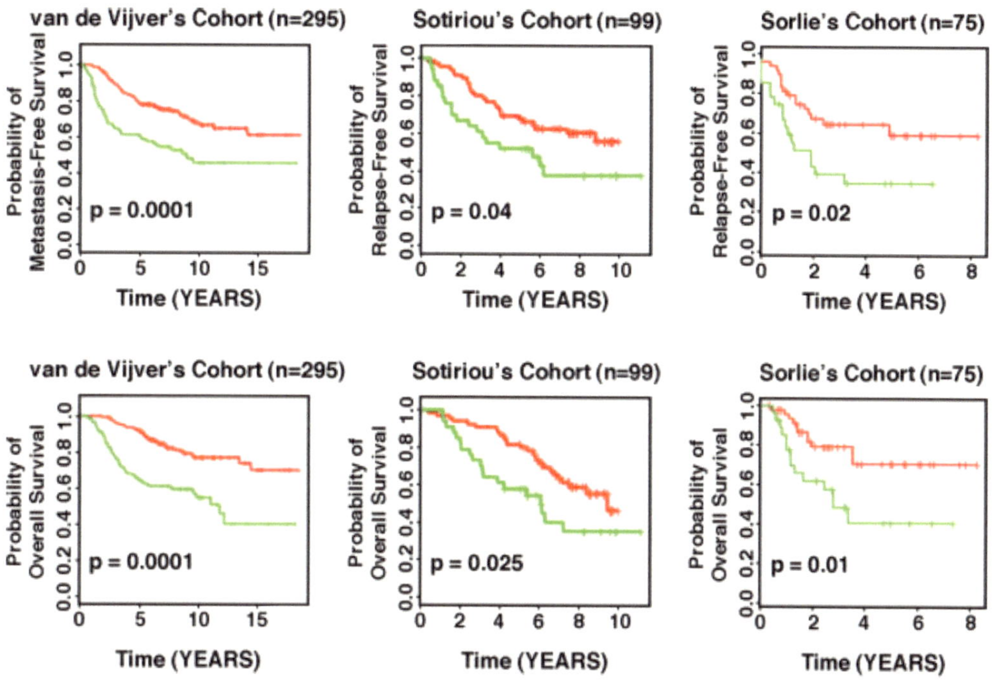

Fig. 7. Applying the 12-gene genomic instability signature for prediction of disease-free and overall survival in independent datasets using Kaplan-Meier analyses. The curves in red reflect carcinoma patients harboring the genomically stable signature, the curves in green the one representing genomic instability. For all examples, statistically significant association of genomic instability with shorter disease-free and overall survival was observed (Habermann et al. 2009).

5. Aneuploidy-associated protein expression

Against the background that nuclear aneuploidy correlates with cancer or cancer subtype-specific chromosomal alterations that impact on gene expression levels, we considered it highly important to elucidate if aneuploidy-associated protein expression patterns can be identified as well. Such protein expression patterns could likely unravel novel targets for improved diagnostics and potentially therapeutic interventions. Two-dimensional gel electrophoresis (2-DE) and mass-spectrometry were applied to assess protein expression profiles of colorectal cancer cell lines of defined ploidy types. Ploidy assessment determined the colorectal cancer cell lines DLD-1, HCT116, and LoVo to be diploid. In contrast, Caco-2,

HT-29, T84, and Colo 201 were classified as aneuploid. Ploidy-type classification of cell lines was further supported by comparative genomic hybridization (CGH) and spectral karyotyping (SKY) analyses (http://www.ncbi.nlm.nih.gov/sky/).

Two independent statistical analyses revealed 38 (ANOVA analysis) and 31 (random forest) protein spots being differentially expressed between the diploid and aneuploid cell lines (Gemoll et al. 2011). Twenty-six spots were identified by peptide mass fingerprinting: eight proteins were higher and 18 lower expressed in the aneuploid than in the diploid cell lines. Based on *Ingenuity Pathways Analysis*, fold changes, molecular functions, and availability of antibodies, YWHAQ, CAPZA1, GNAS, PRDX2, HDAC2, and TXNL1 were selected for downstream analysis. While Western-blot fold changes of all six proteins were in accordance with 2-DE data, only three of the six proteins reached significance ($p < 0.05$) having either lower (TXNL1, CAPZA1) or higher expression (HDAC2) in the aneuploid group.

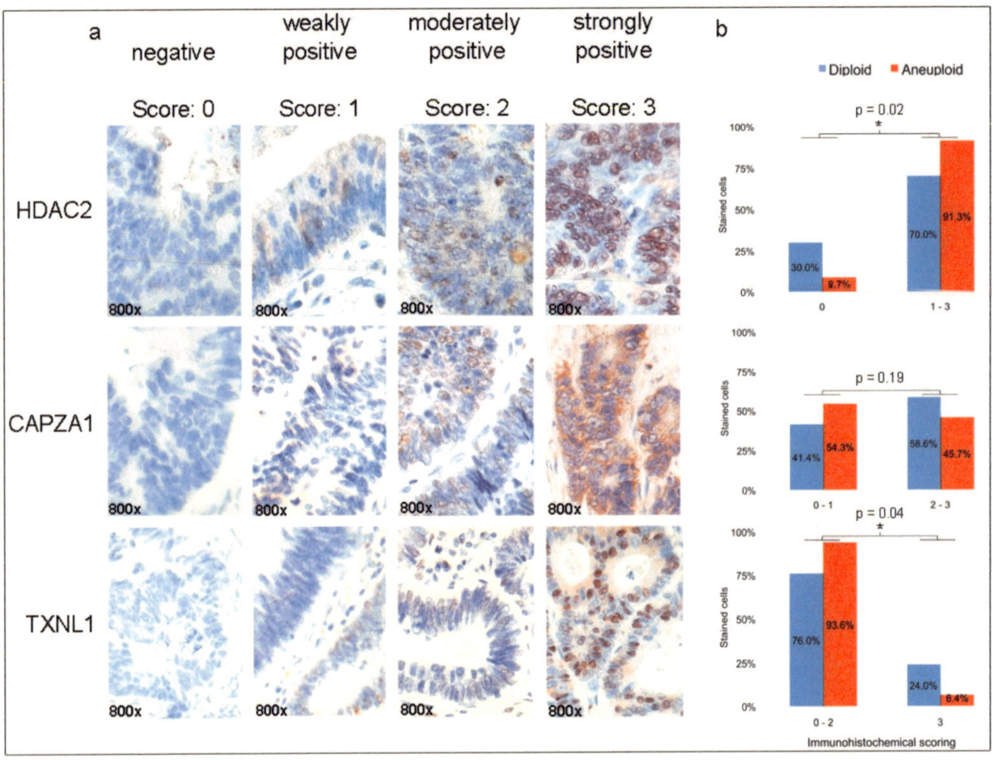

Fig. 8. **(a)** HDAC2, CAPZA1, and TXNL1 immunohistochemical detection in colorectal cancer specimens based on a tissue microarray. Image examples are given at 800-fold magnification. **(b)** Tissue-microarray-based immunohistochemical evaluation of HDAC2, CAPZA1, and TXNL1 comparing diploid versus aneuploid colorectal carcinoma specimens. Immunoreactivity was scored with "0" showing no positivity, "1" presenting up to 20% immunopositive cells, "2" up to 50%, and "3" above 50% stained cells. Barplots of the TMA analysis confirmed HDAC2 and TXNL1 as significantly (asterisk) differentially expressed proteins between diploid and aneuploid tumors (Gemoll et al. 2011).

For proof of clinical relevance we chose those three proteins for tissue microarray (TMA)-based immunohistochemistry assessment. As shown in **Figure 8**, HDAC2 nuclear immunopositivity (score 1, 2, and 3) was more frequently present in aneuploid (91.3%) than in diploid (70%) carcinomas (P = 0.02). For TXNL1, strong nuclear immunoreactivity (score 3) was more frequently observed in diploid (24%) than in aneuploid carcinomas (6.4%, P = 0.04). CAPZA1 immunohistochemistry showed a similar trend as in Western-blot and 2-DE analysis, however, did not reach significance. By comparing immunopositivity between normal adjacent mucosa and all carcinoma specimens irrespective of their ploidy status, we detected significantly stronger immunopositivity in the carcinomas for HDAC2 (P < 0.001) and TXNL1 (P = 0.026).

The *TXNL1* gene encodes a protein that belongs to the thioredoxin family of small redox active proteins. TXNL1 overexpression can increase the transcriptional repressor function through its binding to the transcription factor B-Myb (Kim et al. 2006). Thus, TXNL1 overexpression specifically predisposes to arrest in the G0/G1 phase of the cell cycle. Overexpression in diploid malignancies could therefore help to maintain genomic stability. HDAC2 plays an important role in transcriptional regulation and cell cycle progression (Harms and Chen 2007). HDAC2 is overexpressed in several tumor entities, including colon cancer (Song et al. 2005; Ashktorab et al. 2009). Interestingly, HDAC2 overexpression seems to be induced by APC loss and appears to be sufficient on its own to prevent apoptosis, thus favoring the development of genomic instability and tumor growth (Zhu et al. 2004). The inhibition of HDAC in combination with chemotherapy (doxorubicin) is currently assessed in phase I clinical trials. HDAC2 overexpression in the primary tumor serves as a predictive marker for efficient HDAC inhibition (Munster et al. 2009). Our data show a close correlation of HDAC2 overexpression, aneuploidy, and poor prognosis. It seems therefore reasonable that HDAC2 overexpression is a mere reflection of aneuploidy and that patients, in particular those with aneuploid tumors could benefit from treatment with HDAC-inhibitors. The fact that more than 70% of colorectal cancers are aneuploid makes this even more compelling.

6. Conclusions

DNA aneuploidy is a defining feature of human cancers of epithelial origin, i.e., the carcinomas. Disease-specific chromosomal aneuploidies develop before the transition to invasive disease, e.g., in ulcerative colitis and colorectal adenomas. These early chromosomal alterations are maintained in primary carcinomas and are complemented by additional, recurrent chromosomal aberrations that persist in local and distant metastases. Chromosomal aneuploidy not only has an impact on the expression levels of resident genes but also correlates with protein expression. Such aneuploidy-associated protein expression patterns could reveal novel diagnostic and therapeutic targets. Our general conclusions were supported by the findings of Sinicrope et al., Bosari et al., and Yildirim-Assaf et al. showing that patients with aneuploid tumors had a worse outcome compared to patients with euploid tumors (Sinicrope, Rego, Halling, et al. 2006; Bosari et al. 1992; Yildirim-Assaf et al. 2007). Despite this clear demonstration of an association of aneuploidy and outcome the American Society of Clinical Oncology (ASCO) does not recommend ploidy assessment in clinical routine. In our opinion, this should be reconsidered, also because meta-analysis revealed results clearly indicating the prognostic impact of aneuploidy on colorectal and other cancers (Araujo et al. 2007; Walther, Houlston, and Tomlinson 2008; Schulze and Petersen 2011). Overall, the assessment of nuclear aneuploidy by image cytometry could become routine practice to assist in predicting individual cancer risk and in disease prognostication in solid tumors.

7. Future perspectives

DNA ploidy measurements in premalignant lesions could profoundly improve individual risk assessment for imminent colorectal cancer development. Furthermore, individual risk stratification and survival prognosis in solid malignancies, including colorectal and breast cancer, could benefit from the assessment of nuclear DNA content and the visualization of disease-specific chromosomal aneuploidies. However, large multicenter prospective studies are warranted to further corroborate the value of measurement of aneuploidy for an improved screening and better prognostication in solid malignancies. For this purpose we have initiated the *North German Tumorbank of Colorectal Cancer* (Acronym: ColoNet) that currently comprises patients of the universities and clinics of Hamburg, Lübeck, Rostock, Greifswald, Bad Oldesloe, Berlin-Buch and associated private practices in Northern Germany. Within this network and in collaboration with the *Surgical Center for Translational Oncology-Lübeck* (SCTO-L) as well as the clinical partners at the greater Stockholm area we will investigate the benefit of ploidy measurements for individual risk and prognosis assessment in epithelial malignancies.

8. Acknowledgements

We thank all members of the laboratories of Gert Auer, Jens Habermann, Hans Jörnvall, and Thomas Ried, and all colleagues at the Department of Surgery, Department of Pathology and Unit of Gastroenterology at the University of Lübeck who made these studies possible. In particular, we are indebted to Constanze A. Brucker, Michael J. Difilippantonio, Marco Gerling and Kerstin Heselmeyer-Haddad for their valuable input. Furthermore we gratefully acknowledge the intramural funding of the National Institutes of Health, the Karolinska Institutet, the University of Lübeck and the Werner and Clara Kreitz Foundation, the Ad Infinitum Foundation, the Swedish Cancer Society, the Cancer Society Stockholm, the Swedish Research Council, the King Gustav V Jubilee Fund, the Wallenberg Consortium North, and the Knut and Alice Wallenberg Foundation. These studies were performed in connection with the Surgical Center for Translational Oncology - Lübeck (SCTO-L) and were based on sample collections of the *North German Tumorbank of Colorectal Cancer* (DKH #108446) and the Karolinska Hospital.

9. Abbreviations

2-DE	Two-dimensional gel electrophoresis
aGS	Aneuploid genomically stable
aGU	Aneuploid genomically unstable
ANOVA	Analysis of variance
ASCO	American Society of Clinical Oncology
CDK	Cyclin-dependent kinase
CGH	Comparative genomic hybridization

CI	Confidence intervall
DEG	Differentially expressed gene
dGS	Diploid genomically stable
FISH	Fluorescence in situ hybridization
OR	Odds ratio
SCC	Sporadic colorectal cancer
SKY	Spectral karyotyping
SSI	Stemline Scatter Index
TMA	Tissue microarray
UC	Ulcerative colitis
UCC	Ulcerative colitis-associated colorectal cancer
UICC	Union internationale contre le cancer

10. References

Allshire, R. C. 1997. Centromeres, checkpoints and chromatid cohesion. *Curr Opin Genet Dev* 7 (2):264-73.

Araujo, S. E., W. M. Bernardo, A. Habr-Gama, D. R. Kiss, and I. Cecconello. 2007. DNA ploidy status and prognosis in colorectal cancer: a meta-analysis of published data. *Diseases of the colon and rectum* 50 (11):1800-10.

Ashktorab, H., K. Belgrave, F. Hosseinkhah, H. Brim, M. Nouraie, M. Takkikto, S. Hewitt, E. L. Lee, R. H. Dashwood, and D. Smoot. 2009. Global histone H4 acetylation and HDAC2 expression in colon adenoma and carcinoma. *Dig Dis Sci* 54 (10):2109-17.

Auer, G., E. Eriksson, E. Azavedo, T. Caspersson, and A. Wallgren. 1984. Prognostic significance of nuclear DNA content in mammary adenocarcinomas in humans. *Cancer Res* 44 (1):394-6.

Auer, G., J. Ono, M. Nasiell, T. Caspersson, H. Kato, C. Konaka, and Y. Hayata. 1982. Reversibility of bronchial cell atypia. *Cancer Res* 42 (10):4241-7.

Auer, G. U., T. O. Caspersson, and A. S. Wallgren. 1980. DNA content and survival in mammary carcinoma. *Anal Quant Cytol* 2 (3):161-5.

Aust, D. E., R. F. Willenbucher, J. P. Terdiman, L. D. Ferrell, C. G. Chang, D. H. Moore, 2nd, A. Molinaro-Clark, G. B. Baretton, U. Loehrs, and F. M. Waldman. 2000. Chromosomal alterations in ulcerative colitis-related and sporadic colorectal cancers by comparative genomic hybridization. *Hum Pathol* 31 (1):109-14.

Barrett, J. C., M. Oshimura, N. Tanaka, and T. Tsutsui. 1985. Role of aneuploidy in early and late stages of neoplastic progression of Syrian hamster embryo cells in culture. *Basic Life Sci* 36:523-38.

Bergamaschi, A., Y. H. Kim, P. Wang, T. Sorlie, T. Hernandez-Boussard, P. E. Lonning, R. Tibshirani, A. L. Borresen-Dale, and J. R. Pollack. 2006. Distinct patterns of DNA copy number alteration are associated with different clinicopathological features and gene-expression subtypes of breast cancer. *Genes, chromosomes & cancer* 45 (11):1033-40.

Bomme, L., G. Bardi, N. Pandis, C. Fenger, O. Kronborg, and S. Heim. 1994. Clonal karyotypic abnormalities in colorectal adenomas: clues to the early genetic events in the adenoma-carcinoma sequence. *Genes, Chromosomes & Cancer* 10 (3):190-6.

Bosari, S., A. K. Lee, B. D. Wiley, G. J. Heatley, W. M. Hamilton, and M. L. Silverman. 1992. DNA quantitation by image analysis of paraffin-embedded colorectal adenocarcinomas and its prognostic value. *Modern pathology : an official journal of the United States and Canadian Academy of Pathology, Inc* 5 (3):324-8.

Boveri, T. 1914. Zur Frage der Entstehung maligner Tumoren. *Jena: Gustav Fischer.*

Burmer, G. C., P. S. Rabinovitch, and L. A. Loeb. 1991. Frequency and spectrum of c-Ki-ras mutations in human sporadic colon carcinoma, carcinomas arising in ulcerative colitis, and pancreatic adenocarcinoma. *Environ Health Perspect* 93:27-31.

Cahill, D. P., C. Lengauer, J. Yu, G. J. Riggins, J. K. Willson, S. D. Markowitz, K. W. Kinzler, and B. Vogelstein. 1998. Mutations of mitotic checkpoint genes in human cancers. *Nature* 392 (6673):300-3.

Caspersson, T. O. 1979. Quantitative tumor cytochemistry--G.H.A. Clowes Memorial Lecture. *Cancer Res* 39 (7 Pt 1):2341-5.

Caspersson, T., L. Zech, C. Johansson, and E. J. Modest. 1970. Identification of human chromosomes by DNA-binding fluorescent agents. *Chromosoma* 30 (2):215-27.

Clausen, O. P., S. N. Andersen, H. Stroomkjaer, V. Nielsen, T. O. Rognum, L. Bolund, and S. Koolvraa. 2001. A strategy combining flow sorting and comparative genomic hybridization for studying genetic aberrations at different stages of colorectal tumorigenesis in ulcerative colitis. *Cytometry* 43 (1):46-54.

D'Amours, D., and S. P. Jackson. 2002. The Mre11 complex: at the crossroads of dna repair and checkpoint signalling. *Nat Rev Mol Cell Biol* 3 (5):317-27.

Desper, R., F. Jiang, O. P. Kallioniemi, H. Moch, C. H. Papadimitriou, and A. A. Schaffer. 2000. Distance-based reconstruction of tree models for oncogenesis. *J Comput Biol* 7 (6):789-803.

Donnellan, R., and R. Chetty. 1999. Cyclin E in human cancers. *Faseb J* 13 (8):773-80.

Duesberg, P., C. Rausch, D. Rasnick, and R. Hehlmann. 1998. Genetic instability of cancer cells is proportional to their degree of aneuploidy. *Proc Natl Acad Sci U S A* 95 (23):13692-7.

Fearon, E. R., and B. Vogelstein. 1990. A genetic model for colorectal tumorigenesis. *Cell* 61 (5):759-67.

Forozan, F., R. Karhu, J. Kononen, A. Kallioniemi, and O. P. Kallioniemi. 1997. Genome screening by comparative genomic hybridization. *Trends Genet* 13 (10):405-9.

Fozard, J. B., P. Quirke, M. F. Dixon, G. R. Giles, and C. C. Bird. 1986. DNA aneuploidy in ulcerative colitis. *Gut* 27 (12):1414-8.

Gemoll, T., U. J. Roblick, S. Szymczak, T. Braunschweig, S. Becker, B. W. Igl, H. P. Bruch, A. Ziegler, U. Hellman, M. J. Difilippantonio, T. Ried, H. Jornvall, G. Auer, and J. K. Habermann. 2011. HDAC2 and TXNL1 distinguish aneuploid from diploid colorectal cancers. *Cellular and molecular life sciences : CMLS* 68 (19):3261-74.

Gerling, M., K. F. Meyer, K. Fuchs, B. W. Igl, B. Fritzsche, A. Ziegler, F. Bader, P. Kujath, H. Schimmelpenning, H. P. Bruch, U. J. Roblick, and J. K. Habermann. 2010. High Frequency of Aneuploidy Defines Ulcerative Colitis-Associated Carcinomas: A Comparative Prognostic Study to Sporadic Colorectal Carcinomas. *Annals of surgery* [Epub ahead of print].

Ghadimi, B. M., D. L. Sackett, M. J. Difilippantonio, E. Schrock, T. Neumann, A. Jauho, G. Auer, and T. Ried. 2000. Centrosome amplification and instability occurs exclusively in aneuploid, but not in diploid colorectal cancer cell lines, and correlates with numerical chromosomal aberrations. *Genes, Chromosomes & Cancer* 27 (2):183-90.

Giaretti, W., T. Venesio, C. Prevosto, F. Lombardo, J. Ceccarelli, S. Molinu, and M. Risio. 2004. Chromosomal instability and APC gene mutations in human sporadic colorectal adenomas. *J Pathol* 204 (2):193-9.

Habermann, J. K., C. A. Brucker, S. Freitag-Wolf, K. Heselmeyer-Haddad, S. Kruger, L. Barenboim, T. Downing, H. P. Bruch, G. Auer, U. J. Roblick, and T. Ried. 2011. Genomic instability and oncogene amplifications in colorectal adenomas predict recurrence and synchronous carcinoma. *Mod Pathol* 24 (4):542-55.

Habermann, J. K., J. Doering, S. Hautaniemi, U. J. Roblick, N. K. Bundgen, D. Nicorici, U. Kronenwett, S. Rathnagiriswaran, R. K. Mettu, Y. Ma, S. Kruger, H. P. Bruch, G. Auer, N. L. Guo, and T. Ried. 2009. The gene expression signature of genomic instability in breast cancer is an independent predictor of clinical outcome. *International journal of cancer. Journal international du cancer* 124 (7):1552-64.

Habermann, J. K., U. Paulsen, U. J. Roblick, M. B. Upender, L. M. McShane, E. L. Korn, D. Wangsa, S. Kruger, M. Duchrow, H. P. Bruch, G. Auer, and T. Ried. 2007. Stage-specific alterations of the genome, transcriptome, and proteome during colorectal carcinogenesis. *Genes, Chromosomes & Cancer* 46 (1):10-26.

Habermann, J. K., M. B. Upender, U. J. Roblick, S. Kruger, S. Freitag, H. Blegen, H. P. Bruch, H. Schimmelpenning, G. Auer, and T. Ried. 2003. Pronounced chromosomal instability and multiple gene amplifications characterize ulcerative colitis-associated colorectal carcinomas. *Cancer Genet Cytogenet* 147 (1):9-17.

Habermann, J., C. Lenander, U. J. Roblick, S. Kruger, D. Ludwig, A. Alaiya, S. Freitag, L. Dumbgen, H. P. Bruch, E. Stange, S. Salo, K. Tryggvason, G. Auer, and H. Schimmelpenning. 2001. Ulcerative colitis and colorectal carcinoma: DNA-profile, laminin-5 gamma2 chain and cyclin A expression as early markers for risk assessment. *Scand J Gastroenterol* 36 (7):751-8.

Handa, K., M. Yamakawa, H. Takeda, S. Kimura, and T. Takahashi. 1999. Expression of cell cycle markers in colorectal carcinoma: superiority of cyclin A as an indicator of poor prognosis. *Int J Cancer* 84 (3):225-33.

Harms, K. L., and X. Chen. 2007. Histone deacetylase 2 modulates p53 transcriptional activities through regulation of p53-DNA binding activity. *Cancer Res* 67 (7):3145-52.

Heselmeyer-Haddad, K., N. Chaudhri, P. Stoltzfus, J. C. Cheng, K. Wilber, L. Morrison, G. Auer, and T. Ried. 2002. Detection of chromosomal aneuploidies and gene copy number changes in fine needle aspirates is a specific, sensitive, and objective genetic test for the diagnosis of breast cancer. *Cancer Res* 62 (8):2365-9.

Heselmeyer, K., E. Schrock, S. du Manoir, H. Blegen, K. Shah, R. Steinbeck, G. Auer, and T. Ried. 1996. Gain of chromosome 3q defines the transition from severe dysplasia to invasive carcinoma of the uterine cervix. *Proc Natl Acad Sci U S A* 93 (1):479-84.

Hittelman, W. N. 2001. Genetic instability in epithelial tissues at risk for cancer. *Ann N Y Acad Sci* 952:1-12.

Holzmann, K., B. Klump, F. Borchard, C. J. Hsieh, A. Kuhn, V. Gaco, M. Gregor, and R. Porschen. 1998. Comparative analysis of histology, DNA content, p53 and Ki-ras mutations in colectomy specimens with long-standing ulcerative colitis. *Int J Cancer* 76 (1):1-6.

Holzmann, K., M. Weis-Klemm, B. Klump, C. J. Hsieh, F. Borchard, M. Gregor, and R. Porschen. 2001. Comparison of flow cytometry and histology with mutational screening for p53 and Ki-ras mutations in surveillance of patients with long-standing ulcerative colitis. *Scand J Gastroenterol* 36 (12):1320-6.

Hopman, A. H., F. C. Ramaekers, A. K. Raap, J. L. Beck, P. Devilee, M. van der Ploeg, and G. P. Vooijs. 1988. In situ hybridization as a tool to study numerical chromosome aberrations in solid bladder tumors. *Histochemistry* 89 (4):307-16.

Howard, A., and S. R. Pelc. 1951. Nuclear incorporation of p32 as demonstrated by autoradiographs. *Exp Cell Res* 2:178.

Jallepalli, P. V., and C. Lengauer. 2001. Chromosome segregation and cancer: cutting through the mystery. *Nat Rev Cancer* 1 (2):109-17.

Kallioniemi, A., O. P. Kallioniemi, D. Sudar, D. Rutovitz, J. W. Gray, F. Waldman, and D. Pinkel. 1992. Comparative genomic hybridization for molecular cytogenetic analysis of solid tumors. *Science* 258 (5083):818-21.

Kern, S. E., M. Redston, A. B. Seymour, C. Caldas, S. M. Powell, S. Kornacki, and K. W. Kinzler. 1994. Molecular genetic profiles of colitis-associated neoplasms. *Gastroenterology* 107 (2):420-8.

Kim, K. Y., J. W. Lee, M. S. Park, M. H. Jung, G. A. Jeon, and M. J. Nam. 2006. Expression of a thioredoxin-related protein-1 is induced by prostaglandin E(2). *Int J Cancer* 118 (7):1670-9.

Knudson, A. G., Jr. 1979. Hereditary cancer. *Jama* 241 (3):279.

Knuutila, S., A. M. Bjorkqvist, K. Autio, M. Tarkkanen, M. Wolf, O. Monni, J. Szymanska, M. L. Larramendy, J. Tapper, H. Pere, W. El-Rifai, S. Hemmer, V. M. Wasenius, V. Vidgren, and Y. Zhu. 1998. DNA copy number amplifications in human neoplasms: review of comparative genomic hybridization studies. *Am J Pathol* 152 (5):1107-23.

Kops, G. J., B. A. Weaver, and D. W. Cleveland. 2005. On the road to cancer: aneuploidy and the mitotic checkpoint. *Nature reviews. Cancer* 5 (10):773-85.

Kronenwett, U., S. Huwendiek, C. Ostring, N. Portwood, U. J. Roblick, Y. Pawitan, A. Alaiya, R. Sennerstam, A. Zetterberg, and G. Auer. 2004. Improved grading of breast adenocarcinomas based on genomic instability. *Cancer Res* 64 (3):904-9.

Kronenwett, U., A. Ploner, A. Zetterberg, J. Bergh, P. Hall, G. Auer, and Y. Pawitan. 2006. Genomic instability and prognosis in breast carcinomas. *Cancer epidemiology, biomarkers & prevention : a publication of the American Association for Cancer Research, cosponsored by the American Society of Preventive Oncology* 15 (9):1630-5.

Lengauer, C., K. W. Kinzler, and B. Vogelstein. 1998. Genetic instabilities in human cancers. *Nature* 396 (6712):643-9.

Liao, C., S. Q. Li, X. Wang, S. Muhlrad, A. Bjartell, and D. J. Wolgemuth. 2004. Elevated levels and distinct patterns of expression of A-type cyclins and their associated cyclin-dependent kinases in male germ cell tumors. *Int J Cancer* 108 (5):654-64.

Loeb, K. R., and L. A. Loeb. 1999. Genetic instability and the mutator phenotype. Studies in ulcerative colitis. *Am J Pathol* 154 (6):1621-6.

Loeb, K. R., and L. A. Loeb 2000. Significance of multiple mutations in cancer. *Carcinogenesis* 21 (3):379-85.

Lofberg, R., O. Brostrom, P. Karlen, A. Ost, and B. Tribukait. 1992. DNA aneuploidy in ulcerative colitis: reproducibility, topographic distribution, and relation to dysplasia. *Gastroenterology* 102 (4 Pt 1):1149-54.

Makiyama, K., M. Tokunaga, M. Itsuno, W. Zea-Iriarte, K. Hara, and T. Nakagoe. 1995. DNA aneuploidy in a case of rectosigmoid adenocarcinoma complicated by ulcerative colitis. *J Gastroenterol* 30 (2):258-63.

Munster, P. N., D. Marchion, S. Thomas, M. Egorin, S. Minton, G. Springett, J. H. Lee, G. Simon, A. Chiappori, D. Sullivan, and A. Daud. 2009. Phase I trial of vorinostat and doxorubicin in solid tumours: histone deacetylase 2 expression as a predictive marker. *Br J Cancer* 101 (7):1044-50.

Nigg, E. A. 1996. Cyclin-dependent kinase 7: at the cross-roads of transcription, DNA repair and cell cycle control? *Current opinion in cell biology* 8 (3):312-7.

Nowak, M. A., N. L. Komarova, A. Sengupta, P. V. Jallepalli, M. Shih Ie, B. Vogelstein, and C. Lengauer. 2002. The role of chromosomal instability in tumor initiation. *Proc Natl Acad Sci U S A* 99 (25):16226-31.

Ono, J., G. Auer, T. Caspersson, M. Nasiell, T. Saito, C. Konaka, H. Kato, and Y. Hayata. 1984. Reversibility of 20-methylcholanthrene-induced bronchial cell atypia in dogs. *Cancer* 54 (6):1030-7.

Padilla-Nash, H. M., K. Hathcock, N. E. McNeil, D. Mack, D. Hoeppner, R. Ravin, T. Knutsen, R. Yonescu, D. Wangsa, K. Dorritie, L. Barenboim, Y. Hu, and T. Ried. 2011. Spontaneous transformation of murine epithelial cells requires the early acquisition of specific chromosomal aneuploidies and genomic imbalances. *Genes, chromosomes & cancer* [Epub ahead of print].

Paik, S., S. Shak, G. Tang, C. Kim, J. Baker, M. Cronin, F. L. Baehner, M. G. Walker, D. Watson, T. Park, W. Hiller, E. R. Fisher, D. L. Wickerham, J. Bryant, and N. Wolmark. 2004. A multigene assay to predict recurrence of tamoxifen-treated, node-negative breast cancer. *The New England journal of medicine* 351 (27):2817-26.

Perou, C. M., T. Sorlie, M. B. Eisen, M. van de Rijn, S. S. Jeffrey, C. A. Rees, J. R. Pollack, D. T. Ross, H. Johnsen, L. A. Akslen, O. Fluge, A. Pergamenschikov, C. Williams, S. X. Zhu, P. E. Lonning, A. L. Borresen-Dale, P. O. Brown, and D. Botstein. 2000. Molecular portraits of human breast tumours. *Nature* 406 (6797):747-52.

Ried, T. 2009. Homage to Theodor Boveri (1862-1915): Boveri's theory of cancer as a disease of the chromosomes, and the landscape of genomic imbalances in human carcinomas. *Environmental and molecular mutagenesis* 50 (8):593-601.

Ried, T., K. Heselmeyer-Haddad, H. Blegen, E. Schrock, and G. Auer. 1999. Genomic changes defining the genesis, progression, and malignancy potential in solid human tumors: a phenotype/genotype correlation. *Genes, Chromosomes & Cancer* 25 (3):195-204.

Ried, T., K. E. Just, H. Holtgreve-Grez, S. du Manoir, M. R. Speicher, E. Schrock, C. Latham, H. Blegen, A. Zetterberg, T. Cremer, and et al. 1995. Comparative genomic hybridization of formalin-fixed, paraffin-embedded breast tumors reveals different patterns of chromosomal gains and losses in fibroadenomas and diploid and aneuploid carcinomas. *Cancer Res* 55 (22):5415-23.

Ried, T., R. Knutzen, R. Steinbeck, H. Blegen, E. Schrock, K. Heselmeyer, S. du Manoir, and G. Auer. 1996. Comparative genomic hybridization reveals a specific pattern of chromosomal gains and losses during the genesis of colorectal tumors. *Genes, Chromosomes & Cancer* 15 (4):234-45.

Rowley, J. D. 1973. Letter: A new consistent chromosomal abnormality in chronic myelogenous leukaemia identified by quinacrine fluorescence and Giemsa staining. *Nature* 243 (5405):290-3.

Rubin, C. E., R. C. Haggitt, G. C. Burmer, T. A. Brentnall, A. C. Stevens, D. S. Levine, P. J. Dean, M. Kimmey, D. R. Perera, and P. S. Rabinovitch. 1992. DNA aneuploidy in colonic biopsies predicts future development of dysplasia in ulcerative colitis. *Gastroenterology* 103 (5):1611-20.

Scharf, J. G., and T. Braulke. 2003. The role of the IGF axis in hepatocarcinogenesis. *Hormone and metabolic research = Hormon- und Stoffwechselforschung = Hormones et metabolisme* 35 (11-12):685-93.

Schlegel, J., G. Stumm, H. Scherthan, T. Bocker, H. Zirngibl, J. Ruschoff, and F. Hofstadter. 1995. Comparative genomic in situ hybridization of colon carcinomas with replication error. *Cancer Res* 55 (24):6002-5.

Schrock, E., S. du Manoir, T. Veldman, B. Schoell, J. Wienberg, M. A. Ferguson-Smith, Y. Ning, D. H. Ledbetter, I. Bar-Am, D. Soenksen, Y. Garini, and T. Ried. 1996. Multicolor spectral karyotyping of human chromosomes. *Science* 273 (5274):494-7.

Schulze, S., and I. Petersen. 2011. Gender and ploidy in cancer survival. *Cellular oncology* 34 (3):199-208.

Shay, J. W., and W. E. Wright. 2002. Telomerase: a target for cancer therapeutics. *Cancer Cell* 2 (4):257-65.

Sherr, C. J. 1993. Mammalian G1 cyclins. *Cell* 73 (6):1059-65.

Sinicrope, F. A., R. L. Rego, N. Foster, D. J. Sargent, H. E. Windschitl, L. J. Burgart, T. E. Witzig, and S. N. Thibodeau. 2006. Microsatellite instability accounts for tumor site-related differences in clinicopathologic variables and prognosis in human colon cancers. *The American journal of gastroenterology* 101 (12):2818-25.

Sinicrope, F. A., R. L. Rego, K. C. Halling, N. Foster, D. J. Sargent, B. La Plant, A. J. French, J. A. Laurie, R. M. Goldberg, S. N. Thibodeau, and T. E. Witzig. 2006. Prognostic impact of microsatellite instability and DNA ploidy in human colon carcinoma patients. *Gastroenterology* 131 (3):729-37.

Solinas-Toldo, S., C. Wallrapp, F. Muller-Pillasch, M. Bentz, T. Gress, and P. Lichter. 1996. Mapping of chromosomal imbalances in pancreatic carcinoma by comparative genomic hybridization. *Cancer Res* 56 (16):3803-7.

Song, J., J. H. Noh, J. H. Lee, J. W. Eun, Y. M. Ahn, S. Y. Kim, S. H. Lee, W. S. Park, N. J. Yoo, J. Y. Lee, and S. W. Nam. 2005. Increased expression of histone deacetylase 2 is found in human gastric cancer. *APMIS* 113 (4):264-8.

Sorlie, T., C. M. Perou, R. Tibshirani, T. Aas, S. Geisler, H. Johnsen, T. Hastie, M. B. Eisen, M. van de Rijn, S. S. Jeffrey, T. Thorsen, H. Quist, J. C. Matese, P. O. Brown, D. Botstein, P. Eystein Lonning, and A. L. Borresen-Dale. 2001. Gene expression patterns of breast carcinomas distinguish tumor subclasses with clinical implications. *Proc Natl Acad Sci U S A* 98 (19):10869-74.

Sorlie, T., R. Tibshirani, J. Parker, T. Hastie, J. S. Marron, A. Nobel, S. Deng, H. Johnsen, R. Pesich, S. Geisler, J. Demeter, C. M. Perou, P. E. Lonning, P. O. Brown, A. L. Borresen-Dale, and D. Botstein. 2003. Repeated observation of breast tumor subtypes in independent gene expression data sets. *Proc Natl Acad Sci U S A* 100 (14):8418-23.

Sotiriou, C., S. Y. Neo, L. M. McShane, E. L. Korn, P. M. Long, A. Jazaeri, P. Martiat, S. B. Fox, A. L. Harris, and E. T. Liu. 2003. Breast cancer classification and prognosis based on gene expression profiles from a population-based study. *Proc Natl Acad Sci U S A* 100 (18):10393-8.

Speicher, M. R., S. Gwyn Ballard, and D. C. Ward. 1996. Karyotyping human chromosomes by combinatorial multi-fluor FISH. *Nat Genet* 12 (4):368-75.

Spruck, C. H., K. A. Won, and S. I. Reed. 1999. Deregulated cyclin E induces chromosome instability. *Nature* 401 (6750):297-300.

Strachan, T., and A. P. Read. 1999. In *Human Molecular Genetics*. New York.

Tjio, J. H., and A. Levan. 1956. The chromosome number of man. *Hereditas* 42:1-6.

Upender, M. B., J. K. Habermann, L. M. McShane, E. L. Korn, J. C. Barrett, M. J. Difilippantonio, and T. Ried. 2004. Chromosome transfer induced aneuploidy results in complex dysregulation of the cellular transcriptome in immortalized and cancer cells. *Cancer Res* 64 (19):6941-9.

van 't Veer, L. J., H. Dai, M. J. van de Vijver, Y. D. He, A. A. Hart, M. Mao, H. L. Peterse, K. van der Kooy, M. J. Marton, A. T. Witteveen, G. J. Schreiber, R. M. Kerkhoven, C. Roberts, P. S. Linsley, R. Bernards, and S. H. Friend. 2002. Gene expression profiling predicts clinical outcome of breast cancer. *Nature* 415 (6871):530-6.

van de Vijver, M. J., Y. D. He, L. J. van't Veer, H. Dai, A. A. Hart, D. W. Voskuil, G. J. Schreiber, J. L. Peterse, C. Roberts, M. J. Marton, M. Parrish, D. Atsma, A. Witteveen, A. Glas, L. Delahaye, T. van der Velde, H. Bartelink, S. Rodenhuis, E. T. Rutgers, S. H. Friend, and R. Bernards. 2002. A gene-expression signature as a predictor of survival in breast cancer. *The New England journal of medicine* 347 (25):1999-2009.

Vessey, C. J., C. J. Norbury, and I. D. Hickson. 1999. Genetic disorders associated with cancer predisposition and genomic instability. *Prog Nucleic Acid Res Mol Biol* 63:189-221.

Vogelstein, B., and K. W. Kinzler. 2004. Cancer genes and the pathways they control. *Nat Med* 10 (8):789-99.

Vousden, K. H. 2002. Activation of the p53 tumor suppressor protein. *Biochim Biophys Acta* 1602 (1):47-59.

Walther, A., R. Houlston, and I. Tomlinson. 2008. Association between chromosomal instability and prognosis in colorectal cancer: a meta-analysis. *Gut* 57 (7):941-50.

Willenbucher, R. F., S. J. Zelman, L. D. Ferrell, D. H. Moore, 2nd, and F. M. Waldman. 1997. Chromosomal alterations in ulcerative colitis-related neoplastic progression. *Gastroenterology* 113 (3):791-801.

Yildirim-Assaf, S., A. Coumbos, W. Hopfenmuller, H. D. Foss, H. Stein, and W. Kuhn. 2007. The prognostic significance of determining DNA content in breast cancer by DNA image cytometry: the role of high grade aneuploidy in node negative breast cancer. *Journal of clinical pathology* 60 (6):649-55.

Zetterberg, A., O. Larsson, and K. G. Wiman. 1995. What is the restriction point? *Current opinion in cell biology* 7 (6):835-42.

Zhu, P., E. Martin, J. Mengwasser, P. Schlag, K. P. Janssen, and M. Gottlicher. 2004. Induction of HDAC2 expression upon loss of APC in colorectal tumorigenesis. *Cancer Cell* 5 (5):455-63.

Zindy, F., E. Lamas, X. Chenivesse, J. Sobczak, J. Wang, D. Fesquet, B. Henglein, and C. Brechot. 1992. Cyclin A is required in S phase in normal epithelial cells. *Biochem Biophys Res Commun* 182 (3):1144-54.

6

Aneuploidy and Intellectual Disability

Daisuke Fukushi[1], Seiji Mizuno[2], Kenichiro Yamada[1], Reiko Kimura[1], Yasukazu Yamada[1], Toshiyuki Kumagai[3] and Nobuaki Wakamatsu[1]
[1]*Department of Genetics, Institute for Developmental Research*
[2]*Department of Pediatrics and*
[3]*Department of Pediatric Neurology, Central Hospital, Aichi Human Service Center*
Japan

1. Introduction

Aneuploidy is the presence of an abnormal number of chromosomes in cells. The gain or loss of a chromosome in germ cells is the most common cause of chromosomal aneuploidy. Trisomy 21, trisomy 18, and trisomy 13 are characterized by congenital anomalies with intellectual disability (ID) or short lives. Recently, mosaic variegated aneuploidy (the presence of a different number of chromosomes in some cells) has been reported to be associated with ID and growth retardation, with or without microcephaly and tumors. In the cell cycle, the alignment of sister chromatids at metaphase plates is essential for the equational separation of chromatids. Misaligned chromosomes at metaphase plates, and/or aberration of the mitotic checkpoint, cause a disproportionate separation of chromatids, resulting in aneuploidy. To evaluate the association between aneuploidy and ID, we analyzed the chromosome numbers of over 200 metaphase plates of lymphoblastoid cells in patients with moderate or severe ID, with or without microcephaly. In this chapter, we summarize the previously reported cases and our own cases of patients with ID associated with aneuploidy or severely misaligned chromosomes at metaphase, and discuss the molecular mechanism underlying ID in cases in which aneuploidy is observed.

2. Aneuploidy

The most common forms of chromosomal (complete) aneuploidy are trisomy and monosomy. Trisomy refers to having an extra whole chromosome, and monosomy is the lack of 1 chromosome from a pair of chromosomes. Partial monosomy and partial trisomy, i.e., loss or gain of part of a chromosome, respectively, have preferentially been used instead of partial aneuploidy. Mosaic aneuploidy is the condition in which aneuploidy is detected in a fraction of cells in an individual.

2.1 Trisomy

Trisomy 21, also known as Down syndrome, is the most common chromosomal aneuploidy and a cause of ID. Down syndrome affects up to 1 in 1,000 live births (International Clearinghouse for Birth Defects Monitoring Systems, 1991). Down syndrome is caused by a failure in the proper segregation of chromosome 21 during meiosis. This chromosome 21 nondisjunction is mostly due to maternal meiotic errors; the majority of these errors occur during meiosis I (~80%) (Antonarakis, 1991; Yoon et al., 1996). A recent study has suggested that pericentromeric exchange at meiosis II initiates or exacerbates the susceptibility to the risk of increased maternal age (Oliver et al., 2008). The Down syndrome critical region (DSCR) of human chromosome 21q22 was defined on the basis of analysis of familial cases of partial trisomy 21 (Korenberg et al., 1994; Ronan et al., 2007). One strategy for identifying the genes responsible for ID in Down syndrome is to analyze the genes located in the DSCR. Analyses of 2 unrelated patients with a *de novo* balanced translocation and a patient with a microdeletion within the DSCR demonstrated that *DYRK1A,* encoding the dual-specificity tyrosine phosphorylation-regulated kinase 1A, plays a critical role in brain development (Møller et al., 2008; Yamamoto et al., 2011). Therefore, the dosage of *DYRK1A* is quite important for brain development, and it could be one of the causative genes for ID in Down syndrome. Several studies demonstrated that a normal dosage of *DYRK1A* is critical for normal brain development and function. Transgenic mice overexpressing *Dyrk1A* show marked cognitive deficits and impairment in hippocampal-dependent memory tasks and the generation of both amyloid and tau pathologies, which are observed in early onset Alzheimer disease and Down syndrome (Altafaj et al., 2001; Ahn et al., 2006; Kimura et al., 2007; Park et al., 2007; Ryoo et al., 2008). A recent study showed that Dyrk1A directly interacts with and phosphorylates the regulator of calcineurin 1 (RCAN1) protein at Ser112 and Thr192. *RCAN1* is also located in the DSCR. The phosphorylation of RCAN1 enhances RCAN1 binding to calcineurin, resulting in reduced NFAT transcriptional activity. This activity is important for the outgrowth of embryonic axons (Graef et al., 2003; Jung et al., 2011). Thus, the increased expression of *Dyrk1A* caused by trisomy may cause impaired axon outgrowth during brain development, which may in turn cause ID in Down syndrome.

Other types of common aneuploidy include trisomy 18 (Edwards syndrome), which affects 1 in 6,000 births, and trisomy 13 (Patau syndrome), which affects 1 in 10,000 births. A recent study of the natural outcome of trisomy 13 and trisomy 18 after prenatal diagnosis indicates that the live birth rate is 13% for trisomy 18 and 33% for trisomy 13. Three of 4 live-born infants with trisomy 13 and all 3 trisomy 18 infants died early, within a maximum of 87 postpartum hours. Thus, trisomy 13 and trisomy 18 are associated with a high rate of spontaneous abortion, intrauterine death, and a short life-span (Lakovschek et al., 2011). ID is not clear in these patients because of their short lives.

2.2 Partial aneuploidy (partial monosomy and partial trisomy)

Quite a few reports exist on patients with ID harboring chromosomal microdeletions. This indicates that haploinsufficiency of a gene or genes located in the deletion region are associated with ID. Mutational analysis of the genes located in the deletion region leads the identification of the causal gene(s) of ID, with or without congenital anomalies. Duplications of some chromosomal segments are reported to be associated with ID (1q21.1, Brunetti-Pierri et al., 2008; 3q29, Goobie et al., 2008; Lisi et al., 2008; 16p13.11, Hannes et al., 2009; Xq28, Van Esch et al., 2005). This indicates that increased gene dosage(s) are associated with ID. It is noted that the clinical features of deletions or duplications at the same chromosomal segments are different. There is a tendency for duplications to show milder clinical features than deletions, and autistic features more frequently appear in duplications (Table 1) (Marshall et al., 2008; Sebat et al., 2007).

Chromosomal	Deletion		Duplication		References
location	ID	Syndrome	ID	Clinical features	
5q35	+, ++	Sotos	+	Microcephaly	(1)
7q11.2	+	Williams-Beuren	+	Speech delay	(2)
15q11.2	+/+++	Prader-Will/Angelman	++	Autism	(3)
16p13.3	+++	Rubinstein-Taybi	++	Speech delay	(4)
17p11.2	++	Smith-Magenis	++	ADHD, Autism	(3) (5)
22q11.2	±, +	DiGeorge	−, ±	ADHD, Autism	(6)

Table 1. Clinical features of duplication or deletion at the same chromosomal region. ID, intellectual disability; -, absent; ±, very mild; +, mild; ++, moderate; +++, severe; ADHD, Attention Deficit Hyperactivity Disorder. References: (1) Hunter et al., 2005; (2) Somerville et al., 2005; (3) Keller et al., 2003; (4) Marangi et al., 2008; (5) Potocki et al., 2000; (6) Mukaddes & Herguner, 2007.

2.3 Monosomy

Monosomy is most commonly lethal during prenatal development. X-chromosome monosomy (Turner syndrome) is a commonly observed monosomy that develops without obvious, or with very mild, ID.

2.4 Mosaic aneuploidy

The most common use of the term "mosaic aneuploidy" refers to the condition in which aneuploidy is detected in a fraction of cells, usually in lymphocytes (lymphoblastoid cells), in an individual. Mosaic aneuploidy is observed in 2%-4% of Down syndrome cases, in which 2 types of karyotypes (trisomy 21 and normal) are present (Mikkelsen et al., 1976). In general, individuals who are mosaic for chromosomal aneuploidy tend to have less severe clinical features than those with full trisomy. Therefore, only mosaic patients may survive in many of the chromosomal trisomies.

2.5 Mosaic variegated aneuploidy

Hsu et al. (1970) reported 3 children with sex chromosome mosaicism born to consanguineous parents. The authors suggested that a recessive gene causing mitotic instability is associated with the mosaicism. Tolmie et al. (1988) and Papi et al. (1989) reported male and female siblings with ID, growth retardation, microcephaly, and multiple chromosome mosaicism involving mainly chromosome 18 or chromosomes 7 and 8, respectively. These findings indicate that mutations of autosomal recessive genes are associated with aberrant mitosis causing the observed phenotype. The term "mosaic variegated aneuploidy" (MVA) has been suggested to apply to patients with ID, microcephaly, and the above-mentioned cytogenetic findings (Warburton et al., 1991).

Callier et al. (2005) summarized 28 previously reported cases of MVA and showed that 26 of 28 patients (93%) had microcephaly and 21 of 28 patients (75%) had ID, and in 2 of the 28 cases, clinical features were not described. MVA with premature chromatid separation (PCS) (also called PCS syndrome; Kajii et al., 2001) has been reported (Plaja et al., 2001). Patients with this condition exhibit ID, intrauterine growth retardation, microcephaly, and a characteristic facial appearance; the syndrome is often accompanied by malignancies (Wilms tumor, rhabdomyosarcoma, and acute leukemia). These patients have a variety of aneuploid cells (~40%), but PCS is more apparent (>50%) in these cells. It is noted that healthy parents of patients with MVA with PCS also have PCS (~10%-40%) in their lymphocytes (Kajii et al., 2001). Plaja et al. (2001) summarized 11 previously reported cases of MVA with PCS and showed that all 11 patients (100%) had microcephaly and 8 of 11 patients (73%) had ID, and in 2 of the 11 cases, the ID status was unknown. However, not all patients with MVA have microcephaly (Callier et al., 2005).

A causative gene of MVA, the *BUB1B* gene encoding BUBR1, has been identified in 5 families with MVA, including 2 with embryonal rhabdomyosarcoma (Hanks et al., 2004). These patients have truncating or missense mutations in both alleles of *BUB1B*. BUBR1 is a key protein in the mitotic checkpoint, and its deficiency causes aneuploidy and cancer development. *BUB1B* mutations were also identified in the patients from 7 Japanese families exhibiting MVA with PCS (Matsuura et al., 2006). Eight patients in the 7 families presented with intrauterine growth retardation, microcephaly, and a Dandy-Walker complex. Wilms tumor was also observed, except in 1 patient. Each patient had a loss-of-function mutation of *BUB1B* in one allele; the other allele exhibited a haplotype associated with decreased expression levels of BUBR1 protein. Therefore, a decrease of <50% in BUBR1 function at the mitotic checkpoint is associated with MVA with PCS. Recently, biallelic loss-of-function mutations in *CEP57* were identified in 4 patients with MVA (Snape et al., 2011). All the patients showed random gains and losses of chromosomes in ~25%-50% of the examined cells. It is noteworthy that 2 patients did not have ID and microcephaly, and none had malignancies. The Online Mendelian Inheritance in Man (OMIM) database defines mosaic variegated aneuploidy syndrome 1 (MVA1) (MIM: 257300) as a syndrome caused by homozygous or compound heterozygous mutations in *BUB1B* on chromosome 15q15, and MVA2 (MIM: 614114) as a syndrome caused by homozygous or compound heterozygous mutations in *CEP57* on chromosome 11q21. The proportion of aneuploid cells in MVA is usually >25% (Hanks et al., 2004).

Mitotic checkpoint: The mitotic checkpoint works to ensure accurate chromosome segregation to avoid aneuploidy by regulating the progression from metaphase to anaphase. The checkpoint arrests cells in mitosis, until all chromosomes have aligned at the metaphase plate. Chromosome alignment depends on the attachment of microtubules emanating from the spindle poles to the kinetochores on chromosomes. Once the checkpoint has been satisfied (switched off), the cell proceeds into anaphase and completes the cell cycle (Chan et al., 2005; Musacchio & Salmon, 2007).

3. Microcephaly

Microcephaly is the most common clinical feature (developing in ~1% of the population, Lizarraga et al., 2010) and is usually associated with ID. Microcephaly is defined in persons who have a head circumference (HC) (or occipitofrontal circumference [OFC]) more than 2 standard deviations (-2SD) below the average circumference for the individual's age, sex, race, and period of gestation.

The size of the mammalian neocortex is determined largely by the number of neurons generated at the ventricular zone (VZ) during embryonic neurogenesis. Thus, defects in embryonic neurogenesis decrease the number of neurons in the neocortex, leading to microcephaly and ID. The VZ comprises progenitor cells (mainly radial glial cells); these progenitor cells divide symmetrically to amplify their own cell population before the peak phase of neurogenesis (embryonic days 13–18 in mice). During the peak phase of neurogenesis, progenitor cells divide into a progenitor cell and a neuron, or an intermediate progenitor cell (IPC), by asymmetric division. IPCs continue additional division to generate neurons that migrate into the cortical plate and finally form the cerebral cortex. The term "asymmetric" is used to refer to the generation of either different types of progenitor cells or division (Chenn & McConnell, 1995). A recent study has indicated that asymmetric inheritance of daughter and mother centrosomes regulates the differential behaviors of renewing progenitors and their differentiating progeny (Wang et al., 2009). Therefore, this finding suggests that the centrosomes play essential roles in progenitor cleavage, differentiation, and migration (Higginbotham & Gleeson, 2007).

Centrosome: The centrosome is the microtubule-organizing center responsible for the nucleation and organization of cytoplasmic organelles, primary cilia, and mitotic spindle microtubules. It is located in the cell cytoplasm and contains 2 orthogonally arranged centrioles; each centriole has a barrel-shaped microtubule structure and is surrounded by pericentriolar material (PCM).

3.1 Autosomal recessive microcephaly

Autosomal recessive primary microcephaly (MCPH) is a neurodevelopmental disorder characterized by microcephaly at birth and nonprogressive ID. Its incidence is ~1 in 10,000 in consanguineous populations. The current clinical definition of MCPH is as follows: (1) congenital microcephaly with an HC at least 4SD below age and sex means; (2) ID, but no other neurological findings; and (3) mostly normal height, weight, facial appearance, chromosomal analysis, and brain structure as evaluated by brain MRI (CT) (Woods et al., 2005).

At least 8 MCPH loci exist, and the genes underlying 7 of these have been identified (MCPH1-*MCPH1*, MIM 251200; MCPH2-*WDR62*, MIM 613583; MCPH3-*CDK5RAP2*, MIM 608201; MCPH4-*CEP152*, MIM 613529; MCPH5-*ASPM*, MIM 605481; MCPH6-*CENPJ*, MIM 609279; and MCPH7-*STIL*, MIM 181590). The proteins encoding the causative genes of MCPH are specifically localized at the centrosome during a specific period of the cell cycle (Kumar et al., 2009). Therefore, the failure of proteins associated with the function and/or the structure (maturation) of the centrosome causes MCPH and aneuploidy. Hertwig's anemia (an) mutant (*Cdk5rap2*$^{an/an}$) mice, a mouse model of MCPH3, show reduced neuronal numbers and thinner superficial layers, but preserved cortical layer organization. These mice have a high level of aneuploidy in tissues, and neuronal progenitor cells exhibit mitotic defects with abnormal mitotic spindle pole number and mitotic spindle orientation. The abnormal number of centrosomes might produce abnormal mitosis and aneuploidy that would result in either cell death or cell cycle arrest in cortical progenitor cells (Lizarraga et al., 2010). Taken together, neuronal progenitor cell death, accompanying abnormal mitotic defects and aneuploidy, could be the cause of ID in some types of MCPH. The decreased brain size in MCPH, without a major effect on the cortical layer structure, suggests that the causative genes of MCPH affect the symmetric division of progenitor cells, rather than asymmetric divisions associated with cortical layer formation and subsequent impaired cell functions or apoptosis.

Deficiencies of those proteins (genes) that are reported to be associated with mitotic defects and/or aneuploidy are listed in Table 2.

Mitotic defect: Mitotic defects include disrupted centrosomes, misaligned chromosomes, and spindle misorientation (spindle poles in different focal planes) at metaphase, which result in aneuploidy, lagging chromosomes, and anaphase bridges in dividing cells.

Gene	Cellular location at metaphase	Deficiency of the gene: Misaligned chromosomes	Aneuploidy	Clinical features	References
BUB1B	Kinetochore	++	++	GR, Microcephaly, ID, Cancer	(1) (2)
CEP57	Centrosome	++	++	GR, Microcephaly, ID	(3)
CDK5RAP2 (Cdk5rap2)	Centrosome	+	+	MCPH3, ID	(4) (5)
CENP J	Centrosome	+	ND	MCPH6, ID	(4) (6)
STIL	Pericentrosome	+	ND	MCPH7, ID	(7)
UBE3A	Centrosome	+	ND	Angelman syndrome, ID	(8)
NDE1	Centrosome	+	ND	Microlissencephaly, ID	(9)
ASAP	Centrosome Mitotic spindle	+	ND	ND	(10) (11)
CHD6	Diffuse localization	+	+	ID	(12)
PCNT	Pericentrosome	ND	+	MOPD II	(13)

Table 2. Deficiencies of genes reported to be associated with misaligned chromosomes and/or aneuploidy. +, moderate; ++, severe; ND, not described; ID, intellectual disability; GR, growth retardation. References: (1) Hanks et al., 2004; (2) Matsuura et al., 2006; (3) Snape et al., 2011; (4) Bond et al., 2005; (5) Lizarraga et al., 2010; (6) Cho et al., 2006; (7) Pfaff et al., 2007; (8) Singhmar & Kumar, 2011; (9) Alkuraya et al., 2011; (10) Saffin et al., 2005; (11) Eot-Houllier et al., 2010; (12) Yamada et al., 2010; (13) Rauch et al., 2008.

4. Characterization of aneuploidy in patients with moderate and severe ID

Patients with microcephaly often present with ID, but its etiology is primarily unknown. As described above, recent studies have demonstrated that mitotic dysfunctions in the cell cycle are tightly associated with MCPHs. Although detailed data of aneuploidy in each MCPH are not available, aneuploidy could be found in some types of microcephaly with ID. We analyzed aneuploidy in 10 patients with moderate and severe ID, including 5 solitary cases with microcephaly (HC more than 3SD smaller than the mean) (Table 3). The number of cells exhibiting aneuploidy was determined by counting chromosome numbers in over 200 metaphases derived from lymphoblastoid cells from 5 normal control subjects and 10 patients with ID. Two patients (Lesch-Nyhan syndrome and Rett syndrome) with ID had the same ratio of aneuploidy as normal controls (5%-7%). In contrast, in 3 patients with microcephaly

(S1, S2, and S5), the ratio of aneuploidy increased 2-3 times (13%-21%) as compared with the ratio of aneuploidy in normal controls. This result indicates that there are 2 types of microcephaly with ID, i.e., that with and that without an increased ratio of aneuploidy in lymphoblastoid cells. The findings of the 3 patients with microcephaly and relatively high rates of aneuploidy suggest that these patients have mutations associated with mitotic defects, and the other 2 patients with microcephaly may have other etiologies underlying their ID that are not directly associated with mitotic defects of the cells and aneuploidy.

An increased rate of aneuploidy was also identified in a patient with chromodomain helicase DNA (CHD)-6 haploinsufficiency (S6) and in 2 patients with CHARGE syndrome (manifestations are coloboma of the eye [C], heart anomalies [H], choanal atresia [A], retardation of mental and somatic development [R], genital anomalies [G], and ear abnormalities and/or deafness [E]) caused by haploinsufficiency of CHD7 (S7 and S8), although they did not have microcephaly (Table 3) (Yamada et al., 2010). Both proteins are ATP-dependent chromatin-remodeling enzymes and play important roles in maintaining and regulating chromatin structure. Lymphoblastoid cells from the patients with CHD6 or CHD7 haploinsufficiency, and CHD6 or CHD7 knockdown HeLa cells, display aneuploidy and an increased frequency of misaligned chromosomes, respectively (Fig. 1, Table 3) (Yamada et al., 2010). CHD6 associates with many proteins to form a large protein complex (>2 MDa) (Lutz et al., 2006). This finding and the diffused distribution of CHD6 at metaphase (Yamada et al., 2010) suggest that the protein complex may act as a basis for the formation and/or stabilization of the mitotic spindle structure.

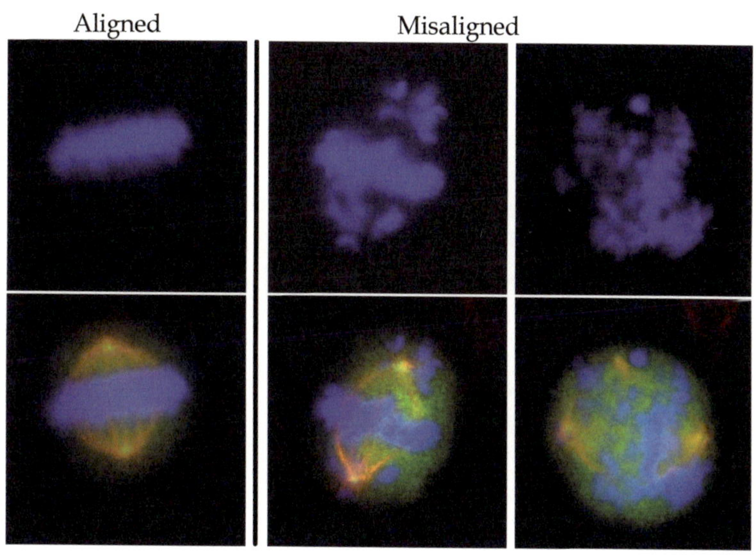

Fig. 1. Misaligned chromosomes observed in RNA interference (RNAi)-mediated knockdown of *CHD6* in metaphase HeLa cells. Aligned chromosomes (left panels, control) and 2 types of misaligned chromosomes – with bipolar centrosomes (middle panels) and with 3 centrosomes (right panels) – caused by knockdown of *CHD6* at metaphase are presented. Cells were fixed and stained with anti-alpha-tubulin (red) and anti-gamma-tubulin (green) antibodies. Chromosomes were stained with 4',6-diamidino-2-phenylindole (DAPI; blue) (upper panels). Lower panels show merged images.

The cytogenetic examination of the chromosomes of patients with ID (Table 3) thus gives us important information as to whether the patients exhibit aneuploidy. Several studies have demonstrated that a high level of aneuploidy (~50%) is a constant feature of human neurons under healthy conditions (Pack et al., 2005; Rehen et al., 2005; Yurov et al., 2005). Moreover, approximately 33% of neural progenitor cells display genetic variability, which is manifested as chromosomal aneuploidy (Kaushal et al., 2003; McConnell et al., 2004; Rehen et al., 2001; Yang et al., 2003). These findings indicate that the brain is a specific region for displaying much aneuploidy caused by genetic variability. We studied the aneuploidy of lymphoblastoid cells and identified increased aneuploidy in some patients with ID. However, it is not clear how increased aneuploidy in lymphoblastoid cells caused by the mutation affect the apoptosis or fate of neuronal progenitor cells. Patients with MVA and MVA with PCS have been shown to have a high incidence of ID (>73%) with increasing aneuploidy (>25%). Such increasing aneuploidy, caused by mutations, adds to the total aneuploidy in the neuronal progenitor cells and may cause the number of aneuploid cells to exceed critical thresholds for ID that is caused by the neuronal death or impaired functions of the progenitor cells. Therefore, it is critical to analyze the aneuploidy of neural progenitor cells in animal models of human diseases known to cause aneuploidy and ID. This study could clarify the relationship of ID and aneuploidy. To perform this kind of study, it is important to accumulate aneuploidy data from patients with ID, with or without microcephaly.

	ID	Microcephaly (HC, at age)	Others	Chromosome numbers				Total metaphase numbers	Aneuploidy (%)	PCS (%)
				<46	46	47	>47			
C1	–	–	Healthy control	21	277	1	1	300	7.7	ND
C2	–	–	Healthy control	14	283	2	1	300	5.7	ND
C3	–	–	Healthy control	20	278	1	1	300	7.3	ND
C4	–	–	Healthy control	14	281	4	1	300	6.3	1.0
C5	–	–	Healthy control	7	188	3	2	200	6.0	1.0
S1	++	-4SD (2y2m)	Epilepsy	21	173	6	0	200	13.5	ND
S2	++	-3.5SD (3y0m)	Epilepsy	20	170	9	1	200	15.0	ND
S3	++	-7SD (2y4m)	Polydactyly, Epilepsy	12	188	0	0	200	6.0	ND
S4	++	-6SD (1y8m)	Cerebellopontine hypoplasia	10	185	5	0	200	7.5	5.5
S5	++	-4.3SD (2y5m)	West syndrome	33	158	7	2	200	21.0	0.5
S6	++	–	CHD6 deficiency	56	329	11	4	400	17.8	–
S7	++	–	CHARGE syndrome, GR	50	333	11	6	400	16.8	–
S8	++	–	CHARGE syndrome, GR	47	338	14	1	400	15.5	1.0
S9	+	–	Lesch-Nyhan syndrome	9	186	4	1	200	7.0	2.0
S10	++	–	Rett syndrome	6	190	3	1	200	5.0	–

Table 3. Chromosome numbers in lymphoblastoid cells from healthy control subjects and patients with moderate and severe ID. ID, intellectual disability; y, year; m, month; ND, not determined; –, absent; +, moderate; ++, severe; HC, head circumference; GR, growth retardation.

5. Conclusion

The amplification of centrosome number and aneuploidy are frequently observed in cancer cells, which may reflect tumorigenesis (Fang & Zhang, 2011). Mitotic defects underlying misaligned chromosomes and/or aneuploidy have also been reported in some patients with ID. Patients with MVA and some types of microcephaly belong to this category. During embryonic neurogenesis, symmetrical and asymmetrical divisions of the progenitor cells are critically important. Impairment of neurogenesis caused by mitotic defects, such as abnormal functioning of centrosomes and/or spindle structures, could result in neuronal loss, with or without abnormal cortical layer formation. Therefore, the study of aneuploidy is important not only for diagnosing mitotic defects but also for analyzing the etiology of patients with ID.

6. Acknowledgments

We are grateful to the patients who participated in this study and their respective families. We would also like to thank Dr. Y. Obara for his useful comments and discussions on this chapter. This study was supported by Takeda Science Foundation and by the Health Labour Sciences Research Grant (to N.W.).

7. References

Ahn, KJ.; Jeong, HK.; Choi, HS.; Ryoo, SR.; Kim, YJ.; Goo, JS.; Choi, SY.; Han, JS.; Ha, I. & Song, WJ. (2006). DYRK1A BAC transgenic mice show altered synaptic plasticity with learning and memory defects. *Neurobiology of Disease*, Vol. 22, No. 3, pp. 463-472, ISSN 0969-9961

Alkuraya, FS.; Cai, X.; Emery, C.; Mochida, GH.; Al-Dosari, MS.; Felie, JM.; Hill, RS.; Barry, BJ.; Partlow, JN.; Gascon, GG.; Kentab, A.; Jan, M.; Shaheen, R.; Feng, Y. & Walsh, CA. (2011). Human mutations in *NDE1* cause extreme microcephaly with lissencephaly [corrected]. *The American Journal of Human Genetics*, Vol. 88, No. 5, pp. 536-547, ISSN 0002-9297

Altafaj, X.; Dierssen, M.; Baamonde, C.; Martí, E.; Visa, J.; Guimerà, J.; Oset, M.; González, JR.; Flórez, J.; Fillat, C. & Estivill, X. (2001). Neurodevelopmental delay, motor abnormalities and cognitive deficits in transgenic mice overexpressing Dyrk1A (minibrain), a murine model of Down's syndrome. *Human Molecular Genetics*, Vol. 10, No. 18, pp. 1915-1923, ISSN 1460-2083

Antonarakis, SE. (1991). Parental origin of the extra chromosome in trisomy 21 as indicated by analysis of DNA polymorphisms. Down Syndrome Collaborative Group. *The New England Journal of Medicine*, Vol., 324, No. 13, pp. 872-876, ISSN 0028-4793

Bond, J.; Roberts, E.; Springell, K.; Lizarraga, SB.; Scott, S.; Higgins, J.; Hampshire, DJ.; Morrison, EE.; Leal, GF.; Silva, EO.; Costa, SM.; Baralle, D.; Raponi, M.; Karbani, G.; Rashid, Y.; Jafri, H.; Bennett, C.; Corry, P.; Walsh, CA. & Woods, CG. (2005). A centrosomal mechanism involving CDK5RAP2 and CENPJ controls brain size. *Nature Genetics*, Vol. 37, No. 4, pp. 353-355, ISSN 1061-4036

Brunetti-Pierri, N.; Berg, JS.; Scaglia, F.; Belmont, J.; Bacino, CA.; Sahoo, T.; Lalani, SR.; Graham, B.; Lee, B.; Shinawi, M.; Shen, J.; Kang, SH.; Pursley, A.; Lotze, T.; Kennedy, G.; Lansky-Shafer, S.; Weaver, C.; Roeder, ER.; Grebe, TA.; Arnold, GL.; Hutchison, T.; Reimschisel, T.; Amato, S.; Geragthy, MT.; Innis, JW.; Obersztyn, E.; Nowakowska, B.; Rosengren, SS.; Bader, PI.; Grange, DK.; Naqvi, S.; Garnica, AD.; Bernes, SM.; Fong, CT.; Summers, A.; Walters, WD.; Lupski, JR.; Stankiewicz, P.; Cheung, SW. & Patel, A. (2008). Recurrent reciprocal 1q21.1 deletions and duplications associated with microcephaly or macrocephaly and developmental and behavioral abnormalities. *Nature Genetics*, Vol. 40, No. 12, pp. 1466-1471, ISSN 1061-4036

Callier, P.; Faivre, L.; Cusin, V.; Marle, N.; Thauvin-Robinet, C.; Sandre, D.; Rousseau, T.; Sagot, P.; Lacombe, E.; Faber, V. & Mugneret, F. (2005). Microcephaly is not mandatory for the diagnosis of mosaic variegated aneuploidy syndrome. *American Journal of Medical Genetics, Part A*, Vol. 137, No. 2, pp. 204-207, ISSN 1552-4833

Chan, GK.; Liu, ST. & Yen, TJ. (2005). Kinetochore structure and function. *Trends in Cell Biology*, Vol. 15, No. 11, PP. 589-598, ISSN 0962-8924

Chenn, A. & McConnell, SK. (1995). Cleavage orientation and the asymmetric inheritance of Notch1 immunoreactivity in mammalian neurogenesis. *Cell*, Vol. 82, No. 4, pp. 631-641, ISSN 0092-8674

Cho, JH.; Chang, CJ.; Chen, CY. & Tang, TK. (2006). Depletion of CPAP by RNAi disrupts centrosome integrity and induces multipolar spindles. *Biochemical and Biophysical Research Communications*, Vol. 339, No. 3, pp. 742-747, ISSN 0006-291X

Eot-Houllier, G.; Venoux, M.; Vidal-Eychenié, S.; Hoang, MT.; Giorgi, D. & Rouquier, S. (2010). Plk1 regulates both ASAP localization and its role in spindle pole integrity. *The Journal of Biochemical Chemistry*, Vol. 285, No. 38, pp. 29556-29568, ISSN 0021-9258

Fang, X. & Zhang, P. (2011). Aneuploidy and tumorigenesis. *Seminars in Cell & Developmental Bioloby*, Vol. 22, No. 6, pp. 595-601, ISSN 1084-9521

Goobie, S.; Knijnenburg, J.; Fitzpatrick, D.; Sharkey, FH.; Lionel, AC.; Marshall, CR.; Azam, T.; Shago, M.; Chong, K.; Mendoza-Londono, R.; den Hollander, NS.; Ruivenkamp, C.; Maher, E.; Tanke, HJ.; Szuhai, K.; Wintle, RF. & Scherer, SW. (2008). Molecular and clinical characterization of de novo and familial cases with microduplication 3q29: guidelines for copy number variation case reporting. *Cytogenetics and Genome Research*, Vol. 123, No. 1-4, pp. 65-78, ISSN 1424-859X

Graef, IA.; Wang, F.; Charron, F.; Chen, L.; Neilson, J.; Tessier-Lavigne, M. & Crabtree, GR. (2003). Neurotrophins and netrins require calcineurin/NFAT signaling to stimulate outgrowth of embryonic axons. *Cell*, Vol. 113, No. 5, pp. 657-670, ISSN 0092-8674

Hanks, S.; Coleman, K.; Reid, S.; Plaja, A.; Firth, H.; Fitzpatrick, D.; Kidd, A.; Méhes, K.; Nash, R.; Robin, N.; Shannon, N.; Tolmie, J.; Swansbury, J.; Irrthum, A.; Douglas, J. & Rahman, N. (2004). Constitutional aneuploidy and cancer predisposition caused by biallelic mutations in *BUB1B*. *Nature Genetics*, Vol. 36, No. 11, pp. 1159-1161, ISSN 1061-4036

Hannes, FD.; Sharp, AJ.; Mefford, HC.; de Ravel, T.; Ruivenkamp, CA.; Breuning, MH.; Fryns, JP.; Devriendt, K.; Van Buggenhout, G.; Vogels, A.; Stewart, H.; Hennekam, RC.; Cooper, GM.; Regan, R.; Knight, SJ.; Eichler, EE. & Vermeesch, JR. (2009). Recurrent reciprocal deletions and duplications of 16p13.11: the deletion is a risk factor for MR/MCA while the duplication may be a rare benign variant. *Journal of Medical Genetics*, Vol. 46, No. 4, pp. 223-232, ISSN 1468-6244

Higginbotham, HR. & Gleeson, JG. (2007). The centrosome in neuronal development. *Trends in Neurosciences*, Vol. 30, No. 6, pp. 276-283, ISSN 0166-2236

Hsu, LYF.; Hirschhorn, K.; Goldstein, A. & Barcinski, MA. (1970). Familial chromosomal mosaicism, genetic aspects. *Annals of Human Genetics*, Vol. 33, No. 4, pp. 343-349, ISSN 0003-4800

Hunter, AG.; Dupont, B.; McLaughlin, M.; Hinton, L.; Baker, E.; Adès, L.; Haan, E. & Schwartz, CE. (2005). The Hunter-McAlpine syndrome results from duplication 5q35-qter. *Clinical Genetics*, Vol. 67, No. 1, pp. 53-60, ISSN 1399-0004

International Clearinghouse for Birth Defects Monitoring Systems. (1991). *Congenital malformations worldwide: a report from the International Clearinghouse for Birth Defects Monitoring Systems*. Amsterdam, Elsevier Science, pp. 157-159, ISBN 0444891374, New York

Jung, MS.; Park, JH.; Ryu, YS.; Choi, SH.; Yoon, SH.; Kwen, MY.; Oh, JY.; Song, WJ. & Chung, SH. (2011). Regulation of RCAN1 activity by DYRK1A-mediated phosphorylation. *The Journal of Biochemical Chemistry*, Vol. 286, No. 46, pp. 40401-40412, ISSN 0021-9258

Kajii, T.; Ikeuchi, T.; Yang, ZQ.; Nakamura, Y.; Tsuji, Y.; Yokomori, K.; Kawamura, M.; Fukuda, S.; Horita, S. & Asamoto, A. (2001). Cancer-prone syndrome of mosaic variegated aneuploidy and total premature chromatid separation: report of five infants. *American Journal of Medical Genetics*, Vol. 104, No. 1, pp. 57-64, ISSN 0148-7299

Kaushal, D.; Contos, JJ.; Treuner, K.; Yang, AH.; Kingsbury, MA.; Rehen, SK.; McConnell, MJ.; Okabe, M.; Barlow, C. & Chun, J. (2003). Alteration of gene expression by chromosome loss in the postnatal mouse brain. *The Journal of Neuroscience*, Vol. 23, No. 13, pp. 5599-5606, ISSN 0270-6474

Keller, K.; Williams, C.; Wharton, P.; Paulk, M.; Bent-Williams, A.; Gray, B.; Ward, A.; Stalker, H.; Wallace, M.; Carter, R. & Zori, R. (2003). Routine cytogenetic and FISH studies for 17p11/15q11 duplications and subtelomeric rearrangement studies in children with autism spectrum disorders. *American Journal of Medical Genetics, Part A*, Vol. 117A, No. 2, pp. 105-111, ISSN 1552-4833

Kimura, R.; Kamino, K.; Yamamoto, M.; Nuripa, A.; Kida, T.; Kazui, H.; Hashimoto, R.; Tanaka, T.; Kudo, T.; Yamagata, H.; Tabara, Y.; Miki, T.; Akatsu, H.; Kosaka, K.; Funakoshi, E.; Nishitomi, K.; Sakaguchi, G.; Kato, A.; Hattori, H.; Uema, T. & Takeda, M. (2007). The *DYRK1A* gene, encoded in chromosome 21 Down syndrome critical region, bridges between beta-amyloid production and tau phosphorylation in Alzheimer disease. *Human Molecular Genetics*, Vol. 16, No. 1, pp. 15-23, ISSN 1460-2083

Korenberg, JR.; Chen, XN.; Schipper, R.; Sun, Z.; Gonsky, R.; Gerwehr, S.; Carpenter, N.; Daumer, C.; Dignan, P.; Disteche, C.; Graham, JM., JR.; Hugdins, L.; Mcgillivray, B.; Miyazaki, K.; Ogasawara, N.; Park, JP.; Pagon, R.; Pueschel, S.; Sack, G.; Say, B.; Schuffenhauer, S.; Soukup, S. & Yamanaka, T. (1994). Down syndrome phenotypes: the consequences of chromosomal imbalance. *Proceedings of the National Academy of Sciences of the United States of America*, Vol. 91, No. 11, pp. 4997-5001, ISSN 1091-6490

Kumar, A.; Girimaji, SC.; Duvvari, MR. & Blanton, SH. (2009). Mutations in *STIL*, encoding a pericentriolar and centrosomal protein, cause primary microcephaly. *The American Journal of Human Genetics*, Vol. 84, No. 2, pp. 286-290, ISSN 0002-9297

Lakovschek, IC.; Streubel, B. & Ulm, B. (2011). Natural outcome of trisomy 13, trisomy 18, and triploidy after prenatal diagnosis. *American Journal of Medical Genetics, Part A*, Vol. 155, No. 11, pp. 2626-2633, ISSN 1552-4833

Lisi, EC.; Hamosh, A.; Doheny, KF.; Squibb, E.; Jackson, B.; Galczynski, R.; Thomas, GH. & Batista, DA. (2008). 3q29 interstitial microduplication: a new syndrome in a three-generation family. *American Journal of Medical Genetics, Part A*, Vol. 146A, No. 5, pp. 601-609, ISSN 1552-4833

Lizarraga, SB.; Margossian, SP.; Harris, MH.; Campagna, DR.; Han, AP.; Blevins, S.; Mudbhary, R.; Barker, JE.; Walsh, CA. & Fleming, MD. (2010). Cdk5rap2 regulates centrosome function and chromosome segregation in neuronal progenitors. *Development*, Vol. 137, No. 11, pp. 1907-1917, ISSN 0950-1991

Lutz, T.; Stöger, R. & Nieto, A. (2006). CHD6 is a DNA-dependent ATPase and localizes at nuclear sites of mRNA synthesis. *FEBS Letters*, Vol. 580, No. 25, pp. 5851-5857, ISSN 0014-5793

Marangi, G.; Leuzzi, V.; Orteschi, D.; Grimaldi, ME.; Lecce, R.; Neri, G. & Zollino, M. (2008). Duplication of the Rubinstein-Taybi region on 16p13.3 is associated with a distinctive phenotype. *American Journal of Medical Genetics, Part A*, Vol. 146A, No. 18, pp. 2313-2317, ISSN 1552-4833

Marshall, CR.; Noor, A.; Vincent, JB.; Lionel, AC.; Feuk, L.; Skaug, J.; Shago, M.; Moessner, R.; Pinto, D.; Ren, Y.; Thiruvahindrapduram, B.; Fiebig, A.; Schreiber, S.; Friedman, J.; Ketelaars, CE.; Vos, YJ.; Ficicioglu, C.; Kirkpatrick, S.; Nicolson, R.; Sloman, L.; Summers, A.; Gibbons, CA.; Teebi, A.; Chitayat, D.; Weksberg, R.; Thompson, A.; Vardy, C.; Crosbie, V.; Luscombe, S.; Baatjes, R.; Zwaigenbaum, L.; Roberts, W.; Fernandez, B.; Szatmari, P. & Scherer, SW. (2008). Structural variation of chromosomes in autism spectrum disorder. *The American Journal of Human Genetics*, Vol. 82, pp. 477-488, ISSN 0002-9297

Matsuura, S.; Matsumoto, Y.; Morishima, K.; Izumi, H.; Matsumoto, H.; Ito, E.; Tsutsui, K., Kobayashi, J.; Tauchi, H.; Kajiwara, Y.; Hama, S.; Kurisu, K.; Tahara, H.; Oshimura, M.; Komatsu, K.; Ikeuchi, T. & Kajii, T. (2006). Monoallelic *BUB1B* mutations and defective mitotic-spindle checkpoint in seven families with premature chromatid separation (PCS) syndrome. *American Journal of Medical Genetics, Part A*, Vol. 140, No. 4, pp. 358-367, ISSN 1552-4833

McConnell, MJ.; Kaushal, D.; Yang, AH.; Kingsbury, MA.; Rehen, SK.; Treuner, K.; Helton, R.; Annas, EG.; Chun, J. & Barlow, C. (2004). Failed clearance of aneuploid embryonic neural progenitor cells leads to excess aneuploidy in the *Atm*-deficient but not the *Trp53*-deficient adult cerebral cortex. *The Journal of Neuroscience*, Vol. 24, No. 37, 8090-8096, ISSN 0270-6474

Mikkelsen, M.; Fischer, G.; Stene, J.; Stene, E. & Petersen, E. (1976). Incidence study of Down's syndrome in Copenhagen, 1960-1971; with chromosome investigation. *Annals of Human Genetics*, Vol. 40, No. 2, pp. 177-182, ISSN 0003-4800

Møller, RS.; Kübart, S.; Hoeltzenbein, M.; Heye, B.; Vogel, I.; Hansen, CP.; Menzel, C.; Ullmann, R.; Tommerup, N.; Ropers, HH.; Tümer, Z. & Kalscheuer, VM. (2008). Truncation of the Down syndrome candidate gene *DYRK1A* in two unrelated patients with microcephaly. *The American Journal of Human Genetics*, Vol. 82, No. 5, pp. 1165-1170, ISSN 0002-9297

Mukaddes, NM. & Herguner, S. (2007). Autistic disorder and 22q11.2 duplication. *The World Journal of Biological Psychiatry*, Vol. 8, No. 2, pp. 127-130, ISSN 1814-1412

Musacchio, A. & Salmon, ED. (2007). The spindle-assembly checkpoint in space and time. *Nature Reviews Molecular Cell Biology*, Vol. 8, No. 5, pp. 379-393, ISSN 1471-0072

Oliver, TR.; Feingold, E.; Yu, K.; Cheung, V.; Tinker, S.; Yadav-Shah, M.; Masse, N. & Sherman, SL. (2008). New insights into human nondisjunction of chromosome 21 in oocytes. *PLoS Genetics*, Vol. 4, No. 3, e1000033, ISSN 1553-7404

Pack, SD.; Weil, RJ.; Vortmeyer, AO.; Zeng, W.; Li, J.; Okamoto, H.; Furuta, M.; Pak, E.; Lubensky, IA.; Oldfield, EH. & Zhuang, Z. (2005). Individual adult human neurons display aneuploidy: detection by fluorescence in situ hybridization and single neuron PCR. *Cell Cycle*, Vol. 4, No. 12, pp. 1758-1760, ISSN 1538-4101

Papi, L.; Montali, E.; Marconi, G.; Guazzelli, R.; Bigozzi, U.; Maraschio, P. & Zuffardi, O. (1989). Evidence for a human mitotic mutant with pleiotropic effect. *Annals of Human Genetics*, Vol. 53, part 3, pp. 243-248, ISSN 0003-4800

Park, J.; Yang, EJ.; Yoon, JH. & Chung, KC. (2007). Dyrk1A overexpression in immortalized hippocampal cells produces the neuropathological features of Down syndrome. *Molecular and Cellular Neuroscience*, Vol. 36, No. 2, pp. 270-279, ISSN 1044-7431

Pfaff, KL.; Straub, CT.; Chiang, K.; Bear, DM.; Zhou, Y. & Zon, LI. (2007). The zebra fish *cassiopeia* mutant reveals that SIL is required for mitotic spindle organization. *Molecular and Cellular Biology*, Vol. 27, No. 16, pp. 5887-5897, ISSN 1098-5549

Plaja, A.; Vendrell, T.; Smeets, D.; Sarret, E.; Gili, T.; Catalá, V.; Mediano, C. & Scheres, JM. (2001). Variegated aneuploidy related to premature centromere division (PCD) is expressed in vivo and is a cancer-prone disease. *American Journal of Medical Genetics*, Vol. 98, No. 3, pp. 216-223, ISSN 0148-7299

Potocki, L.; Chen, KS.; Park, SS.; Osterholm, DE.; Withers, MA.; Kimonis, V.; Summers, AM.; Meschino, WS.; Anyane-Yeboa, K.; Kashork, CD.; Shaffer, LG. & Lupski, JR. (2000). Molecular mechanism for duplication 17p11.2- the homologous recombination reciprocal of the Smith-Magenis microdeletion. *Nature Genetics*, Vol. 24, No. 1, pp. 84-87, ISSN 1061-4036

Rauch, A.; Thiel, CT.; Schindler, D.; Wick, U.; Crow, YJ.; Ekici, AB.; van Essen, AJ.; Goecke, TO.; Al-Gazali, L.; Chrzanowska, KH.; Zweier, C.; Brunner, HG.; Becker, K.; Curry, CJ.; Dallapiccola, B.; Devriendt, K.; Dörfler, A.; Kinning, E.; Megarbane, A.; Meinecke, P.; Semple, RK.; Spranger, S.; Toutain, A.; Trembath, RC.; Voss, E.; Wilson, L.; Hennekam, R.; de Zegher, F.; Dörr, HG. & Reis, A. (2008). Mutaions in the pericentrin (*PCNT*) gene cause primordial dwarfism. *Science*, Vol. 319, No. 5864, pp. 816-819, ISSN 0036-8075

Rehen, SK.; McConnell, MJ.; Kaushal, D.; Kingsbury, MA.; Yang, AH. & Chun, J. (2001). Chromosomal variation in neurons of the developing and adult mammalian nervous system. *Proceedings of the National Academy of Sciences of the United States of America*, Vol. 98, No. 23, pp. 13361-13366, ISSN 1091-6490

Rehen, SK.; Yung, YC.; McCreight, MP.; Kaushal, D.; Yang, AH.; Almeida, BS.; Kingsbury, MA.; Cabral, KM.; McConnell, MJ.; Anliker, B.; Fontanoz, M. & Chun, J. (2005). Constitutional aneuploidy in the normal human brain. *The Journal of Neuroscience*, Vol. 25, No. 9, pp. 2176-2180, ISSN 0270-6474

Ronan, A.; Fagan, K.; Christie, L.; Conroy, J.; Nowak, NL. & Turner, G. (2007). Familial 4.3 Mb duplication of 21q22 sheds new light on the Down syndrome critical region. *Journal of Medical Genetics*, Vol. 44, No. 7, pp. 448-451, ISSN 1468-6244

Ryoo, SR.; Cho, HJ.; Lee, HW.; Jeong, HK.; Radnaabazar, C.; Kim, YS.; Kim, MJ.; Son, MY.; Seo, H.; Chung, SH. & Song, WJ. (2008). Dual-specificity tyrosine(Y)-phosphorylation regulated kinase 1A-mediated phosphorylation of amyloid precursor protein: evidence for a functional link between Down syndrome and Alzheimer's disease. *Journal of Neurochemistry*, Vol. 104, No. 5, pp. 1333-1344, ISSN 1471-4159

Saffin, JM.; Venoux, M.; Prigent, C.; Espeut, J.; Poulat, F.; Giorgi, D.; Abrieu, A. & Rouquier, S. (2005). ASAP, a human microtubule-associated protein required for bipolar spindle assembly and cytokinesis. *Proceedings of the National Academy of Sciences of the United States of America*, Vol. 102, No. 32, pp. 11302-11307, ISSN 1091-6490

Sebat, J.; Lakshmi, B.; Malhotra, D.; Troge, J.; Lese-Martin, C.; Walsh, T.; Yamrom, B.; Yoon, S.; Krasnitz, A.; Kendall, J.; Leotta, A.; Pai, D.; Zhang, R.; Lee, YH.; Hicks, J.; Spence, SJ.; Lee, AT.; Puura, K.; Lehtimäki, T.; Ledbetter, D.; Gregersen, PK.; Bregman, J.; Sutcliffe, JS.; Jobanputra, V.; Chung, W.; Warburton, D.; King, MC.; Skuse, D.; Geschwind, DH.; Gilliam, TC.; Ye, K. & Wigler, M. (2007). Strong association of de novo copy number mutations with autism. *Science*, Vol. 316, No. 5823, pp. 445-449, ISSN 0036-8075

Singhmar, P. & Kumar, A. (2011). Angelman syndrome protein UBE3A interacts with primary microcephaly protein ASPM, localizes to centrosomes and regulates chromosome segregation. *PLoS One*, Vol. 6, No. 5, e20397, ISSN 1932-6203

Snape, K.; Hanks, S.; Ruark, E.; Barros-Núñez, P.; Elliott, A.; Murray, A.; Lane, AH.; Shannon, N.; Callier, P.; Chitayat, D.; Clayton-Smith, J.; Fitzpatrick, DR.; Gisselsson, D.; Jacquemont, S.; Asakura-Hay, K.; Micale, MA.; Tolmie, J.;

Turnpenny, PD.; Wright, M.; Douglas, J. & Rahman, N. (2011). Mutations in CEP57 cause mosaic variegated aneuploidy syndrome. *Nature Genetics*, Vol. 43, No. 6, pp. 527-529, ISSN 1061-4036

Somerville, MJ.; Mervis, CB.; Young, EJ.; Seo, EJ.; del Campo, M.; Bamforth, S.; Peregrine, E.; Loo, W.; Lilley, M.; Pérez-Jurado, LA.; Morris, CA.; Scherer, SW. & Osborne, LR. (2005). Severe expressive-language delay related to duplication of the Williams-Beuren locus. *The New England Journal of Medicine*, Vol. 353, No. 16, pp. 1694-1701, ISSN 1533-4406

Tolmie, JL.; Boyd, E.; Batstone, P.; Ferguson-Smith, ME.; al Room, L. & Connor, JM. (1988). Siblings with chromosome mosaicism, microcephaly, and growth retardation: the phenotypic expression of human mitotic mutant? *Human Genetics*, Vol. 80, No. 2, pp. 197-200, ISSN 0340-6717

Van Esch, H.; Bauters, M.; Ignatius, J.; Jansen, M.; Raynaud, M.; Hollanders, K.; Lugtenberg, D.; Bienvenu, T.; Jensen, LR.; Gecz, J.; Moraine, C.; Marynen, P.; Fryns, JP. & Froyen, G. (2005). Duplication of the *MECP2* region is a frequent cause of severe mental retardation and progressive neurological symptoms in males. *The American Journal of Human Genetics*, Vol. 77, No. 3, pp. 442-453, ISSN 0002-9297

Wang, X.; Tsai, JW.; Imai, JH.; Lian, WN.; Vallee, RB. & Shi, SH. (2009). Asymmetric centrosome inheritance maintains neural progenitors in neocortex. *Nature*, Vol. 461, No. 7266, pp. 947-955, ISSN 0028-0836

Warburton, D.; Anyane-Yeboa, K.; Taterka, P.; Yu, CY. & Olsen, D. (1991). Mosaic variegated aneuploidy with microcephaly: a new human mitotic mutant? *Annales de Génétique*, Vol. 34, No. 3-4, pp. 287-292, ISSN 0003-3995

Woods, CG.; Bond, J. & Enard, W. (2005). Autosomal recessive primary microcephaly (MCPH): a review of clinical, molecular, and evolutionary findings. *The American Jounal of Human Genetics*, Vol. 76, No. 5, pp. 717-728, ISSN 0002-9297

Yamada, K.; Fukushi, D.; Ono, T.; Kondo, Y.; Kimura, R.; Nomura, N.; Kosaki, KJ.; Yamada, Y.; Mizuno, S. & Wakamatsu, N. (2010). Characterization of a de novo balanced t(4;20)(q33;q12) translocation in a patient with mental retardation. *American Journal of Medical Genetics, Part A*, Vol. 152A, No. 12, pp. 3057-3067, ISSN 1552-4833

Yamamoto, T.; Shimojima, K.; Nishizawa, T.; Matsumoto, M.; Ito, M. & Imai, K. (2011). Clinical manifestations of the deletion of Down syndrome critical region including *DYRK1A* and *KCNJ6*. *American Journal of Medical Genetics, Part A*, Vol. 155, No. 1, pp. 113-119, ISSN 1552-4833

Yang, AH.; Kaushal, D.; Rehen, SK.; Kriedt, K.; Kingsbury, MA.; McConnell, MJ.& Chun, J. (2003). Chromosome segregation defects contribute to aneuploidy in normal neural progenitor cells. *The Journal of Neuroscience*, Vol. 23, No. 32, 10454-10462, ISSN 0270-6474

Yoon, PW.; Freeman, SB.; Sherman, SL.; Taft, LF.; Gu, Y.; Pettay, D.; Flanders, W.; Khoury, MJ. & Hassold, TJ. (1996). Advanced maternal age and the risk of Down syndrome characterized by the meiotic stage of chromosomal error: a population-based study. *The American Journal of Human Genetics*, Vol. 58, No. 3, pp.628-633, ISSN 0002-9297

Yurov, YB.; Iourov, IY.; Monakhov, VV.; Soloviev, IV.; Vostrikov, VM. & Vorsanova, SG. (2005). The variation of aneuploidy frequency in the developing and adult human brain revealed by an interphase FISH study. *Journal of Histochemistry & Cytochemistry*, Vol. 53, No. 3, pp. 385-390, ISSN 0022-1554

7

Sex Chromosome Aneuploidies

Eliona Demaliaj[1], Albana Cerekja[2] and Juan Piazze[3]
[1]*Department of Obstetric-Gynecology, Faculty of Medicine, University of Tirana Hospital "Mbreteresha Geraldine", Tirane*
[2]*Gynecology and Obstetrics Ultrasound Division, ASL Roma B, Rome*
[3]*Ultrasound Division, Ospedale di Ceprano/Ospedale SS. Trinità di Sora, Frosinone*
[1]*Albania*
[2,3]*Italy*

1. Introduction

Sex chromosome aneuploidy is defined as a numeric abnormality of an X or Y chromosome, with addition or loss of an entire X or Y chromosome. Sex chromosome mosaicism, in which one or more populations of cells have lost or gained a sex chromosome, also is common. The most commonly occurring sex chromosome mosaic karyotypes include 45,X/46XX, 46XX/47,XXX, and 46,XY/47,XXY. Less frequent are those sex chromosome abnormalities where addition of more than one sex chromosome or a structural variant of an X or Y chromosome occur.

The X chromosome is one of the two sex-determining chromosomes in many animal species, including mammals and is common in both males and females. It is a part of the XY and X0 sex-determination system. The X chromosome in humans represents about 2000 out of 20,000 - 25,0000 genes. Normal human females have 2 X-chromosomes (XX), for a total of nearly 4000 "sex-tied" genes (many of which have nothing to do with sex, other than being attached to the chromosome that is believed to cause sexual bimorphism (or polymorphism if you count more rare variations). Men have, depending on the study, 1400-1900 fewer genes, as the Y chromosome is thought to have only the remaining genes down from an estimated 1438 --2000 (Graves 2004).

The Y chromosome is the other sex-determining chromosome in most mammals, including humans. The Y chromosome likely contains between 70 and 200 genes. Because only males have the Y chromosome, the genes on this chromosome tend to be involved in male sex determination and development. Sex is determined by the SRY gene, which triggers embryonic development as a male if present. Other genes on the Y chromosome are important for male fertility. Many genes are unique to the Y chromosome, but genes in areas known as pseudoautosomal regions are present on both sex chromosomes. As a result, men and women each have two functional copies of these genes. Many genes in the pseudoautosomal regions are essential for normal development.

Given that the X chromosome carries more than one thousand genes it is surprising that individuals with X chromosome aneuploidies survive and may reproduce. The reason appears to be that, according to the Lyon hypothesis, one of the two X chromosomes in each female somatic cell is inactivated genetically early in embryonic life (on or about day 16), that means that genes are expressed from only one of the two X chromosomes. This can be understood as "dosage compensation" between males and females that ensures that genes on the X are expressed to approximately the same extent in either sex.

Whether the maternal or paternal X is inactivated, usually is a random event within each cell at the time of inactivation; that same X then remains inactive in all descendant cells. The result of X inactivation is that all normal females are mosaics with regard to this chromosome, meaning that they are composed of some cells that express genes only from the maternal X chromosome and others that express genes only from the paternal X chromosome.

It is hypothesized that there is an autosomally-encoded 'blocking factor' which binds to the X chromosome and prevents its inactivation. The model postulates that there is a limiting blocking factor, so once the available blocking factor molecule binds to one X chromosome the remaining X chromosome(s) are not protected from inactivation. This model is supported by the existence of a single Xa in cells with many X chromosomes and by the existence of two active X chromosomes in cell lines with twice the normal number of autosomes.

The rule is that one X remains active, and extra X's are inactivated. Why then does the absence or presence of an extra X have any effect? The explanation appears to be that the small class of genes that is present on both X and Y chromosomes in the pseudoautosomal regions is protected from inactivation on the inactive X in females. Again this can be seen as a compensatory mechanism ensuring equivalence of gene dosage in males (XY) and females (XX). But when the number of sex chromosomes is increased above two or decreased to one, it is the genes that are present on both the X and the Y that are abnormally expressed.

Thus the phenomena of sex chromosome aneuploidy point to the selective involvement of X-Y homologous genes: the features of Klinefelter's and Turner's syndrome etc are attributable to this small class. For example the changes in stature are almost certainly due to the expression of three doses of a growth factor gene located within the pseudo-autosomal (exchange) region in Klinefelter's syndrome and one dose in Turner's syndrome.

2. Klinefelter syndrome and Klinefelter variants

2.1 Definition

The term Klinefelter syndrome describes a group of chromosomal disorder in which there is at least one extra X chromosome to a normal male karyotype, 46,XY (Visootsak et al 2006 bis). The classic form is the most common chromosomal disorder, in which there is one extra X chromosome resulting in the karyotype of 47,XXY. XXY aneuploidy is the most common disorder of sex chromosomes in humans, with prevalence of one in 500 males (Nielsen et al 1991).

2.2 Background

In 1942, Klinefelter et al published a report on 9 men who had enlarged breasts, sparse facial and body hair, small testes, and an inability to produce sperm. At that time it was believed (Klinefelter et al 1942) to be an endocrine disorder of unknown etiology. In 1959, these men with Klinefelter syndrome were discovered to have an extra sex chromosome (genotype

XXY) instead of the usual male sex complement (genotype XY) (Jacobs et al 1959). The extra X chromosome in 47,XXY results sporadically from either meiotic nondisjunction where a chromosome fails to separate during the first or second division of gametogenesis *or* from mitotic nondisjunction in the developing zygote. The likelihood of X chromosome nondisjunction increases with advancing maternal age. The addition of more than one extra X chromosome to a male karyotype results in variable physical and cognitive abnormalities. In general, the extent of phenotypic abnormalities, including mental retardation, is directly related to the number of supernumerary X chromosomes. As the number of X chromosomes increases, somatic and cognitive development are more likely to be affected. Each extra X is associated with an IQ decrease of approximately 15-16 points, with language most affected, particularly expressive skills (Linden et al 1995).

Postfertilization nondisjunction is responsible for mosaicism, which is seen in approximately 10% of Klinefelter syndrome patients. Men with mosaicism are less affected and are often not diagnosed (Paduch et al 2008). The androgen receptor (AR) gene encodes the androgen receptor, which is located on the X chromosome. The AR gene contains a highly polymorphic trinucleotide (CAG) repeat sequence in exon 1, and the length of this CAG repeat is inversely correlated with the functional response of the androgen receptor to androgens. Thus, a short AR CAG repeat sequence correlates with a marked effect of androgens. In individuals with Klinefelter syndrome, the X chromosome with the shortest AR CAG repeat has been demonstrated to be preferentially inactivated; this process is called skewed or nonrandom X-chromosome inactivation. Individuals with short AR CAG repeats have been found to respond better to androgen therapy, to form more stable partnerships, and to achieve a higher level of education compared with individuals with long CAG repeats (Zitzmann et al 2004 , Bojesen et al 2007). Conversely, long AR CAG repeat lengths are associated with increased body height and arm span, decreased bone density, decreased testicular volume, and gynecomastia. Nonrandom X-chromosome inactivation, which preferentially leaves the allele with the longest AR CAG repeat active, may actually contribute to the hypogonadal phenotype found in Klinefelter syndrome and may also explain some of the diverse physical appearances observed in affected individuals.

In boys with Klinefelter syndrome, the paternal origin of the supernumerary X chromosome is associated with later onset of puberty and longer CAG repeats of the androgen receptor, with later pubertal reactivation of the pituitary-testicular axis.

2.3 Physical characteristics

If the diagnosis is not made prenatally, 47,XXY males may present with a variety of subtle clinical signs that are age-related.

Infants and children achieve normal height, weight, and head circumference. Height velocity increases by age 5 years, and adults with Klinefelter syndrome are usually taller than adults who do not have the syndrome. Affected individuals also have disproportionately long arms and legs (Ratcliffe et al 1999, Schibler et al 1974). About 25% have clinodactyly.

Boys with 47,XXY have variable phenotypic characteristics and do not have obvious facial dysmorphology; thus, they are indistinguishable from other boys with normal karyotypes (Caldwell et al 1972). Many 47,XXY boys appear to enter puberty normally with a tendency for testosterone concentrations to decline at late adolescence and early adulthood. With a decrease in androgen production, secondary sexual characteristics do not completely develop, and features of eunuchoidism and gynecomastia can develop. This also results in sparse facial, body, and sexual hair (Robinson et al).

About 40% of patients have taurodontism, which is characterized by enlargement of the molar teeth by an extension of the pulp. The incidence rate is about 1% in healthy XY individuals.

2.4 Fertility

Androgen deficiency causes eunuchoid body proportions; sparse or absent facial, axillary, pubic, or body hair; decreased muscle mass and strength; feminine distribution of adipose tissue; gynecomastia; small testes and penis; diminished libido; decreased physical endurance; and osteoporosis. The loss of functional seminiferous tubules and Sertoli cells results in a marked decrease in inhibin B levels, which is presumably the hormone regulator of the follicle-stimulating hormone (FSH) level. The hypothalamic-pituitary-gonadal axis is altered in pubertal patients with Klinefelter syndrome.

Although most patients with Klinefelter syndrome are infertile, there have been a few patients with reports of pregnancy without assisted medical technology, typically in mosaic cases. With the introduction of intracytoplasmic sperm injection, which involves the use of sperm extraction from deep within the testicles of patients with nonmosaic Klinefelter syndrome, some XXY men will have an increased chance of fathering a child (Kaplan et al 1963, Okada et al 1999, Ron-El et al 2000, Schiff et al 2005, Paduch et al 2009).

Guidelines for the assessment and treatment of people with fertility problems have been established (Guideline 2004).

2.5 Intelligence

Contrary to other genetic syndromes that arise from chromosomal trisomy (eg, Down syndrome, trisomy 18), the general cognitive ability of patients with Klinefelter syndrome is not typically in the intellectual disability range (Boada et al 2009). A wide range of intelligence quotient (IQ) has been noted and extends from well below average to well above average. Several longitudinal studies of males with 47,XXY have revealed a tendency in about 70% of patients for language deficits that often causes academic difficulties during the school years, delayed speech and language acquisition, diminished short-term memory, decreased data-retrieval skills, reading difficulties, dyslexia, and attention deficit disorder.

2.6 Psychological aspects

Patients may exhibit behavioral problems and psychological distress. This may be due to poor self-esteem and psychosocial development or a decreased ability to deal with stress. Most 47,XXY boys have a lag in language skills with mildly delayed expression of single words. These individuals also demonstrate that the production of expressive language is affected more than that of comprehension or receptive skills (Graham et al 1988).

The personalities of 47,XXY males are variable. One study characterized 47,XXY males as timid, immature, and reserved, with difficulty relating to their peer group, whereas other studies described 47,XXY subjects as friendly, kind, helpful, and relates well with other people. Most are described to be quiet, sensitive, and unassertive. The majority of 47,XXY males rate themselves as more sensitive, apprehensive, and insecure than their peers. An increased incidence of anxiety, depression, neurosis, psychosis and substance abuse is reported in adolescents with 47,XXY (Bender et al 1995). The language difficulty experienced by these males possibly contributes to the challenges in behavioral and social domains (Bancroft et al 1982, Jimenez 1991).

2.7 Complications

Associated endocrine complications include diabetes mellitus, hypothyroidism, and hypoparathyrodism (Hsueh et al 1978). Autoimmune diseases, such as systemic lupus erythematosus, Sjogren syndrome, and rheumatoid arthritis, are more common in Klinefelter syndrome, with frequencies similar to those found in 46,XX females. Development of varicose veins and leg ulcers may result from venous stasis (Campbell et al 1981). Decreased bone density occurs in 25% of patients with Klinefelter syndrome, possibly reflecting the impact of decreased bone formation, increased bone resorption and/or hypogonadism (Horowitz et al 1992).

Risk of acquiring breast carcinoma in 47,XXY is relatively increased, with relative risk exceeding 200 times (Swerdlow et al 2005). The cause may result from the estradiol to testosterone ratio being severalfold higher than that of karyotypically normal men or possibly due to an increased peripheral conversion of testosterone to estradiol in men with Klinefelter syndrome (Swerdlow et al 2005). Patients may have an increased frequency of extragonadal germ cell tumors such as embryonal carcinoma, teratoma, and primary mediastinal germ cell tumor.

The mortality rate is not significantly higher than in healthy individuals.

2.8 Diagnosis

Klinefelter syndrome goes undiagnosed in most affected males; among males with known Klinefelter syndrome, many do not receive the diagnosis until they are adults. Infertility and gynecomastia are the 2 most common symptoms that lead to diagnosis in patients with Klinefelter syndrome.

A karyotype analysis of peripheral blood is the gold standard. Follicle stimulating hormone (FSH), luteinizing hormone (LH) and estradiol are elevated, and testosterone level are low to low-normal without testosterone therapy. Urinary gonadotropins are increased due to abnormal Leydig cell function. The decline in testosterone production is progressive over the life span, and not all men suffer from hypogonadism (Vorona et al 2007).

2.9 Differential diagnosis

The physical manifestations of Klinefelter syndrome are often variable. When the following features: small testes, infertility, gynecomastia, long legs and arms, developmental delay, speech and language deficits, learning disabilities or academic issues, psychosocial difficulties, behavioral issues are present in an undiagnosed male, a karyotype analysis may be indicated. Other causes of hypogonadism need to be considered, such as Kallmann syndrome. Fragile X Syndrome and Marfan Syndrome should also be differentiated.

2.10 Genetic counseling

The recurrence risk is not increased above that of the general population. There is no evidence to suggest that a chromosomal nondisjunction process is likely to repeat itself in a particular family.

2.11 Antenatal diagnosis

Klinefelter syndrome can be detected prenatally by chorionic villous sampling and amniocentesis. Prenatal test consists in chorionic villous sampling (CVS) or amniocentesis. Currently available methods for rapid aneuploidy detection (RAD) include fluorescence in situ hybridization (FISH) and quantitative fluorescence polymerase chain reaction (QF-PCR). Multiplex ligation-dependent probe amplification (MLPA) is a newer technology under investigation that is proving to, have similar sensitivity and specificity to full cytogenetic karyotyping (the current "gold standard") for the detection of fetal aneuploidy (for chromosomes 13, 18, and 21 and the sex chromosomes) (Sparkes et al 2008).

Parents should be counseled based on recent prospective and unbiased information. About 40% of concepti with Klinefelter syndrome survive the fetal period.

2.12 Management

Androgen replacement therapy should begin at puberty, around age 12 years, in increasing dosage sufficient to maintain age appropriate serum concentrations of testosterone, estradiol, FSH, and LH. Androgen replacement promotes normalization of body proportions or development of normal secondary sex characteristics, but does not treat infertility, gynecomastia, and small testes. Testosterone replacement also results in general improvement in behavior and work performance (Nielsen et al 1988). Testosterone also has beneficial long-term effects that might reduce the risk of osteoporosis, autoimmune disease, and breast cancer (Kocar et al 2000).

Early identification and anticipatory guidance are important in boys with 47,XXY. Early speech/language therapy is particularly essential in helping the child to develop skills in the understanding and production of more complex language. Physical therapy should be considered for boys who have hypotonia or delayed in gross motor skills which may impact the muscle tone, balance, and coordination.

3. Klinefelter variants

3.1 48,XXYY

Much less frequent are 48,XXYY and 48,XXXY being present in 1 per 17,000 to 1 per 50,000 male births (Linden et al 1995). Extra copies of genes from the pseudoautosomal region of the extra X and Y chromosome contribute to the signs and symptoms of 48,XXYY syndrome; however, the specific genes have not been identified. Males with 48,XXYY are often tall, with an adult height above 6 feet. They may have an eunuchoid habitus with long legs, sparse body hair, small testicles and penis, hypergonadotropic hypogonadism, and gynecomastia. Peripheral vascular disease may result in leg ulcers and varicosities. Their IQ level is in the range of 60–80, with delayed speech and they are at risk for academic, behavioral, and social deficits. They are usually shy but can be aggressive and impulsive (Linden et al 1995, Visootsak et al 2001, Visootsak et al 2006). In a study of 16 males with 48,XXYY compared to 9 males with 47,XXY between the ages of 5 and 20, findings indicate that 48,XXYY males have verbal and full scale IQ's significantly lower than males with 47,XXY (Tartaglia et al 2005).

48,XXYY males are also prone to have problems with hyperactivity, aggression, conduct, and depression compared to males with 47,XXY. Their mean scores in these areas are in the clinically significant range and males with 47,XXY have scores in the average range. Furthermore, 48,XXYY males have significantly lower adaptive functioning than males with 47,XXY (Tartaglia et al 2005).

3.2 48,XXXY

Males with 48,XXXY chromosome karyotype can be of average or tall stature , have abnormal face (epicanthal folds, hypertelorism, protruding lips with ocular hypertelorism, flat nasal bridge), radioulnar synostosis, fifth-finger clinodactyly, gynecomastia (33-50%) and hypoplastic penis and testicles with hypergonadotropic hypogonadism, infertility and benefit from testosterone therapy. They typically have mild-to-moderate mental retardation and their IQs are usually between 40 and 60, with severely delayed speech. They present slow motor development, poor coordination. Their behavior is often immature and consistent with their IQ level, and they are typically described as passive, cooperative, and not particularly aggressive (Linden et al, Visootsak et al 2001, Visootsak et al 2006).

3.3 49,XXXXY

The incidence of 49,XXXXY is 1 per 85,000 to 100,000 male births (Linden et al 1995). Males with 49,XXXXY are severely affected. The classic triad is mild-to-moderate mental retardation, radioulnar synostosis, and hypergonadotropic hypogonadism. Other clinical features include severely impaired language, behavioral problems, low birthweight, short stature in some individuals, abnormal face (round face in infancy, coarse features in older age, hypertelorism, flat nasal bridge, upslanting palpebral fissures, epicanthal folds, prognathism), short or broad neck, gynecomastia (rare), congenital heart defects (patent ductus arteriosus is most common), skeletal anomalies (genu valgus, pes cavus, fifth finger clinodactyly), muscular hypotonia, hyperextensible joints, hypoplastic genitalia, and cryptorchidism. Pea-sized testes, hypoplastic penis, and infantile secondary sex characteristics are characteristic in patients with 49,XXXXY. Their IQ ranges between 20 to 60. They tend to be shy and friendly, with occasional irritability and temper tantrums, low frustration tolerance, and difficulty changing routines (Linden et al 1995, Visootsak et al 2001, Visootsak et al 2006).

3.4 49,XXXYY

This is a rare aneuploidy and only a few cases of liveborn males have been described. Patients typically have moderate-to-severe mental retardation with passive but occasionally aggressive behavior and temper tantrums, tall stature, dysmorphic facial features, gynecomastia, and hypogonadism (Linden et al 1995).

3.5 46,XX male

XX male syndrome occurs when the affected individual appears as a normal male, but has a female genotype. XX male syndrome occurs in approximately 1/20000 -1/25000 individuals. XX male syndrome can occur in any ethnic background and usually occurs as a sporadic event, not inherited from the person's mother of father. However, some exceptions of more than one affected family member have been reported.

46,XX male chromosomal karyotype is caused by translocation of Y material including sex determining region (SRY) to the X chromosome during paternal meiosis. Two types of XX male syndrome can occur: those with detectable SRY gene and those without detectable SRY.

In XX male syndrome where the SRY gene is *detectable*, a translocation between the X chromosome and Y chromosome causes the condition. In XX male syndrome, the tip of the Y chromosome that includes SRY is translocated to the X chromosome. As a result, an embryo with XX chromosomes with a translocated SRY gene will develop the physical characteristics of a male. Typically, a piece of the Y chromosome in the pseudoautosomal region exchanges with the tip of the X chromosome. In XX male syndrome, this crossover includes the SRY portion of the Y.

Males with SRY positive XX male syndrome look like and identify as males. They have normal male physical features including normal male body, genitals, and testicles, but hypospadia or cryptochidism may be seen (Yencilek et al 2005). Males with 46,XX have decreased testosterone level with high levels of LH and FSH and infertility may be present (Yencilek et al 2005).

In individuals with XX male syndrome that *do not have an SRY gene detectable* in their cells, the cause of the condition is not known. Scientists assert that one or more genes that are involved in the development of the sex of an embryo are mutated or altered and cause physical male characteristics in a chromosomally female person. These genes could be located on the X chromosome or on one of the 22 pairs of autosomes that males and females have in common. As of 2001, no genes have been found to explain the female to male sex reversal in people affected with XX male syndrome that are SRY negative. Approximately 20% of XX males do not have a known cause and are SRY negative. It is thought that SRY is a switch point, and the protein that is made by SRY regulates the activity of one or more genes (likely on an autosomal chromosome) that contribute to sex development.

4. Other sex chromosomal aneuploidies

4.1 47,XYY

There are three plausible mechanisms by which an extra Y chromosome can be generated: 1) non-disjunction at male meiosis II following a normal chiasmate meiosis I (MI) in which recombination occurs between the X and Y chromosomes within the Xp/Yp pseudoautosomal region (MII-C); 2) non-disjunction at male meiosis II (MII) following a meiosis I in which recombination between the X and Y chromosomes does not occur (MII-NC) or 3) postzygotic mitotic (PZM) non-disjunction. One in 800 to 100 males has an extra Y chromosome (Nielsen et al 1991).

Males with 47,XYY syndrome have one X chromosome and two Y chromosomes in each cell, for a total of 47 chromosomes. This arises through nondisjunction at paternal meiosis II. It is unclear why an extra copy of the Y chromosome is associated with tall stature, learning problems, and other features in some boys and men.

Physical phenotype is normal (Robinson et al 1979), with tall stature (75th percentile) by adolescence. There are no problems associated with puberty or fertility. Among the 39 boys followed prospectively, full-scale IQ averaged 105 (range 65-129). Speech delay was noted in approximately half of the boys, and half of the sample needed part-time or fulltime educational intervention. There was no consistent behavioral phenotype. Several investigators reported an increase in temper tantrums and distractibility among boys. Aggression was not frequently observed in children and adolescents (Linden et al 2002).

The condition is clearly variable. Most blend into the population as normal individuals. Better outcomes seem to be associated with a supportive, stable environment.

4.2 47,XXX

Normal females possess two X chromosomes, and in any given cell one chromosome will be active (designated as Xa) and one will be inactive (Xi). However, studies of individuals with extra copies of the X chromosome show that in cells with more than two X chromosomes there is still only one Xa, and all the remaining X chromosomes are inactivated. This indicates that the default state of the X chromosome in females is inactivation, but one X chromosome is always selected to remain active.

Trisomy X is a sex chromosome anomaly with a variable phenotype caused by the presence of an extra X chromosome in females (47,XXX instead of 46,XX). The 47,XXX karyotype originally described as the "superfemale" in 1959 (Jacobs et al 1959 bis) in a 35-year-old woman with normal intellectual abilities who presented with secondary amenorrhea at 19 years of age, is known as triple X or triplo-X. Its incidence is approximately 1/1000 (Tartaglia et al 2010). It is estimated that only approximately 10% of cases are diagnosed (Nielsen 1990).

Although rare, 48,XXXX and 49,XXXXX females exist. There is no consistent phenotype. The risk of intellectual disability and congenital anomalies increases markedly when there are more than three X chromosomes. The genetic imbalance in early embryonic life may cause anomalous development

4.3 Etiology

Trisomy X occurs from a nondisjunction event, in which the X chromosomes fail to properly separate during cell division either during gametogenesis (resulting in a trisomic conceptus), or after conception (known as post-zygotic nondisjunction). Similar to other trisomies, trisomy X has been shown to have a statistically significant correlation with advancing maternal age, as the likelihood of nondisjunction events during meiosis increases with increasing maternal age.

4.4 Physical characteristics

Significant facial dysmorphology or striking physical features are not commonly associated with 47,XXX, however, minor physical findings can be present in some individuals including epicanthal folds, hypertelorism, upslanting palpebral fissures, clinodactyly, overlapping digits, pes planus, and pectus excavatum. Hypotonia and joint hyperextensibility may also be present (Linden et al 1988).

Length and weight at birth is usually normal for gestational age, however, stature typically increases in early childhood, and by adolescence most girls with 47,XXX are at or above the 75th percentile for height (Linden et al 1988). A few cases have been ascertained due to tall stature, and current evaluation of tall stature in females should include karyotype analysis to evaluate for 47,XXX. Cases of short stature have also been described (unrelated to a known 45,X mosaicism). Body segment proportions typically show long legs, with a short sitting height. Studies of bone age have shown no significant differences from 46,XX females (Webber et al 1982). The average head circumference is below the 50th percentile, however, there is a lot of individual variation.

4.5 Clinical characteristics

Although major medical problems are not present in most cases, other medical problems may be associated with trisomy X. The most common are genitourinary abnormalities, congenital heart defects, seizure disorders and EEG abnormalities in approximately 15% of cases with good responses to standard anticonvulsant treatments (Roubertie et al 2006). Gastrointestinal problems, including constipation and abdominal pain, are also common.

Pubertal onset and sexual development are usually normal in trisomy X, however, there have been cases of ovarian or uterine dysgenesis described in children and young adults with trisomy X. Premature ovarian failure (POF) is a condition in which the ovarian functions of hormone production and oocyte development become impaired before the typical age for menopause.

There have been no direct studies of fertility in trisomy X, however, many reports of successful pregnancies have been described, and fertility is likely normal in most cases unless complicated by a genitourinary malformation or POF as described above (Linden et al 1988).

4.6 Psychological characteristics

There is significant variability in the developmental and psychological features of children and adults with trisomy X, ranging from those with minimal involvement to those with clinically significant problems requiring comprehensive intervention services.

Infants and toddlers are at increased risk for early developmental delays, especially in speech-language development and motor development related to hypotonia. Average age at walking independently is 16.2 months (range 11-22 months), and for first words is 18.5 months (range 12 - 40 months) (Linden et al 1988). Expressive language may be more impaired than receptive language, with a pattern described as developmental dyspraxia in some patients. Speech and language deficits may continue throughout childhood into adulthood.

Studies on cognitive abilities in trisomy X also show a wide range of cognitive skills, with full scale IQ's ranging from 55-115. While there are clearly many girls with trisomy X with cognitive skills in the average to above average range, cognitive deficits and learning disabilities are more common than in the general population and when compared to sibling controls.

Motor skill deficits may also be present. Walking may be delayed, and decreased muscle tone and lack of coordination are often clinically significant. (Linden et al 1988). Attentional problems, poor executive function, and decreased adaptive functioning skills may also impact educational and home functioning. There is a paucity of research on mental health problems in trisomy X, however, increased rates of anxiety, depression/dysthymia and adjustment disorders have been described in previous studies (Linden et al 1988, Bender et al 1995). Anxiety concerns are mostly related to social avoidance, generalized anxiety and separation anxiety, and can present in the early school age years or in adolescence. Language deficits may also impact social adjustment in some children when they have difficulty communicating with playmates and when self-expression is limited in older children and adolescents. Again, the variability in the phenotype needs to be emphasized, since many females with trisomy X have minimal cognitive, social, or emotional difficulties.

4.7 Diagnosis

Karyotype analysis of peripheral blood is the most standard test used to make the diagnosis. Prenatal amniocentesis or CVS also identify a percentage of patients with trisomy X, however, confirmation studies are recommended after birth via FISH to study 50+ cells in order to evaluate for mosaicism. It is also important to identify mosaicism with a Turner syndrome (45,X) cell line in order to determine appropriate medical evaluations and treatments needed for Turner syndrome.

4.8 Prognosis and genetic counseling

The prognosis of trisomy X is variable. As noted, there is significant variability in developmental delays, learning disabilities and psychological characteristics in trisomy X. Couples should be informed of the high frequency of trisomy X and that most girls go undiagnosed, in order to support them in understanding and accepting that their diagnosis is not an isolated case with a predetermined outcome (Warwick et al 1999).

5. 45,X

Turner syndrome is most commonly the result of an absence of an entire X chromosome resulting in a 45,X karyotype. The Turner phenotype can also be produced by various partial X deletions or other structural abnormalities. No cause has been identified for Turner syndrome.

Turner syndrome (TS) affects1:2500 live females (Tan et al 2009) and thus it occurs considerably less frequently than the other sex chromosome aneuploidies. At least 99% of all 45,X pregnancies are aborted spontaneously in early pregnancy. Usually, the phenotype is obvious in infancy and childhood, and thus most cases are identified at an early age (Vakrilova et al 2010).

5.1 Physical characteristics

Short stature is a hallmark of Turner syndrome. These females are usually small at birth, do not experience an adolescent growth spurt, and reach an adult height of approximately 4'6"

(144cm, below the fifth percentile). Using current therapy, most of these girls can now be treated with recombinant human growth hormone injections, usually beginning in childhood, and can expect to reach an average height of at least4'11" (150 cm, fifth percentile).

Patients with deletions of the distal segment of the short arm of X chromosome (Xp-) including haplo insufficiency of the SHOX (short stature homeobox) have, more often, short stature, skeletal abnormalities and hearing impairments (Oliveria et al 2011).

5.2 Fertility

The other significant feature of Turner syndrome is gonadal dysgenesis. Therefore, 45,X women are usually infertile, and in very rare cases have spontaneous menses followed by early menopause. Only 2% of the women have natural pregnancies, with high rates of miscarriages, stillbirths and malformed babies. Their pregnancy rate in oocyte donation programs is 24-47%, but even these pregnancies have a high rate of miscarriage, probably due to uterine factors. A possible future prospect is cryopreservation of ovarian tissue containing immature follicles before the onset of early menopause, but methods of replantation and in-vitro maturation still need to be developed. Should these autologous oocytes indeed be used in the future, affected women would need to undergo genetic counseling before conception, followed by prenatal assessment (Abir et al 2001).

5.3 Other somatic features

These can include cardiac and kidney abnormalities, webbed neck and lymphedema. Congenital heart disease was found in 26%. When compared with the general population a higher incidence was present for all types of congenital heart diseases observed. Among cardiac anomalies in Turner's patients, aortic malformations (aortic coarctation and bicuspid aorta) were the most frequent, followed by patent ductus arterious and pulmonary valve stenosis. We have observed that the most severe malformations were preferably found with the 45,X karyotype. Pulmonary valve stenosis was found in a mosaicism 45,X/46,XX case (Couceiro et al 1996).

Aortic dilation and dissection is reported in patients with Turner's syndrome, both with and without cardiovascular risk factors. The bicuspid aortic valve is closely associated with dilated aortic root, although expression of aortic dilation is variable. The determinants for variable expression of aortic dilation in individuals with Turner's syndrome, however, are unknown. A primary mesenchymal defect is prevalent in individuals with Turner's syndrome, suggested by having abnormalities in bone matrix, and lymphatic and peripheral blood vessels. The studies are hypothesized that an abnormal intrinsic elastic property of aorta is a forerunner of aortic dilation in Turner's syndrome (Sharma et al 2009).

Renal/collecting system anomalies are found in 29.3% of patients with Turner's syndrome who underwent ultrasonography. Among them, duplication of the collecting system and hydronephrosis (25% each) and horseshoe kidney (21.2%) were the most frequent (Carvalho et al 2010).

These females are at an increased risk of otitis media, cardiovascular disease, hypertension, diabetes mellitus, thyroid disorders, and obesity. Careful medical management can assist in identifying and treating most of these problems.

5.4 Intelligence and psychological issues

Genetic, hormonal, and medical problems associated with TS are likely to affect psychosexual development of female adolescent patients, and thus influence their psychological functioning, behavior patterns, social interactions and learning ability.

Mental retardation is not prevalent in Turner syndrome, and most girls have normal IQ's. Usually, verbal IQ is significantly greater than performance IQ, resulting in a visual-spatial deficit. Many investigators have noted deficits in left-right orientation, copying shapes, handwriting, and solving math problems.

Girls with Turner syndrome did not differ on untimed arithmetic calculations or problem verification accuracy, but they had limited mastery of counting skills and longer response times to complete the problem verification task (Murphy et al 2008).

In general, speech is normal, but expression can be compromised if recurrent otitis media has not been treated successfully. These women have a high occurrence of ear and hearing problems, and neurocognitive dysfunctions, including reduced visual-spatial abilities; it is assumed that estrogen deficiency is at least partially responsible for these problems.

The results of TEOAE, ABR and speech recognition scores in noise were all indicative of cochlear dysfunction as the cause of the sensorineural impairment. Phase audiometry, a test for sound localization, showed mild disturbances in the Turner women compared to the reference group, suggesting that auditory-spatial dysfunction is another facet of the recognized neurocognitive phenotype in Turner women (Hederstierna et al 2009).

Motor skills can be delayed slightly, and poor gross and fine motor coordination has been observed frequently.

Turner syndrome occurs approximately threefold more frequently in female schizophrenics compared to the general female population. A polymorphism of the HOPA gene within Xq13 termed HOPA(12bp) is associated with schizophrenia, mental retardation, and hypothyroidism. Interestingly, Xq13 is the X-chromosome region that contains the X-inactivation center and a gene escaping X-inactivation whose gene product may be involved in the X-inactivation process as well as in the pathogenesis of sex chromosome anomalies such as Turner syndrome. These genes that escape X-inactivation may produce their gene products in excess, influencing normal brain growth and differentiation (Roser et al 2010).

5.5 Treatment

Women with Turner's syndrome should be carefully followed throughout life. Growth hormone therapy should be started at age 2-5 years. Early treatment with r-hGH helps to prevent natural evolution towards short stature in most girls with TS. IGF1 levels and glucose metabolism should be monitored routinely during r-hGH therapy (Linglart et al 2011). Hormone replacement therapy for the development of normal female sexual characteristics should be started at age 12-15 years and continued for the long term to prevent coronary artery disease and osteoporosis.

Although TS constitutes a chronic medical condition, with possible physical, social and psychological complications in a woman's life, hormonal and estrogen replacement therapy and assisted reproduction, are treatments that can be helpful for TS patients and improve their quality of life (Christopoulos et al 2008).

6. Mosaicism

Sex chromosome mosaic karyotypes are most often 45,X/46,XX, 46,XX/47,XXX or 46,XY/47,XXY, but many other combinations are possible. In general, the presence of a normal 46,XX or 46,XY cell line tends to modify the effects of the aneuploid cells. Twenty-two mosaics have been followed prospectively, including 11 45,X mosaics, six 47,XXY mosaics, and five 47,XXX mosaics (Linden et al 1996). On evaluations of intelligence, educational intervention, motor skills, and behavioral problems, those with mosaicism scored similarly to controls, and no significant differences were determined. Fertility may vary, depending on the chromosomal constitution. Although 46,XX/47,XXX females usually can be assumed to be fertile, the prognosis for 45,X/46,XX mosaics and 46,XY/47XXY mosaics is less definitive. Although many may have normal reproductive competency, appropriate tests must be performed at puberty or later to establish fertility status. The international investigators have long recognized that an element of the self-fulfilling prophecy could affect the study results. In question is whether early identification and disclosure of a sex chromosome aneuploidy to parents, physicians and affected individuals would influence development and behavior over the course of infancy and into adulthood.

7. Discussion

Aneuploidies of the sex chromosomes are present in the general population with a frequency of approximately 1 in a 1000 for each syndrome. The effects of X/Y chromosome anomalies are not as severe as those from analogous autosomal anomalies. Females with 3 X chromosomes often appear normal physically and mentally and are fertile. In contrast, all known autosomal trisomies have devastating effects. Similarly, whereas the absence of one X chromosome leads to a specific syndrome (Turner's syndrome), the absence of an autosome is invariably lethal.

While sex chromosome aneuploidies can include a variety of abnormalities of the sex chromosomes, by far the most commonly occurring SCA involve the deletion (45,X or partial X monosomy) or addition (47,XXY, 47,XYY, 47,XXX) of an X or Y chromosome. Often these individuals are unaware of their disorder. Of these conditions, only Turner syndrome, caused by the loss of all or part of an X chromosome, results in an easily identifiable physical phenotype. Subtle language, neuromotor, and learning difficulties have been identified in most forms of SCA, however.

Sex chromosome anomalies are common and cause syndromes that include a range of congenital and developmental anomalies. They are rarely suspected prenatally but may be incidentally discovered if karyotyping is done for other reasons. They are often hard to recognize at birth and may not be diagnosed until puberty.

The prognosis of sexual aneuploidies is variable, with some individuals doing extremely well with minimal manifestations of the disorder, and others with more significant physical, endocrine, cognitive and psychological involvement as described above and it is not yet possible to predetermine which child will exhibit any or all of these concerns.

It is evident that prevention or reduction of deviation from the normal range in mental development in children with sex chromosome abnormalities is possible if educational and social resources are available, early intervention is offered and the parents are well informed and counseled regularly. Parents having a child with a sex chromosome abnormality need information, counseling, and assistance. The type and magnitude of this assistance depend on the individual child, the specific sex chromosome abnormality, and the parents' own resources, psychologically, socially, and otherwise.

8. References

Abir R, Fisch B, Nahum R, Orvieto R, Nitke S, Ben Rafael Z. Turner's syndrome and fertility: current status and possible putative prospects. Hum Reprod Update 2001;7:603-10.

Bancroft J, Axworthy D, Ratcliffe S. The personality and psycho-sexual development of boys with 47,XXY chromosome constitution. J Child Psychol Psychiatry 1982;23:169–180.

Bender BG, Harmon RJ, Linden MG. Psychosocial adaptation of 39 adolescents with sex chromosome abnormalities. Pediatrics 1995;96:302–308.

Boada R, Janusz J, Hutaff-Lee C, Tartaglia N. The cognitive phenotype in Klinefelter syndrome: a review of the literature including genetic and hormonal factors. Dev Disabil Res Rev. 2009;15:284-94.

Bojesen A, Gravholt CH. Klinefelter syndrome in clinical practice. Nat Clin Pract Urol. 2007;4:192-204

Campbell WA, Price WH. Venous thromboembolic disease in Klinefelter's syndrome. Clin Genet 1981;19:275–280.

Carvalho AB, Guerra Júnior G, Baptista MT, de Faria AP, Marini SH, Guerra AT. Cardiovascular and renal anomalies in Turner syndrome. Rev Assoc Med Bras 2010;56:655-9.

Christopoulos P, Deligeoroglou E, Laggari V, Christogiorgos S, Creatsas G, Psychological and behavioural aspects of patients with Turner syndrome from childhood to adulthood: a review of the clinical literature. J Psychosom Obstet Gynaecol 2008;29:45-51

Couceiro Gianzo JA, Pérez Cobeta R, Fuster Siebert M, Barreiro Conde J, Pombo Arias M.The Turner syndrome and cardiovascular change, An Esp Pediatr 1996;44;242-4.

Ferguson-Smith MA. X-Y chromosomal interchange in the aetiology of true hermaphroditism and of XX Klinefelter's syndrome. Lancet. 1966;2:475-6.

Guideline. National Collaborating Centre for Women's and Children's Health. Fertility: assessment and treatment for people with fertility problems. Feb 2004;216-225.

Graham JM, Jr, Bashir AS, Stark RE, Silbert A, Walzer S. Oral and written language abilities of XXY boys: implications for anticipatory guidance. Pediatrics. 1988;81:795–806.

Graves J.A.M. "The degenerate Y chromosome—can conversion save it?". Reproduction, Fertility and Development 2004;16:527–534.

Hederstierna C, Hultcrantz M, Rosenhall U. A longitudinal study of hearing decline in women with Turner syndrome Hear Res. 2009;252:3-8.

Horowitz M, Wishart JM, O'Loughlin PD, Morris HA, Need AG, Nordin BE. Osteoporosis and Klinefelter's syndrome. Clin Endocrinol. 1992;36:113–118.

Hsueh WA, Hsu TH, Federman DD. Endocrine features of Klinefelter's syndrome. Medicine. 1978;57:447–461.

Jacobs PA, Strong JA. A case of human intersexuality having possible XXY sex-determining mechanism. Nature. 1959;2:164–167.

Jacobs P, Baikie A, Brown W, Macgregor T, Maclean N, Harnden D: Evidence for the existence of the human "superfemale". Lancet 1959, 2:423-425 (bis)

Jimenez SB. Individuals with sex chromosomal aneuploidies: Does the Phenotype Reflect the Genotype? NEXUS 1991;9:Iss.1,Article 9.

Kaplan H, Aspillaga M, Shelley TF, Gardner LI. Possible fertility in Klinefelter's syndrome. Lancet. 1963;1:506.

Klinefelter HF, Reifenstein EC, Albright F. Syndrome characterized by gynecomastia aspermatogenes without A-Leydigism and increased excretion of follicle stimulating hormone. J Clin Endocrinol Metab. 1942;2:615–627.

Kocar IH, Yesilova Z, Ozata M, Turan M, Sengul A, Ozdemir I. The effect of testosterone replacement treatment on immunological features of patients with Klinefelter's syndrome. Clin Exp Immunol. 2000;121:448–452.

Linden MG, Bender BG, Harmon RJ, Mrazek DA, Robinson A: 47,XXX: what is the prognosis? Pediatrics 1988 , 82:619-30.

Linden MG, Bender BG, Robinson A. Sex chromosome tetrasomy and pentasomy. Pediatrics. 1995;96:672–682.

Linden MG, Bender BG, Robinson A. "Intrauterine diagnosis of sex chromosome aneuploidy." Obstet Gynecol. 1996;87:468-475.

Linden MG, Bender BG. Fifty-one prenatally diagnosed children and adolescents with sex chromosome abnormalities. Am J Med Genet. 2002;110:11-8.

Linglart A, cabrol S, Berlier P, Stuckens C, Wagner K, de kerdenet M, Limoni C, Carel JC. Growth hormone treatment before the age of 4 years prevents short stature in young girls with Turner syndrome. Eur J Endocrinol 2011;164:891-7.

Murphy MM, Mazzocco MM. Mathematics learning disabilities in girls with fragile X. J Learn Disabil. 2008;41:29-46.

Nielsen J, Pelsen B, Sorensen K. Follow-up of 30 Klinefelter males treated with testosterone. Clin Genet. 1988;33:262–269.

Nielsen J. Sex Chromosome Abnormalities found among 34,910 newborn children: results from a 13-year incidence study in Arhus, Denmark. Birth Defects Orig Artic Ser 1990,26:209-23.

Nielsen J, Wohlert M. Sex chromosome abnormalities found among 34,910 newborn children: results from a 13-year incidence study in Arthus, Denmark. In: Evans JA, Hamerton JL, editor. Children and Young Adults with Sex Chromosome Aneuploidy Birth Defects: Original Article Series. Vol. 26. New York: Wiley-Liss, for the March of Dimes Birth Defects Foundation; 1991. pp. 209–223.

Oliveira CS, Alves C The role of the SHOX gene in the pathophysiology of Turner syndrome. Endocrinol Nutr 2011; Sep 16. [Epub ahead of print].

Paduch DA, Fine RG, Bolyakov A, Kiper J. New concepts in Klinefelter syndrome. Curr Opin Urol. 2008;18:621-7.

Paduch et al DA, Bolyakov A, Cohen P, Travis A. Reproduction in men with Klinefelter syndrome: the past, the present, and the future. Semin Reprod Med. Mar 2009;27:137-48.

Ratcliffe S. Long-term outcome in children of sex chromosome abnormalities. Arch Dis Child. 1999;80:192–195.

Robinson, A., Lubs HA, Bergsma D. Sex chromosome aneuploidy: Prospective studies on children. Birth Defects 1979;15: 261-6.

Robinson A, Bender B, Linden MG. Summary of clinical findings in children and young adults with sex chromosome anomalies. In: Evans JA, Hamerton JL, editor. Children and Young Adults with Sex Chromosome Aneuploidy Birth Defects: Original Article Series. Vol. 26. New York: Wiley-Liss, for the March of Dimes Birth Defect Foundation; 1991:225–228.

Ron-El R, Strassburger D, Gelman-Kohan S, Friedler S, Raziel A, Appelman Z. 47,XXY fetus conceived after ICSI of spermatozoa from a patient with non-mosaic Klinefelter's syndrome. Hum Reprod. 2000;15:1804–1806.

Roser P, Kawohl W. Turner syndrome and schizophrenia: a further hint for the role of the X-chromosome in the pathogenesis of schizophrenic disorders. World J BIol Psychiatry 2010;11(2 Pt 2):239-42.

Roubertie A, Humbertclaude V, Leydet J, Lefort G, Echenne B: Partial epilepsy and 47,XXX karyotype: report of four cases. Pediatr Neurol 2006 ,35:69-74

Rovenský J. Rheumatic diseases and Klinefelter's syndrome. Autoimmun Rev. Nov 2006;6:33-6

Smyth CM, Bremner WJ. Klinefelter syndrome. Arch Intern Med. 1998;158:1309–1314.

Schibler D, Brook CG, Kind HP, Zachmann M, Prader A. Growth and body proportions in 53 boys and men with Klinefelter's syndrome. Helv Paediat Acta. 1974;29:325–333.

Schiff JD, Palermo GD, Veeck LL, Goldstein M, Rosenwaks Z, Schlegel PN. Success of testicular sperm injection and intracytoplasmic sperm injection in men with Klinefelter syndrome. J Clin Endocrinol Metab. 2005;90:6263-7.

Seo JT, Lee JS, Oh TH, Joo KJ. The clinical significance of bone mineral density and testosterone levels in Korean men with non-mosaic Klinefelter's syndrome. BJU Int.2007;99:141-6.

Sharma J, Friedman D, Dave-Sharma S, Harbison M. Aortic distensibility and dilation in Turner's syndrome. Cardiol Young. 2009;19:568-72.

Sparkes R, Johnson JA, Langlois S. New molecular techniques for the prenatal detection of chromosomal aneuploidy. Obstet Gynaecol Can 2008;30:617–621

Swerdlow AJ, Schoemaker MJ, Higgins CD, Wright AF, Jacobs PA, UK Clinical Cytogenetics Group Cancer incidence and mortality in men with Klinefelter syndrome: a cohort study. J Natl Cancer Inst 2005;97:1204–1210.

Tan KB, Yeo GS. Pattern of Turner syndrome in Singapore (1999-2004), Singapore Med J 2009;50:587-90.

Tartaglia N, Reynolds A, Visootsak J, Gronly S, Hansen R, Hagerman R. Behavioral phenotypes of males with sex chromosomal aneuploidy. J Dev Behav Pediatr. 2005;26:464–465.

Tartaglia NR, Howell S, Sutherland A, Wilson R, Wilson L. A review of trisomy X (47/XXX). Orphanet Journal of Rare Diseases 2010,5:8doi:10.1186/1750-1172-5-8.

Vakrilova L, Dimitrova V, Sluncheva B, Jarukova N, Pramatarova T, Shishkova R, Emilova Z. Early diagnosis of Turner syndrome in a newborn, Akush Ginekol 2010; 4991:63-7.

Visootsak J, Aylstock M, Graham JM. Klinefelter syndrome and its variants: an update and review for the primary pediatrician. Clin Pediatr. 2001;40:639–651.

Visootsak J, Rosner B, Dykens E, Tartaglia N, Graham JM. Jr. Adaptive and Maladaptive Behavior of Males with Sex Chromosome Aneuploidy. J Investig Med. 2006;54:S280.

Visootsak J, Graham JM Jr. Klinefelter syndrome and other sex chromosomal aneuploidies Orphanet J Rare Dis. 2006;1: 42. Published online 2006 October 24. doi:10.1186/1750-1172-1-42 PMCID: PMC1634840 (bis)

Vorona E, Zitzmann M, Gromoll J, Schuring AN, Nieschlag E. Clinical, endocrinological, and epigenetic features of the 46,XX male syndrome, compared with 47,XXY Klinefelter patients. J Clin Endocrinol Metab. 2007;92:3458-65.

Warwick MM, Doody GA, Lawrie SM, Kestelman JN, Best JJ, Johnstone EC. Volumetric magnetic resonance imaging study of the brain in subjects with sex chromosome aneuploidies. J Neurol Neurosurg Psychiatry 1999,66:628-32.

Webber ML, Puck MH, Maresh MM, Goad WB, Robinson A: Short communication: skeletal maturation of children with sex chromosome abnormalities. Pediatr Res. 1982,16:343-6.

Yencilek F, Baykal C. 46,XX male syndrome: a case report. Clin Exp Obst Gyn. 2005;32:263–264.

Zitzmann M, Depenbusch M, Gromoll J, Nieschlag E. X-chromosome inactivation patterns and androgen receptor functionality influence phenotype and social characteristics as well as pharmacogenetics of testosterone therapy in Klinefelter patients. J Clin Endocrinol Metab. 2004;89:6208-17.

8

Human Male Meiosis and Sperm Aneuploidies

María Vera[1], Vanessa Peinado[1], Nasser Al-Asmar[1,2], Jennifer Gruhn[3], Lorena Rodrigo[1], Terry Hassold[3] and Carmen Rubio[1,2]

[1]Iviomics
[2]Instituto Valenciano de Infertilidad (IVI Valencia)
[3]Center for Reproductive Biology
School of Molecular Biosciences
Washington State University
[1,2]Spain
[3]USA

1. Introduction

Infertility affects 15% of couples of reproductive age (De Krester, 1997; reviewed by O'Flynn O'Brien et al., 2010). For years most reproductive problems were attributed to women, but recent research has shown that between 30 and 50% of infertility cases result from male factor (Lipshultz & Howards, 1997; reviewed by Stahl et al., 2011).

Reports indicate that infertile males, especially those with low sperm count, have an increase in chromosomally-abnormal spermatozoa, therefore the study of these individuals is critical for the field of assisted reproduction. Importantly, aneuploid sperm remain able to fertilize eggs, often resulting in repetitive intracytoplasmic sperm injection (ICSI) failure, recurrent miscarriage, and offspring with increased genetic risk. Most numerical chromosomal abnormalities, especially monosomies, are inviable and result in spontaneous abortion. However, a subset of chromosomal abnormalities can result in live birth, including trisomies 13, 18, and 21 and sex chromosome aneuploidies. Offspring with these aneuploidies typically display physical disabilities, mental retardation, infertility, etc. (reviewed by Martin, 2008). Thus, effective diagnostic methods to detect sperm aneuploidy are of great interest.

An estimated 5% (minimally) of pregnancies are aneuploid. However, in assisted reproductive technology (ART), estimates are as high as 25% or more. Aneuploid conceptions often derive from aneuploid gametes: the incidence of aneuploidy in human oocytes is about 20-25%, and is more than 2% in sperm (reviewed by Hassold & Hunt, 2001). Aneuploidy in gametes is intimately associated with meiotic errors. This chapter focuses on the etiology of aneuploidy in the human male gamete, particularly examining male meiosis, meiotic errors, and their possible relationship with aneuploidy. We also describe aneuploidy rates in fertile and infertile men and their reproductive outcomes.

2. Male meiosis

2.1 Generalities

Meiosis in humans varies considerably between males and females (Fig. 1). In females, meiosis begins somewhat synchronously in all oocytes during fetal development, but then arrests before birth. Resumption of meiosis occurs asynchronously at or after puberty, at the time of ovulation, but arrests again until fertilization. In contrast, male meiosis does not begin until puberty and occurs continuously and asynchronously throughout adulthood. Primary spermatocytes divide into two secondary spermatocytes through meiosis I (MI), and each secondary spermatocyte divides into two spermatids, which will differentiate and maturate into sperm. The main difference between the male and female production of gametes is that oogenesis only leads to the production of one final ovum from each primary oocyte, in contrast in males four sperm are originated from each primary spermatocyte.

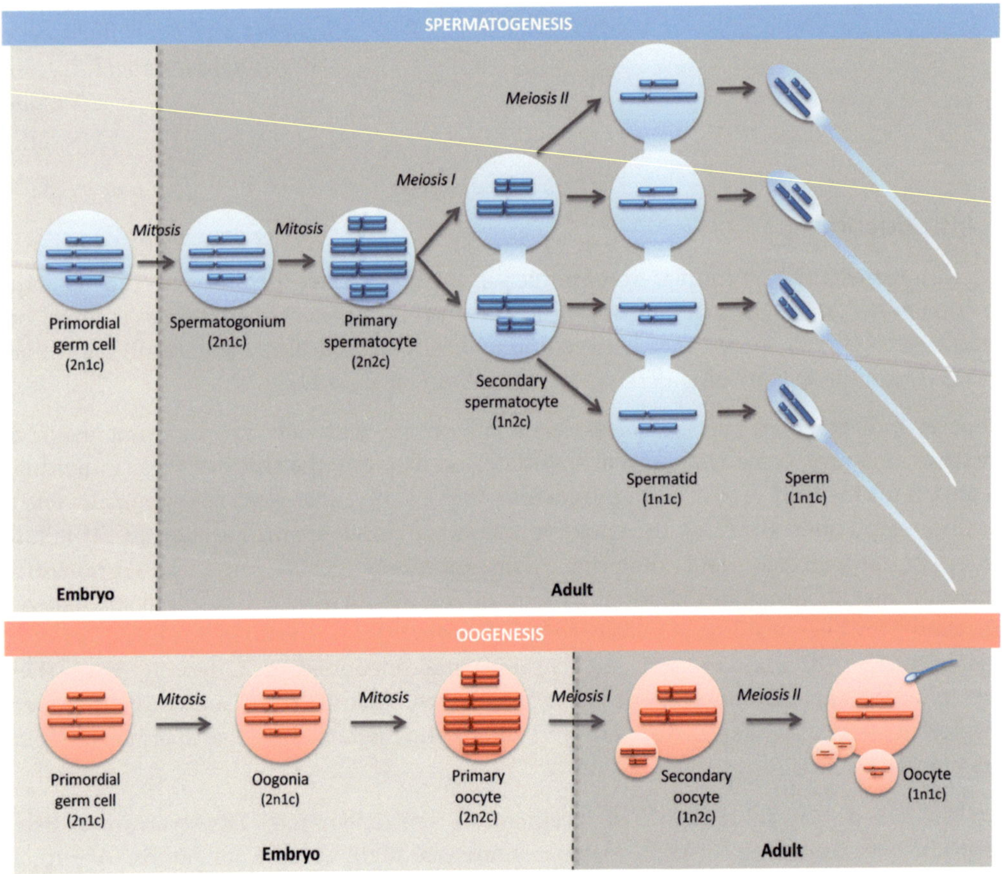

Fig. 1. Gamete formation in males (spermatogenesis) and females (oogenesis).

Meiosis is characterized by an extended prophase followed by two divisions that produce haploid gametes. Prior to meiosis, during S phase, DNA is replicated and sister chromatids remain connected through proteins called cohesins. Meiosis begins with prophase I, arguably the most critical stage thanks to two key events: synapsis and recombination (explained in detail later). Prophase I is divided into four stages: leptotene, zygotene, pachytene, and diplotene. During leptotene, homologous chromosomes begin to condense and approach each other to align, but do not yet pair. With the aid of cohesins (e.g., REC8 and SMC1B), a chromosomal scaffold—the synaptonemal complex (SC)—begins to form via assembly of axial elements composed of SC-specific proteins [e.g., synaptonemal complex protein 2 (SYCP2) and SYCP3]. Additionally, DNA double-strand breaks (DSB) are induced by the protein SPO11; this is the initiating event of recombination, or DNA exchange between homologous chromosomes. During zygotene chromosomes continue condensing and homologues pair and begin synapsis (reviewed by Handel & Schimenti, 2010). Axial elements become lateral elements and, joined by the transverse filaments (e.g., SYCP1), form the SC to maintain synapsis. Subsequently, during pachytene—the longest stage of prophase I—synapsis is completed and DSB are repaired by DNA break repair machinery; a small subset of DSB are repaired as crossovers (chiasmata). Finally, during diplotene the SC is disassembled. Each pair of homologues (bivalents) begins to separate, but they remain temporarily joined at chiasmata (reviewed by Burgoyne et al., 2009).

Following prophase I, germ cells continue into the first meiotic metaphase, in which axial elements are disassembled and cohesins are removed, except those located at centromeres. In this phase, homologous pairs of chromosomes migrate to the equatorial plane of the spindle, with their centromeres facing different poles, forming the metaphase plate. In anaphase I, homologous chromosomes separate. Finally, cell division at telophase I results in two secondary spermatocytes with haploid chromosomes, but with two chromatids per chromosome.

The second meiotic division is an equational division similar to mitosis except that, in this case, the parent cells are haploid. Four spermatids are thus generated from one pre-meiotic germ cell; each should contain 23 chromosomes, with a single chromatid for each chromosome.

Three events can lead to aneuploidy during MI: failure to resolve chiasmata, resulting in a true non-disjunction; no chiasma formation or early disappearance of one, resulting in an achiasmate non-disjunction; and, finally, a premature separation of sister chromatids. In meiosis II (MII) the only cause of aneuploidy is non-disjunction of sister chromatids (reviewed by Hassold & Hunt, 2001).

The importance of MI versus MII errors varies among chromosomes. For example, trisomy 16 is caused by MI errors, while trisomy 18 is usually caused by non-disjunction in MII (reviewed by Hassold & Hunt, 2001). In male, the chromosome with the highest estimated frequency of non-disjunction in MI is the XY bivalent and in MII is the Y chromosome (reviewed by Hall et al., 2006). Further, autosomal trisomies are usually maternal in origin, while sex chromosome aneuploidies are more frequently paternal in origin (reviewed by Templado et al., 2011).

The critical events of meiosis are reflected in two series of specific processes: First, pairing, synapsis, and formation of the SC between homologues establish and regulate cohesion between sister chromatids. Second, recombination between homologous chromosomes and proper orientation of the two centromeres of each bivalent must be completed. Both sets of events are controlled by a pachytene checkpoint, which induces delay or arrest of cells that have not completed these steps to avoid aberrant chromosome segregation and formation of defective gametes (reviewed by Roeder & Bailis, 2000). However, a failure in any of these steps together with a checkpoint failure can result in aneuploidy or segregation failure.

2.2 Synapsis

The SC is a protein structure that mediates pairing, synapsis, and recombination between homologous chromosomes during meiosis. The SC is formed by two parallel lateral elements and a central element that links them with transverse filaments. Three protein components of the SC have been identified: SYCP1, forming the central element, and SYCP2 and SYCP3, which are recruited to the chromosomal cores to form the axial elements (reviewed by Handel & Schimenti, 2010). These structures have been visualized using monoclonal antibodies, particularly against SYCP3, in immunocytogenetic assays. As the first component to localize to the forming SC, SYCP3 can be used to monitor its assembly and disassembly during prophase I. Indeed, SYCP3 distribution varies greatly during prophase (Fig. 2): in leptotene SYCP3 appears as small linear fragments; in zygotene the axial elements begin to elongate and synapse; in pachytene synapsis is complete revealing 22 structures (one for each bivalent) and one sex vesicle (XY bivalent); and, finally, in diplotene each pair of sister chromatids starts to separate, visualized as forks in the SC.

It has been observed that the synaptic initiation occurs in subtelomeric regions and not in the telomeres as initially was thought. Furthermore it has been seen that the centromere avoids spreading the synapsis from q-arm to p-arm and vice versa (Brown et al., 2005).

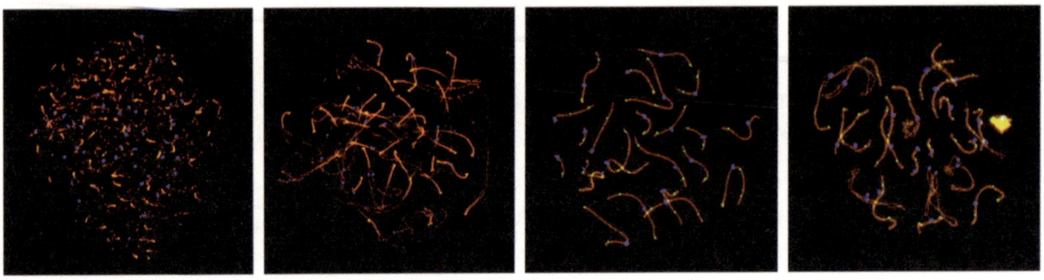

Fig. 2. SYCP3, MLH1, and CREST (stained in orange, green, and blue respectively) distribution in prophase I stages (from left to right: leptotene, zygotene, pachytene, and diplotene).

Synapsis fidelity can be measured by observing the frequency of certain anomalies: gaps, splits, and lack of crossovers. Gaps are discontinuities in the SC and occur often in normal males. Splits are misaligned chromosomal regions that form looplike structures; these occur less commonly than gaps. Finally, SCs without crossovers are detected by absence of MutL protein homolog 1 (MLH1) foci on the bivalent. This anomaly is less common than gaps and even splits. The existence of gaps is reported to correlate with the location of the MLH1 protein. Further, recombination frequency is reduced on SCs with gaps, but not those with splits, which suggests that the nature of splits and gaps differs (Sun et al., 2005, 2007).

2.3 Recombination

Proper recombination between homologous chromosomes is required for normal meiosis and segregation of chromosomes. Chiasmata, physical structures corresponding to crossover points between homologous chromosomes, keep homologues joined until anaphase I. The distribution of these points is not entirely random; rather, there are genomic regions that exhibit much higher rates of recombination, called hot spots, and other locations that rarely have recombination events, called cold spots. For example, centromeres seem to be cold spots, while subtelomeric regions seem to be hot spots with an excess of recombination points. Several studies of human chromosomes have shown that at least one crossover occurs in each arm, except in short arms of acrocentric chromosomes, where crossovers occur infrequently. Further, the existence of a crossover inhibits the formation of another in a nearby region, a phenomenon known as "interference" (Brown et al., 2005; reviewed by Lynn et al., 2004; Sun et al., 2004a).

Antibodies against MLH1, a DNA mismatch-repair protein involved in crossing-over, are used to localize recombination sites. Applying this method in human spermatocytes, groups have described inter-individual variations in MLH1 frequency (Hassold et al., 2004; Lynn et al., 2002; Sun et al., 2005, 2006). Additional findings demonstrated that patient age does not affect meiotic recombination frequency (Lynn et al., 2002). Further, a role for the SC in mediating recombination levels was observed, with a correlation between the number of MLH1 foci and chromosome arm lengths (Lynn et al., 2002; Sun et al., 2004a). Despite these advances, the basis of crossover formation remains incompletely understood, e.g., why crossovers form at a particular site. This indicates the importance of continued efforts toward revealing the mechanistic basis of recombination.

2.4 Methods for studying critical events of meiosis

Male meiosis can be studied using indirect methods, like linkage mapping, or direct assays such as cytogenetics and immunocytogenetics.

Linkage maps, also called genetic or meiotic maps, are derived from genotype data in families by examining heredity of short tandem repeat polymorphisms to detect all recombination events per meiosis. This type of assay provides high resolution, but has some disadvantages. First, at least three generations need to be examined, and second, only half of all recombination events can be observed since only two of the four chromatids are involved in the exchange process (reviewed by Lynn et al., 2004).

Direct assays, although they forfeit some resolution, can help combat these disadvantages. For example, analysis of diakinesis/metaphase I stage cells by conventional cytogenetic techniques is used to directly observe crossovers. However, because diakinesis and metaphase I have a short duration, finding these cells can be difficult. Additionally, material for this kind of study requires testicular biopsy. Finally, chromosomes are highly condensed, making it difficult to identify them correctly (reviewed by Lynn et al., 2004; reviewed by Vallente et al., 2006). This last problem can be solved by adding M-FISH (Multiplex-fluorescent *in situ* hybridization), which allows the identification of individual bivalents. Unfortunately, this technique is costly and quite laborious, prohibiting its application in clinical practice (Sarrate et al., 2004).

Another, more recently developed direct assay uses immunocytogenetics to study prophase I, particularly pachytene, germ cells. Antibodies against lateral element proteins (SYCP3) and transverse filament proteins (SYCP1) are used to visualize the SC, anti-MLH1 antibodies are used to detect recombination sites, and the centromere can be localized with

CREST sera (calcinosis-Raynaud's phenomenon-esophageal dysfunction-sclerodactyly-telangiectasia) (Fig. 2). This assay allows the study of meiotic progression, synaptic defects, recombination rates, etc. Additionally, immunocytogenetics can be combined with FISH to analyze recombination rates and crossover placement in individual chromosomes. While this assay also requires testicular biopsies to obtain material, pachytene has a long duration and nuclei are not as condensed as in diakinesis (Gonsalves et al., 2004, 2005; Judis et al., 2004; Lynn et al., 2002; Ma et al., 2006; Sun et al., 2004a, 2004b, 2006, 2007, 2008a, 2008b).

3. Male meiosis abnormalities

Different types of meiotic abnormalities have been described, and they are not mutually exclusive. One type of abnormality is meiotic arrest, which occurs when spermatogenesis stops at any stage of maturation of the germ line (spermatogonia, primary spermatocyte, secondary spermatocyte, or spermatid). Arrest can be partial, affecting only some germline cells and causing oligozoospermia, or complete, affecting all germline cells and causing azoospermia. In 74% of cases, meiotic arrest is caused by *synaptic defects*, which are due to a decrease in the number of exchanges (chiasmata) between homologous chromosomes in prophase I. This can induce abnormal chromosome segregation in MI, resulting in secondary spermatocytes with an altered chromosome complement (reviewed by Egozcue et al., 2005).

Importantly, a decrease in the total number of crossovers can result from homologues devoid of recombination sites. This, in turn, could cause misalignment of chromosomes on the metaphase plate and, subsequently, improper segregation (reviewed by Martin et al., 2008). The XY bivalent is particularly susceptible to this phenomenon, since only a small region of homology exists between the X and Y chromosomes, and, thus, the pair has only a single recombination site (Shi & Martin, 2000; Thomas & Hassold, 2003). In fact, several studies have demonstrated that sex chromosomes have the highest frequency of achiasmate bivalents (Sun et al., 2006).

In addition to altered frequency of recombination, abnormal crossover distribution can also occur. In a recent study was found an altered MLH1 distribution in one of four infertile males, these could have negative consequences as aneuploid sperm (Ferguson et al., 2009).

3.1 Abnormal meiosis in infertile males

Reports indicate that up to 8% of the general infertile population exhibit meiotic defects (reviewed by Egozcue et al., 2005). Studies of patients with obstructive azoospermia (OA) are typically used to define normal meiosis, since, in these cases, the absence of sperm in semen is due exclusively to a physical barrier (reviewed by Vallente et al., 2006). In fact, recent studies in testicular sperm from OA patients did not show differences in aneuploidy rates compared to testicular control subjects (Rodrigo et al., 2011). Further, recombination levels showed a similar pattern in all patients, with a mean recombination level of 49.5±0.7 crossovers (MLH1 foci) (Al-Asmar et al., 2010, 2011).

On the other hand, in most non-obstructive azoospermic (NOA) patients the cause of testicular damage is idiopathic (Judis et al., 2004). In these individuals various meiotic abnormalities have been observed. Indeed, several studies have reported a significant decrease in recombination levels in NOA, with averages of 32.7-42.7 MLH1 foci versus 46.0-

48.5 for controls (Sun et al., 2004b, 2007). Additionally, one report described a NOA patient with a significant increase (73% vs. 4.5% in controls) in cells with at least one autosomal bivalent without an MLH1 focus (Sun et al., 2004b). Further, NOA samples may have altered distributions of germ cells in meiotic stages. In particular, leptotene and zygotene stage cells are more common in azoospermic patients than in controls (7.95% vs. 2.30% and 9.75% vs. 1.45% respectively), with corresponding decreases in pachytene stage cells (75.30% vs. 96.25% in controls). This phenomenon may reflect meiotic arrest in the earlier stages of prophase (Tassistro et al., 2009). In fact, complete meiotic arrest was observed in one case of NOA (Judis et al., 2004), in which the blockage was at zygotene/pachytene stage and no evidence was detected for synapsis or crossovers between homologues. Another study reported a partial or complete arrest during zygotene in 4 of 40 NOA patients (Gonsalves et al., 2004).

Other types of meiotic abnormalities have been observed in NOA patients. For example, SC discontinuities are more frequent in these patients than in controls (Sun et al., 2004b; Tassistro et al., 2009). In addition, differences have been detected in the frequency of asynapsis events between NOA and control populations (7.97% vs. 2.95%) (Tassistro et al., 2009).

Meiotic abnormalities have also been found in other patients. In a study with oligoasthenozoospermic patients, 17.5% of individuals had an increased incidence of meiotic anomalies (reviewed by Egozcue et al., 2000; Vendrell et al., 1999). Additionally, in a retrospective study of 500 patients with different types of infertility or sterility, the incidence of synaptic abnormalities was inversely proportional to the quantitative level of spermatogenesis. Specifically, altered or incomplete meiosis was found in 24% of azoospermic males, 33% of asthenoteratozoospermic males, 51.5% of oligoastheno-teratozoospermia (OAT) patients, and in 90% of NOA males (García et al., 2005).

Furthermore, genetic studies have identified mutations for proteins involved in meiosis in infertile males. For example, mutations in SCP3, MLH1, SPO11 -a protein involved in the formation of DSB- and RAD54 -a protein that participates in recombination and DNA repair- have been found (reviewed by Sanderson et al., 2008). Otherwise, variations in DNA sequence and their relationship with an increase or decrease in the recombination rate have been described (Kong et al., 2008).

3.2 Abnormal meiosis and reproductive outcomes

Alterations in meiosis do not necessarily lead to azoospermia. Indeed, meiotic errors can produce abnormal sperm that retain fertilization capabilities, resulting in abnormal embryos and either recurrent miscarriage or abnormal offspring. Aran et al. (2004) observed a high number o chromosomal abnormalities (42.5%) in embryos from ICSI cycles for males with meiotic abnormalities (Aran et al., 2004). Furthermore, it has been reported that approximately 50% of individuals with Klinefelter syndrome (47,XXY) have resulted from paternal non-disjunction. Indeed, paternal origin has been associated with a decrease in recombination for sex chromosomes (reviewed by Martin et al., 2008).

3.3 Correlation with sperm aneuploidy

Both aberrant meiosis and increased frequency of sperm aneuploidy have been described in infertile men. However, very few studies have examined meiosis and chromosomal abnormalities in the same patients. One study to determine the relationship between frequency of recombination in pachytene cells and frequency of sperm aneuploidy in six fertile men did not find a significant correlation (Sun et al., 2008b). Other studies observed that recombination frequency in 24,XY spermatozoa was significantly lower than in normal sperm (25.3 vs. 38.3%) (Shi et al., 2001) and that 67.1% of those XY bivalents were achiasmate (Thomas & Hassold, 2003). Also, in one infertile male with extremely high sperm aneuploidy rates, a correlation was observed between low recombination frequency in pachytene cells for chromosomes 13, 21, and the sex chromosomes and a high aneuploidy frequency for the same chromosomes (Ma et al., 2006).

A study in testicular tissue of seven NOA patients reported an increase in the frequency of pachytene cells with at least one achiasmate bivalent compared with controls (12.4% vs. 4.2% respectively). The same patients exhibited an increase in the frequency of aneuploidies, specifically more sperm disomy than controls for chromosomes 21 (1.00% vs. 0.24%), X, (0.16% vs. 0.03%), and Y (0.12% vs. 0.03%). Further, a significant correlation was found between cells with sex vesicles lacking MLH1 foci and sex chromosome disomy in sperm (Sun et al., 2008a).

Another recent study by Peinado and colleagues (2011) analyzed testicular biopsies of 11 NOA patients and compared these with a control group of 10 patients with obstructive azoospermia post-vasectomy. NOA patients had a mean of 44.9±3.6 MLH1 foci versus 48.2±2.1 in controls. This decrease in recombination levels resulted from a significant increase in the percentage of SC without exchanges (1.1% vs. 0.4%) and with one exchange (19.4% vs. 14.6%) and a significant decrease in complexes with three (19.7% vs. 22.8%) and four exchanges (3.6% vs. 5.5%) compared to the control group. In the same study using FISH analysis, NOA patients displayed an increase in sex chromosome disomies (0.39% vs. 0.18%) and a three-fold increase in disomy for chromosomes 13 (0.4% vs. 0.09%) and 21 (0.3% vs. 0.09%) as well as in diploidy rates (0.13% vs. 0.05%). These findings corroborate the correlation between both parameters, recombination frequency and synapsis defects, and higher aneuploidy risk for offspring in NOA patients (Peinado et al., 2011).

4. Sperm aneuploidies in males

In recent years, the use of ICSI has significantly improved the fertility prognosis of infertile couples affected by severe oligozoospermia (Palermo et al., 1992; Van Steirteghem et al., 1993) or azoospermia, in the latter case using spermatozoa retrieved from the epididymis (Tournaye et al., 1994) or testicle (Devroey et al., 1995; Gil-Salom et al., 1995a, 1995b, 1996, 2000); Schoysman et al., 1993). However, prenatal diagnosis (i.e., preimplantation genetic diagnosis, PGD) following ICSI has shown statistically significant increases in *de novo* sex chromosome abnormalities and structural autosomal aberrations (Bonduelle et al., 2002; Van Steirteghem et al., 2002), most of which seem to have a paternal origin (Meschede et al., 1998; Van Opstal et al., 1997). This finding emphasizes the importance of a strict genetic evaluation of ICSI candidates.

4.1 Approaches to studying aneuploidy in sperm samples

The first chromosomal studies of spermatozoa were developed in 1970, with differential staining of concrete regions of chromosomes (Barlow & Vosa, 1970; Pearson & Bobrow, 1970). These showed that 1.4% of sperm have aneuploidies for sex chromosomes. Other authors published an individual chromosomal aneuploidy rate of 2% and a global aneuploidy rate of 38% (Pawlowitzki & Pearson, 1972). However, this method was later demonstrated to be non-specific, resulting in over-reporting of aneuploidy. Thus, more reliable techniques were needed.

A later technique introduced spermatozoa to hamster oocytes (Yanagimachi et al., 1976) to directly study human sperm chromosomes (Rudak et al., 1978). After incubating spermatozoa with several hamster eggs, cells were fixed and stained using karyotyping methods to observe metaphase nuclei and analyze numerical and structural chromosome abnormalities. However, this method could not test samples from men with severe male factor because their sperm were not able to capacitate and penetrate zona-free oocytes. Additionally, this technique allowed analysis of only a limited number of sperm (reviewed by Carrell, 2008). Finally, the time and animals required limited the use of this technique in clinical practice (reviewed by Martin, 2008).

In the 1990s, the first FISH assays were developed, offering a faster, easier, and less costly method to detect aneuploidies in human spermatozoa (reviewed by Martin, 2008). This technique uses fluorescent nucleic acid probes complementary to DNA to visualize regions of interest. This approach permits analysis of a large number of sperm from the same sample. However, FISH cannot be performed for all chromosomes of a single sperm nucleus because the sperm head is too small and signals overlap. Therefore, FISH is typically performed for just five chromosomes (13, 18, 21, X, and Y—aneuploidies for these chromosomes can result in live offspring), and resulting aneuploidy rates refer only to those chromosomes analyzed (Fig. 3) (reviewed by Templado et al., 2011). Despite the drawbacks, FISH remains the most widely used technique to detect aneuploidies.

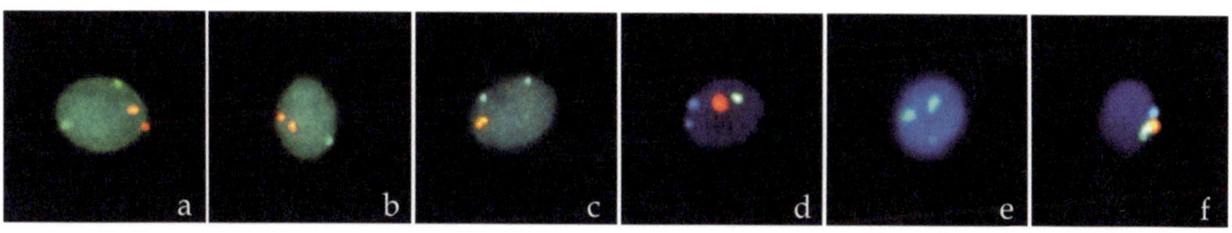

Fig. 3. FISH assays in human spermatozoa. a: diploid spermatozoon (13,13,21,21), b: disomy for chromosome 21 (13,21,21), c: disomy for chromosome 13 (13,13,21), d: diploid spermatozoon (X,Y,18,18), e: disomy for chromosome X (X,X,18), f: disomy for sex chromosomes (X,Y,18).

Recently, an automated tool for the analysis of sperm aneuploidy has been developed. This system has several advantages over manual FISH. First, automated FISH reduces the time required from 10-20 hours to 1 hour. Additionally, the software is able to store all images captured under microscopy. However, this system is costly (reviewed by Carrell, 2008; reviewed by Templado et al., 2011) and is less efficient in identifying diploid sperm than manual analysis (i.e., manual analysis found higher diploidy rates than automatic analysis, Molina et al., 2009).

4.2 Incidence of aneuploidy in fertile males

The detection of alterations in aneuploidy rates first requires establishment of normal parameters. Such values must be based on sperm from normozoospermic males with proven fertility to establish the baseline levels of human sperm aneuploidy. Notably, baseline sperm aneuploidy rates may be subject to inter-individual and intra-individual variability. Studies published to date show considerable variability in aneuploidy rates in fertile men. However, it is unclear whether this variability is real or is due to different methodologies used in each laboratory (reviewed by Templado et al., 2011). One study on intra-individual and inter-individual variability indicates that unknown life events may sporadically or consistently affect sperm aneuploidy rates (Tempest et al., 2009). Despite these factors, a recent review analyzed 32 studies that described aneuploidy rates from normal men. The authors found that total aneuploidy frequency in sperm is about 4.5%. However, disomy rates for autosomes were highly variable, ranging from 0.03% for chromosome 8 to 0.47% for chromosome 22. Sex chromosomes, the most commonly analyzed, exhibited a disomy rate of 0.27% (reviewed by Templado et al., 2011).

4.3 Incidence of aneuploidy in infertile males

FISH studies reveal a significantly increased incidence of numerical chromosomal abnormalities in sperm from infertile males, mainly in sex chromosomes, and in sperm from OAT patients (Aran et al., 1999; Bernardini et al., 1998, 2000; Calogero et al., 2001a,b; Colombero et al., 1999; Martin et al., 2003; Moosani et al., 1995; Nishikawa et al., 2000; Pang et al., 1999; Pfeffer et al., 1999; Rubio et al., 2001; Ushijima1 et al., 2000; Vegetti et al., 2000). Indeed, Rubio et al. observed statistically significant differences in disomies for chromosome 21 and sex chromosomes and in diploidy in OAT males compared to normozoospermic (Normo), asthenozoospermic (Astheno), teratozoospermic (Terato), and asthenoteratozoospermic (AT) males (Table 1).

	Normo (n=14)	Astheno (n=14)	Terato (n=8)	AT (n=6)	OAT (n=21)
% sex chromosome disomy	0.44	0.36	0.42	0.29	0.68[a]
% disomy 13	0.14	0.09	0.07	0.11	0.17
% disomy 18	0.02	0.04	0.03	0.02	0.05
% disomy 21	0.17	0.12	0.10	0.08	0.24[b]
% diploidy	0.10	0.11	0.15	0.06	0.25[a]

Table 1. Percentage of chromosome aneuploidies. [a]$p<0.0001$, [b]$p=0.0423$ (Rubio et al., 2001).

Additionally, at a lower sperm concentration aneuploidy rates were higher. The highest percentage of abnormal FISH results was found at concentrations $<1x10^6$ sperm/mL (severe oligozoospermia)—57% of these patients presented some kind of chromosomal abnormality (Fig. 4).

Although some studies have found similar incidences of chromosomal abnormalities in testicular sperm from NOA patients (Martin et al., 2000) and OA patients (Viville et al., 2000) compared to ejaculated sperm from fertile males, most FISH studies report a higher incidence of chromosomal abnormalities in testicular spermatozoa, particularly in NOA patients (Bernardini et al., 2000; Burrello et al., 2002; Levron et al., 2001; Mateizel et al., 2002; Palermo et al., 2002) than in ejaculated spermatozoa from normozoospermic donors. This difference seems to be more appreciable in sex chromosomes (Rodrigo et al., 2004).

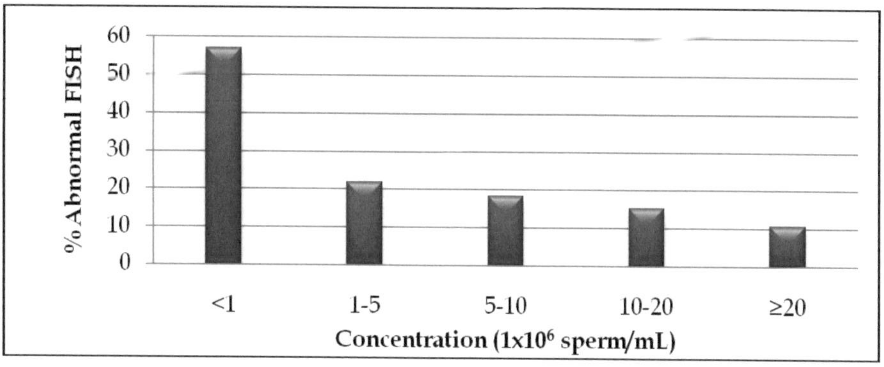

Fig. 4. Percentage of abnormal FISH for different sperm concentration (Rodrigo, L. Unpublished data).

A recent study examined sperm aneuploidy rates in NOA and OA patients (Rodrigo et al., 2011). Importantly, this study used two control groups: one group included ejaculated sperm samples from normozoospermic donors with proven fertility (ejaculated control group, EC); the other included testicular sperm samples of males with proven fertility, for whom a testicular sperm aspiration was performed at the time of vasectomy (testicular control group, TC) because the endocrine environment of the testis had not been altered. In control samples, testicular sperm showed higher incidences of aneuploidies than ejaculated sperm. For azoospermic patients (both NOA and OA), the differences were greater when compared to EC than to TC. Additionally, these differences were greater in NOA than in OA patients. Therefore, to better assess NOA patients, testicular sperm from controls should be used for statistical comparisons.

5. Sperm aneuploidies and reproductive outcomes

5.1 Sperm aneuploidies in ART/infertile populations

Sperm aneuploidies can impact reproductive outcome at different stages: fertilization, embryo development, pregnancy, or birth. Several studies have analyzed the clinical consequences of aneuploidies during *in vitro* fertilization (IVF) cycles.

Fertilization rate

Chromosomally abnormal sperm have been related to repetitive ICSI failures in a prospective study. The authors found a higher aneuploidy rate in those with unsuccessful ICSI outcome, especially for chromosome 18 and the sex chromosomes (Nicopoullos et al., 2008).

Embryo development

Sperm aneuploidies can also result in abnormal embryos. A FISH study in couples with abnormal sperm detected a significant decrease in the number of normal embryos and a significant increase in mosaic embryos (Rodrigo et al., 2003). A similar study in couples with abnormal FISH and low sperm concentration (<5X10^6 sperm/mL) also found a significant increase in abnormal embryos, especially in mosaic embryos -embryos with cells with different chromosome complement- and sex chromosome aneuploidies (Pehlivan et al.,

2003). Mosaicism rate as high as 53% has been reported in patients with NOA (Silber et al., 2003). These findings could be explained by fertilization with sperm carrying multiple chromosomal alterations or centrosome abnormalities. Sperm defective centrosomes impede the formation of asters or lead to an abnormal spindle, with an abnormal distribution of chromosomes, resulting in aneuploid embryos (Chatzimeletiou et al., 2008). In addition, an abnormal number of male centrioles in the centrosome has been related with the production of haploid, poliploid, or mosaic embryos (Munne et al., 2002; Silber et al., 2003).

Sanchez-Castro et al. (2009) studied sperm aneuploidy rates and embryo chromosomal abnormalities in couples with oocyte donation. They found more abnormal embryos in the study group compared to the control group. Further, oligozoospermic patients showed a higher proportion of abnormal embryos (Sanchez-Castro et al., 2009). Recently, an increase in sperm chromosomal abnormalities has been reported to directly affect chromosomal constitution of preimplantation embryos. This study showed that an increase in disomy for sex chromosomes is associated with an elevated risk of generating potentially viable embryos whose sex chromosomes are affected. Additionally, they observed that an increase in diploid sperm results in a higher incidence of triploid embryos, which are associated with more spontaneous abortions (Rodrigo et al., 2010).

Implantation rate

Oocyte fertilization by a chromosomally abnormal sperm is believed to cause implantation failure (Pang et al., 1999). A study in patients with three or more implantation failures reported an increase in sex chromosome disomies in 31.6% of males (Rubio et al., 2001). Further, later studies correlated abnormal FISH in spermatozoa with a decrease in pregnancy and implantation rates in ICSI cycles (Burrello et al., 2003; Nicopoullos et al., 2008).

Miscarriage

Abnormal sperm has also been related to recurrent miscarriage. A study in sperm samples from couples with recurrent miscarriage showed that sex chromosome disomy was significantly increased compared to internal controls. Further, in a subset of seven couples who underwent oocyte donation, mean frequencies for sex chromosome disomy were even higher and diploidy was also significantly increased (Rubio et al., 1999). These results suggest an implication of sperm chromosome abnormalities in some cases of recurrent pregnancy loss. Later, other studies corroborated this hypothesis, reporting an increase in sex chromosome disomies and diploid spermatozoa in couples with recurrent miscarriage (Al-Hassan et al., 2005; Bernardini et al., 2004; Giorlandino et al., 1998; Rubio et al., 2001). Finally, a recent study described that approximately 66% of abnormal karyotypes from miscarriages originate from male factor (Kim et al., 2010).

5.2 Sperm aneuploidies and abnormal offspring

Although most embryonic abnormalities end in implantation failure or spontaneous abortion, a variable percentage of abnormal offspring has been reported and associated with the presence of aneuploid spermatozoa in the father.

Down syndrome

Blanco et al. (1998) studied two fathers of children with Down syndrome who had a paternally-derived extra chromosome 21. FISH sperm studies showed elevated incidences of spermatozoa with disomy 21. Further, in one patient, an increase in diploid sperm and disomy for sex chromosomes was observed (Blanco et al., 1998). Later chromosomes 4, 13, and 22 were analyzed in the same patients; an increase in disomies for chromosomes 13 and 22 was reported (Soares et al., 2001).

Sex chromosomes

Several studies of sperm samples in fathers of children with sex chromosome abnormalities have described higher rates of sex chromosome aneuploidy in sperm, especially related to Klinefelter syndrome (47,XXY) and Turner syndrome (X0). Moosani et al. (1999) performed FISH in sperm from males with normal karyotypes whose children had Klinefelter syndrome. They observed a higher percentage of XY disomy in sperm from these patients compared to fertile donors (Moosani et al., 1999). In another study the incidence of sperm with XY disomy was compared among males with children with Klinefelter syndrome of paternal or maternal origin. A significant increase in disomic sperm was detected in the paternal origin group (Eskenazi et al., 2002).

One study of males having children with Turner syndrome (45,X0) of paternal origin analyzed aneuploidy incidence for sex chromosomes. An increase in disomies and nullisomies for sex chromosomes was observed compared to the control group. Oocyte fertilization by sperm with nullisomy for sex chromosomes can produce a (45,X0) embryo (Martinez-Pasarell et al., 1999). Later, aneuploidy incidences for chromosomes 4, 13, 21, and 22 were assessed in ejaculated sperm from the same four males. A significant increase in chromosomes 13 and 22 disomies was observed in one male and in chromosome 21 in two other males (Soares et al., 2001). Another group studied the incidence of sex chromosomal aneuploidies in a male with a previous miscarriage with Turner syndrome of paternal origin. This study reported a significant increase in sex chromosomal disomies and nullisomies compared to the control group (Tang et al., 2004).

6. Conclusion

Many couples with infertility receive a diagnosis of "male origin". Thus, the study of male gametogenesis and accurate evaluation of male gametes are extremely important.

As a key step of spermatogenesis, meiosis has been the focus of many recent studies. These studies often use immunocytogenetic assays to detect relevant proteins for recombination and synapsis. Thanks to this technique, meiotic abnormalities in infertile males have been well-described, especially for NOA males. Importantly, meiotic abnormalities can result in abnormal chromosome segregation; in fact, a correlation between meiotic abnormalities and sperm aneuploidy has already been described.

Chromosome abnormalities are increasingly found in sperm of many infertile men. This makes the direct analysis of sperm aneuploidy of clinical relevance, since male infertility is now treated by ICSI, which has the implicit risk of transmitting chromosomal aberrations from paternal side. Therefore, in IVF settings, the analysis of sperm chromosomal aneuploidies by FISH is of great interest. Using sperm FISH analysis, an increased incidence of sex chromosome disomies has been described in patients with impaired sperm parameters and in patients with recurrent spontaneous abortions. In this regard, an inverse correlation between sperm quality and sperm aneuploidy rates has been reported.

Another important issue is how sperm aneuploidy may influence ICSI outcome in infertile patients. The studies published so far suggest that sperm aneuploidy may be associated with implantation failure and/or early fetal loss. For these couples at risk, several treatment options has been postulated that range from regular ICSI cycles, to genetic diagnosis or donor sperm. Genetic screening studies in male factor infertility have reported a higher incidence of chromosome abnormalities in embryos from infertile men with altered sperm parameters. In azoospermic patients, higher rates of mosaic and chromosomally abnormal embryos have been reported, most frequently for sex chromosomes.

Therefore, accurate detection of sperm aneuploidies by FISH could be an useful tool for reproductive counseling in couples with male infertility.

7. Acknowledgment

Special thanks go to author's colleagues who contributed to the research and clinical work, presented in this chapter.

8. List of abbreviations

ART	Assisted reproductive technology
CREST	Calcinosis-Raynaud's phenomenon-esophageal dysfunction sclerodactyly-telangiectasia
DSB	Double-strand breaks
EC	Ejaculated control
FISH	Fluorescent in situ hybridization
ICSI	Intracytoplasmic sperm injection
IVF	In vitro fertilization
M-FISH	Multiplex-fluorescent in situ hybridization
MI	Meiosis I
MII	Meiosis II
MLH1	MutL protein homolog 1
NOA	Non-obstructive azoospermia
OA	Obstructive azzospermia
OAT	Oligoasthenoteratozoospermia
RAD54	DNA repair and recombination protein RAD54-like
REC8	Meiotic recombination protein REC8 homolog
SC	Synaptonemal complex
SMC1B	Structural maintenance of chromosomes protein 1B
SPO11	Meiotic recombination protein SPO11
SYCP	Synaptonemal complex protein
TC	Testicular control

9. References

Al-Asmar, N., Peinado, V., Gruhn, J., Susiarjo, M., Gil-Salom, M., Martínez-Jabaloyas, J.M., Pellicer, A., Remohí, J., Rubio, C., Hassold, T. (2010). Sperm aneuploidy and meiotic recombination in patients with post-vasectomy obstructive azoospermia,

Proceedings in 26th Annual Meeting of the European Society of Human Reproduction and Embryology, Rome, Italy, June 27-30, 2010

Al-Asmar, N., Peinado, V., Gruhn, J., Gil-Salom, M., Martínez-Jabaloyas, J.M., Pellicer, A., Remohí, J., Hassold, T., Rubio, C., (2011). Meiotic recombination, crossover placement and sperm aneuploidy in fertile post-vasectomy patients, *Proceedings in 8th European Cytogenetics Conference*, Porto, Portugal, July 2-5, 2011

Al-Hassan, S., Hellani, A., Al-Shahrani, A., Al-Deery, M., Jaroudi, K. & Coskun, S. (2005). Sperm chromosomal abnormalities in patients with unexplained recurrent abortions. *Arch.Androl.*, Vol.51, No.1, pp. 69-76

Aran, B., Blanco, J., Vidal, F., Vendrell, J. M., Egozcue, S., Barri, P. N., Egozcue, J. & Veiga, A. (1999). Screening for abnormalities of chromosomes X, Y, and 18 and for diploidy in spermatozoa from infertile men participating in an in vitro fertilization-intracytoplasmic sperm injection program. *Fertil.Steril.*, Vol.72, No.4, pp. 696-701

Aran, B., Veiga, A., Vidal, F., Parriego, M., Vendrell, J. M., Santalo, J., Egozcue, J. & Barri, P. N. (2004). Preimplantation genetic diagnosis in patients with male meiotic abnormalities. *Reprod.Biomed.Online*, Vol.8, No.4, pp. 470-476

Barlow, P. & Vosa, C. G. (1970). The Y chromosome in human spermatozoa. *Nature*, Vol.226, No.5249, pp. 961-962

Bernardini, L., Borini, A., Preti, S., Conte, N., Flamigni, C., Capitanio, G. L. & Venturini, P. L. (1998). Study of aneuploidy in normal and abnormal germ cells from semen of fertile and infertile men. *Hum.Reprod.*, Vol.13, No.12, pp. 3406-3413

Bernardini, L., Gianaroli, L., Fortini, D., Conte, N., Magli, C., Cavani, S., Gaggero, G., Tindiglia, C., Ragni, N. & Venturini, P. L. (2000). Frequency of hyper-, hypohaploidy and diploidy in ejaculate, epididymal and testicular germ cells of infertile patients. *Hum.Reprod.*, Vol.15, No.10, pp. 2165-2172

Bernardini, L. M., Costa, M., Bottazzi, C., Gianaroli, L., Magli, M. C., Venturini, P. L., Francioso, R., Conte, N. & Ragni, N. (2004). Sperm aneuploidy and recurrent pregnancy loss. *Reprod.Biomed.Online*, Vol.9, No.3, pp. 312-320

Blanco, J., Gabau, E., Gomez, D., Baena, N., Guitart, M., Egozcue, J. & Vidal, F. (1998). Chromosome 21 disomy in the spermatozoa of the fathers of children with trisomy 21, in a population with a high prevalence of Down syndrome: increased incidence in cases of paternal origin. *Am.J.Hum.Genet.*, Vol.63, No.4, pp. 1067-1072

Bonduelle, M., Liebaers, I., Deketelaere, V., Derde, M. P., Camus, M., Devroey, P. & Van Steirteghem, A. (2002). Neonatal data on a cohort of 2889 infants born after ICSI (1991-1999) and of 2995 infants born after IVF (1983-1999). *Hum.Reprod.*, Vol.17, No.3, pp. 671-694

Brown, P. W., Judis, L., Chan, E. R., Schwartz, S., Seftel, A., Thomas, A. & Hassold, T. J. (2005). Meiotic synapsis proceeds from a limited number of subtelomeric sites in the human male. *Am.J.Hum.Genet.*, Vol.77, No.4, pp. 556-566

Burgoyne, P. S., Mahadevaiah, S. K. & Turner, J. M. (2009). The consequences of asynapsis for mammalian meiosis. *Nat.Rev.Genet.*, Vol.10, No.3, pp. 207-216

Burrello, N., Calogero, A. E., De Palma, A., Grazioso, C., Torrisi, C., Barone, N., Pafumi, C., D'Agata, R. & Vicari, E. (2002). Chromosome analysis of epididymal and testicular spermatozoa in patients with azoospermia. *Eur.J.Hum.Genet.*, Vol.10, No.6, pp. 362-366

Burrello, N., Vicari, E., Shin, P., Agarwal, A., De Palma, A., Grazioso, C., D'Agata, R. & Calogero, A. E. (2003). Lower sperm aneuploidy frequency is associated with high pregnancy rates in ICSI programmes. *Hum.Reprod.,* Vol.18, No.7, pp. 1371-1376

Calogero, A. E., De Palma, A., Grazioso, C., Barone, N., Romeo, R., Rappazzo, G. & D'Agata, R. (2001a). Aneuploidy rate in spermatozoa of selected men with abnormal semen parameters. *Hum.Reprod.,* Vol.16, No.6, pp. 1172-1179

Calogero, A. E., De Palma, A., Grazioso, C., Barone, N., Burrello, N., Palermo, I., Gulisano, A., Pafumi, C. & D'Agata, R. (2001b). High sperm aneuploidy rate in unselected infertile patients and its relationship with intracytoplasmic sperm injection outcome. *Hum.Reprod.,* Vol.16, No.7, pp. 1433-1439

Carrell, D. T. (2008). The clinical implementation of sperm chromosome aneuploidy testing: pitfalls and promises. *J.Androl.,* Vol.29, No.2, pp. 124-133

Chatzimeletiou, K., Morrison, E. E., Prapas, N., Prapas, Y. & Handyside, A. H. (2008). The centrosome and early embryogenesis: clinical insights. *Reprod.Biomed.Online,* Vol.16, No.4, pp. 485-491

Colombero, L. T., Hariprashad, J. J., Tsai, M. C., Rosenwaks, Z. & Palermo, G. D. (1999). Incidence of sperm aneuploidy in relation to semen characteristics and assisted reproductive outcome. *Fertil.Steril.,* Vol.72, No.1, pp. 90-96

De Kretser, D. M. (1997). Male infertility. *Lancet,* Vol.349, No.9054, pp. 787-790

Devroey, P., Liu, J., Nagy, Z., Goossens, A., Tournaye, H., Camus, M., Van Steirteghem, A. & Silber, S. (1995). Pregnancies after testicular sperm extraction and intracytoplasmic sperm injection in non-obstructive azoospermia. *Hum.Reprod.,* Vol.10, No.6, pp. 1457-1460

Egozcue, S., Vendrell, J. M., Garcia, F., Veiga, A., Aran, B., Barri, P. N. & Egozcue, J. (2000). Increased incidence of meiotic anomalies in oligoasthenozoospermic males preselected for intracytoplasmic sperm injection. *J.Assist.Reprod.Genet.,* Vol.17, No.6, pp. 307-30

Egozcue, J., Sarrate, Z., Codina-Pascual, M., Egozcue, S., Oliver-Bonet, M., Blanco, J., Navarro, J., Benet, J. & Vidal, F. (2005). Meiotic abnormalities in infertile males. *Cytogenet.Genome Res.,* Vol.111, No.3-4, pp. 337-342

Eskenazi, B., Wyrobek, A. J., Kidd, S. A., Lowe, X., Moore, D.,2nd, Weisiger, K. & Aylstock, M. (2002). Sperm aneuploidy in fathers of children with paternally and maternally inherited Klinefelter syndrome. *Hum.Reprod.,* Vol.17, No.3, pp. 576-583

Ferguson, K. A., Leung, S., Jiang, D. & Ma, S. (2009). Distribution of MLH1 foci and inter-focal distances in spermatocytes of infertile men. *Hum.Reprod.,* Vol.24, No.6, pp. 1313-1321

García, F., Egozuce, S., López Teijón, M.L., Olivares, R., Serra, O., Aura, M., Moragas, M., Rabanal, A., Egozuce, J. (2005). Meiosis en biopsia testicular y patrón espermatogenico, *Proceedings in XII Congreso Nacional de Andrologia,* A Coruña, España, April 14-16, 2005

Gil-Salom, M., Minguez, Y., Rubio, C., De los Santos, M. J., Remohi, J. & Pellicer, A. (1995a). Efficacy of intracytoplasmic sperm injection using testicular spermatozoa. *Hum.Reprod.,* Vol.10, No.12, pp. 3166-3170

Gil-Salom, M., Minguez, Y., Rubio, C., Remohi, J. & Pellicer, A. (1995b). Intracytoplasmic testicular sperm injection: an effective treatment for otherwise intractable obstructive azoospermia. *J.Urol.,* Vol.154, No.6, pp. 2074-2077

Gil-Salom, M., Romero, J., Minguez, Y., Rubio, C., De los Santos, M. J., Remohi, J. & Pellicer, A. (1996). Pregnancies after intracytoplasmic sperm injection with cryopreserved testicular spermatozoa. *Hum.Reprod.*, Vol.11, No.6, pp. 1309-1313

Gil-Salom, M., Romero, J., Rubio, C., Ruiz, A., Remohi, J. & Pellicer, A. (2000). Intracytoplasmic sperm injection with cryopreserved testicular spermatozoa. *Mol.Cell.Endocrinol.,* Vol.169, No.1-2, pp. 15-19

Giorlandino, C., Calugi, G., Iaconianni, L., Santoro, M. L. & Lippa, A. (1998). Spermatozoa with chromosomal abnormalities may result in a higher rate of recurrent abortion. *Fertil.Steril.,* Vol.70, No.3, pp. 576-577

Gonsalves, J., Sun, F., Schlegel, P. N., Turek, P. J., Hopps, C. V., Greene, C., Martin, R. H. & Pera, R. A. (2004). Defective recombination in infertile men. *Hum.Mol.Genet.,* Vol.13, No.22, pp. 2875-2883

Gonsalves, J., Turek, P. J., Schlegel, P. N., Hopps, C. V., Weier, J. F. & Pera, R. A. (2005). Recombination in men with Klinefelter syndrome. *Reproduction,* Vol.130, No.2, pp. 223-229

Hall, H., Hunt, P. & Hassold, T. (2006). Meiosis and sex chromosome aneuploidy: how meiotic errors cause aneuploidy; how aneuploidy causes meiotic errors. *Curr.Opin.Genet.Dev.,* Vol.16, No.3, pp. 323-329

Handel, M. A. & Schimenti, J. C. (2010). Genetics of mammalian meiosis: regulation, dynamics and impact on fertility. *Nat.Rev.Genet.,* Vol.11, No.2, pp. 124-136

Hassold, T. & Hunt, P. (2001). To err (meiotically) is human: the genesis of human aneuploidy. *Nat.Rev.Genet.,* Vol.2, No.4, pp. 280-291

Hassold, T., Judis, L., Chan, E. R., Schwartz, S., Seftel, A. & Lynn, A. (2004). Cytological studies of meiotic recombination in human males. *Cytogenet.Genome Res.,* Vol.107, No.3-4, pp. 249-255

Judis, L., Chan, E. R., Schwartz, S., Seftel, A. & Hassold, T. (2004). Meiosis I arrest and azoospermia in an infertile male explained by failure of formation of a component of the synaptonemal complex. *Fertil.Steril.,* Vol.81, No.1, pp. 205-209

Kim, J. W., Lee, W. S., Yoon, T. K., Seok, H. H., Cho, J. H., Kim, Y. S., Lyu, S. W. & Shim, S. H. (2010). Chromosomal abnormalities in spontaneous abortion after assisted reproductive treatment. *BMC Med.Genet.,* Vol.11, pp. 153

Kong, A., Thorleifsson, G., Stefansson, H., Masson, G., Helgason, A., Gudbjartsson, D. F., Jonsdottir, G. M., Gudjonsson, S. A., Sverrisson, S., Thorlacius, T., Jonasdottir, A., Hardarson, G. A., Palsson, S. T., Frigge, M. L., Gulcher, J. R., Thorsteinsdottir, U. & Stefansson, K. (2008). Sequence variants in the RNF212 gene associate with genome-wide recombination rate. *Science,* Vol.319, No.5868, pp. 1398-1401

Levron, J., Aviram-Goldring, A., Madgar, I., Raviv, G., Barkai, G. & Dor, J. (2001). Studies on sperm chromosomes in patients with severe male factor infertility undergoing assisted reproductive technology treatment. *Mol.Cell.Endocrinol.,* Vol.183 Suppl 1, pp. S23-8

Lipshultz L.I., Howards, S. S. (1997). *Infertility in the male* (3), Mosby, ISBN 0815155018, 9780815155010, USA

Lynn, A., Koehler, K. E., Judis, L., Chan, E. R., Cherry, J. P., Schwartz, S., Seftel, A., Hunt, P. A. & Hassold, T. J. (2002). Covariation of synaptonemal complex length and mammalian meiotic exchange rates. *Science,* Vol.296, No.5576, pp. 2222-2225

Lynn, A., Ashley, T. & Hassold, T. (2004). Variation in human meiotic recombination. *Annu.Rev.Genomics Hum.Genet.*, Vol.5, pp. 317-349

Ma, S., Arsovska, S., Moens, P., Nigro, M. & Chow, V. (2006). Analysis of early meiotic events and aneuploidy in nonobstructive azoospermic men: a preliminary report. *Fertil.Steril.*, Vol.85, No.3, pp. 646-652

Martin, R. H., Greene, C., Rademaker, A., Barclay, L., Ko, E. & Chernos, J. (2000). Chromosome analysis of spermatozoa extracted from testes of men with non-obstructive azoospermia. *Hum.Reprod.*, Vol.15, No.5, pp. 1121-1124

Martin, R. H., Greene, C., Rademaker, A. W., Ko, E. & Chernos, J. (2003). Analysis of aneuploidy in spermatozoa from testicular biopsies from men with nonobstructive azoospermia. *J.Androl.*, Vol.24, No.1, pp. 100-103

Martin, R. H. (2008). Meiotic errors in human oogenesis and spermatogenesis. *Reprod.Biomed.Online*, Vol.16, No.4, pp. 523-531

Martinez-Pasarell, O., Nogues, C., Bosch, M., Egozcue, J. & Templado, C. (1999). Analysis of sex chromosome aneuploidy in sperm from fathers of Turner syndrome patients. *Hum.Genet.*, Vol.104, No.4, pp. 345-349

Mateizel, I., Verheyen, G., Van Assche, E., Tournaye, H., Liebaers, I. & Van Steirteghem, A. (2002). FISH analysis of chromosome X, Y and 18 abnormalities in testicular sperm from azoospermic patients. *Hum.Reprod.*, Vol.17, No.9, pp. 2249-2257

Meschede, D., Lemcke, B., Exeler, J. R., De Geyter, C., Behre, H. M., Nieschlag, E. & Horst, J. (1998). Chromosome abnormalities in 447 couples undergoing intracytoplasmic sperm injection--prevalence, types, sex distribution and reproductive relevance. *Hum.Reprod.*, Vol.13, No.3, pp. 576-582

Molina, O., Sarrate, Z., Vidal, F. & Blanco, J. (2009). FISH on sperm: spot-counting to stop counting? Not yet. *Fertil.Steril.*, Vol.92, No.4, pp. 1474-1480

Moosani, N., Pattinson, H. A., Carter, M. D., Cox, D. M., Rademaker, A. W. & Martin, R. H. (1995). Chromosomal analysis of sperm from men with idiopathic infertility using sperm karyotyping and fluorescence in situ hybridization. *Fertil.Steril.*, Vol.64, No.4, pp. 811-817

Moosani, N., Chernos, J., Lowry, R. B., Martin, R. H. & Rademaker, A. (1999). A 47,XXY fetus resulting from ICSI in a man with an elevated frequency of 24,XY spermatozoa. *Hum.Reprod.*, Vol.14, No.4, pp. 1137-1138

Munne, S., Sandalinas, M., Escudero, T., Marquez, C. & Cohen, J. (2002). Chromosome mosaicism in cleavage-stage human embryos: evidence of a maternal age effect. *Reprod.Biomed.Online*, Vol.4, No.3, pp. 223-232

Nicopoullos, J. D., Gilling-Smith, C., Almeida, P. A., Homa, S., Nice, L., Tempest, H. & Ramsay, J. W. (2008). The role of sperm aneuploidy as a predictor of the success of intracytoplasmic sperm injection? *Hum.Reprod.*, Vol.23, No.2, pp. 240-250

Nishikawa, N., Murakami, I., Ikuta, K. & Suzumori, K. (2000). Sex chromosomal analysis of spermatozoa from infertile men using fluorescence in situ hybridization. *J.Assist.Reprod.Genet.*, Vol.17, No.2, pp. 97-102

O'Flynn O'Brien, K. L., Varghese, A. C. & Agarwal, A. (2010). The genetic causes of male factor infertility: a review. *Fertil.Steril.*, Vol.93, No.1, pp. 1-12

Palermo, G., Joris, H., Devroey, P. & Van Steirteghem, A. C. (1992). Pregnancies after intracytoplasmic injection of single spermatozoon into an oocyte. *Lancet*, Vol.340, No.8810, pp. 17-18

Palermo, G. D., Colombero, L. T., Hariprashad, J. J., Schlegel, P. N. & Rosenwaks, Z. (2002). Chromosome analysis of epididymal and testicular sperm in azoospermic patients undergoing ICSI. *Hum.Reprod.*, Vol.17, No.3, pp. 570-575

Pang, M. G., Hoegerman, S. F., Cuticchia, A. J., Moon, S. Y., Doncel, G. F., Acosta, A. A. & Kearns, W. G. (1999). Detection of aneuploidy for chromosomes 4, 6, 7, 8, 9, 10, 11, 12, 13, 17, 18, 21, X and Y by fluorescence in-situ hybridization in spermatozoa from nine patients with oligoasthenoteratozoospermia undergoing intracytoplasmic sperm injection. *Hum.Reprod.*, Vol.14, No.5, pp. 1266-1273

Pawlowitzki, I. H. & Pearson, P. L. (1972). Chromosomal aneuploidy in human spermatozoa. *Humangenetik*, Vol.16, No.1, pp. 119-122

Pearson, P. L. & Bobrow, M. (1970). Fluorescent staining of the Y chromosome in meiotic stages of the human male. *J.Reprod.Fertil.*, Vol.22, No.1, pp. 177-179

Pehlivan, T.S., Rodrigo, L., Simón, C., Remohí, J., Pellicer, A., Rubio, C. (2003). Chromosomal abnormalities in day 3 embryos from severe oligozoospermic patients, *Proceedings in 59th Annual Meeting of the American Society for Reproductive Medicine*, Texas, USA, October, 2003

Peinado, V., Al-Asmar, N., Gruhn, J., Rodrigo, L., Gil-Salom, M., Martinez, J.M., Pellicer, A., Remohi, J., Hassold, T.J., Rubio, C. Relationship between meiotic recombination and sperm aneuploidy and diploidy in non-obstructive azoospermic males, *Proceedings in 8th European Cytogenetics Conference*, Porto, Portugal, July 2-5, 2011

Pfeffer, J., Pang, M. G., Hoegerman, S. F., Osgood, C. J., Stacey, M. W., Mayer, J., Oehninger, S. & Kearns, W. G. (1999). Aneuploidy frequencies in semen fractions from ten oligoasthenoteratozoospermic patients donating sperm for intracytoplasmic sperm injection. *Fertil.Steril.*, Vol.72, No.3, pp. 472-478

Rodrigo, L., Rubio, C., Gil-Salom, M., Mateu, E., Pérez-Cano, I., Herrer, R., Simon, C., Remohí, J., Pellicer, A. (2003). Sperm chromosomal abnormalities: a new indication for preimplantational genetic diagnosis?, *Proceedings in 19th Annual Meeting of the European Society of Human Reproduction and Embryology*, Madrid, Spain, June-July, 2003

Rodrigo, L., Rubio, C., Mateu, E., Simon, C., Remohi, J., Pellicer, A. & Gil-Salom, M. (2004). Analysis of chromosomal abnormalities in testicular and epididymal spermatozoa from azoospermic ICSI patients by fluorescence in-situ hybridization. *Hum.Reprod.*, Vol.19, No.1, pp. 118-123

Rodrigo, L., Peinado, V., Mateu, E., Remohi, J., Pellicer, A., Simon, C., Gil-Salom, M. & Rubio, C. (2010). Impact of different patterns of sperm chromosomal abnormalities on the chromosomal constitution of preimplantation embryos. *Fertil.Steril.*, Vol.94, No.4, pp. 1380-1386

Rodrigo, L., Rubio, C., Peinado, V., Villamon, R., Al-Asmar, N., Remohi, J., Pellicer, A., Simon, C. & Gil-Salom, M. (2011). Testicular sperm from patients with obstructive and nonobstructive azoospermia: aneuploidy risk and reproductive prognosis using testicular sperm from fertile donors as control samples. *Fertil.Steril.*, Vol.95, No.3, pp. 1005-1012

Roeder, G. S. & Bailis, J. M. (2000). The pachytene checkpoint. *Trends Genet.*, Vol.16, No.9, pp. 395-403

Rubio, C., Simon, C., Blanco, J., Vidal, F., Minguez, Y., Egozcue, J., Crespo, J., Remohi, J. & Pellicer, A. (1999). Implications of sperm chromosome abnormalities in recurrent miscarriage. *J.Assist.Reprod.Genet.*, Vol.16, No.5, pp. 253-258

Rubio, C., Gil-Salom, M., Simon, C., Vidal, F., Rodrigo, L., Minguez, Y., Remohi, J. & Pellicer, A. (2001). Incidence of sperm chromosomal abnormalities in a risk population: relationship with sperm quality and ICSI outcome. *Hum.Reprod.*, Vol.16, No.10, pp. 2084-2092

Rudak, E., Jacobs, P. A. & Yanagimachi, R. (1978). Direct analysis of the chromosome constitution of human spermatozoa. *Nature*, Vol.274, No.5674, pp. 911-913

Sanchez-Castro, M., Jimenez-Macedo, A. R., Sandalinas, M. & Blanco, J. (2009). Prognostic value of sperm fluorescence in situ hybridization analysis over PGD. *Hum.Reprod.*, Vol.24, No.6, pp. 1516-1521

Sanderson, M. L., Hassold, T. J. & Carrell, D. T. (2008). Proteins involved in meiotic recombination: a role in male infertility? *Syst.Biol.Reprod.Med.*, Vol.54, No.2, pp. 57-74

Sarrate, Z., Blanco, J., Egozcue, S., Vidal, F. & Egozcue, J. (2004). Identification of meiotic anomalies with multiplex fluorescence in situ hybridization: Preliminary results. *Fertil.Steril.*, Vol.82, No.3, pp. 712-717

Schoysman, R., Vanderzwalmen, P., Nijs, M., Segal, L., Segal-Bertin, G., Geerts, L., van Roosendaal, E. & Schoysman, D. (1993). Pregnancy after fertilisation with human testicular spermatozoa. *Lancet*, Vol.342, No.8881, pp. 1237

Shi, Q. & Martin, R. H. (2000). Aneuploidy in human sperm: a review of the frequency and distribution of aneuploidy, effects of donor age and lifestyle factors. *Cytogenet.Cell Genet.*, Vol.90, No.3-4, pp. 219-226

Shi, Q., Spriggs, E., Field, L. L., Ko, E., Barclay, L. & Martin, R. H. (2001). Single sperm typing demonstrates that reduced recombination is associated with the production of aneuploid 24,XY human sperm. *Am.J.Med.Genet.*, Vol.99, No.1, pp. 34-38

Silber, S., Escudero, T., Lenahan, K., Abdelhadi, I., Kilani, Z. & Munne, S. (2003). Chromosomal abnormalities in embryos derived from testicular sperm extraction. *Fertil.Steril.*, Vol.79, No.1, pp. 30-38

Soares, S. R., Templado, C., Blanco, J., Egozcue, J. & Vidal, F. (2001). Numerical chromosome abnormalities in the spermatozoa of the fathers of children with trisomy 21 of paternal origin: generalised tendency to meiotic non-disjunction. *Hum.Genet.*, Vol.108, No.2, pp. 134-139

Stahl, P. J., Stember, D. S. & Goldstein, M. (2011). Contemporary Management of Male Infertility. *Annu.Rev.Med.* Vol 63, No.18, pp. 1-16

Sun, F., Oliver-Bonet, M., Liehr, T., Starke, H., Ko, E., Rademaker, A., Navarro, J., Benet, J. & Martin, R. H. (2004a). Human male recombination maps for individual chromosomes. *Am.J.Hum.Genet.*, Vol.74, No.3, pp. 521-531

Sun, F., Kozak, G., Scott, S., Trpkov, K., Ko, E., Mikhaail-Philips, M., Bestor, T. H., Moens, P. & Martin, R. H. (2004b). Meiotic defects in a man with non-obstructive azoospermia: case report. *Hum.Reprod.*, Vol.19, No.8, pp. 1770-1773

Sun, F., Oliver-Bonet, M., Liehr, T., Starke, H., Trpkov, K., Ko, E., Rademaker, A. & Martin, R. H. (2005). Discontinuities and unsynapsed regions in meiotic chromosomes have a cis effect on meiotic recombination patterns in normal human males. *Hum.Mol.Genet.*, Vol.14, No.20, pp. 3013-3018

Sun, F., Oliver-Bonet, M., Liehr, T., Starke, H., Turek, P., Ko, E., Rademaker, A. & Martin, R. H. (2006). Variation in MLH1 distribution in recombination maps for individual chromosomes from human males. *Hum.Mol.Genet.*, Vol.15, No.15, pp. 2376-2391

Sun, F., Turek, P., Greene, C., Ko, E., Rademaker, A. & Martin, R. H. (2007). Abnormal progression through meiosis in men with nonobstructive azoospermia. *Fertil.Steril.*, Vol.87, No.3, pp. 565-571

Sun, F., Mikhaail-Philips, M., Oliver-Bonet, M., Ko, E., Rademaker, A., Turek, P. & Martin, R. H. (2008a). Reduced meiotic recombination on the XY bivalent is correlated with an increased incidence of sex chromosome aneuploidy in men with non-obstructive azoospermia. *Mol.Hum.Reprod.*, Vol.14, No.7, pp. 399-404

Sun, F., Mikhaail-Philips, M., Oliver-Bonet, M., Ko, E., Rademaker, A., Turek, P. & Martin, R. H. (2008b). The relationship between meiotic recombination in human spermatocytes and aneuploidy in sperm. *Hum.Reprod.*, Vol.23, No.8, pp. 1691-1697

Tang, S. S., Gao, H., Robinson, W. P., Ho Yuen, B. & Ma, S. (2004). An association between sex chromosomal aneuploidy in sperm and an abortus with 45,X of paternal origin: possible transmission of chromosomal abnormalities through ICSI. *Hum.Reprod.*, Vol.19, No.1, pp. 147-151

Tassistro, V., Ghalamoun-Slami, R., Saias-Magnan, J. & Guichaoua, M. R. (2009). Chronology of meiosis & synaptonemal complex abnormalities in normal & abnormal spermatogenesis. *Indian J.Med.Res.*, Vol.129, No.3, pp. 268-278

Tempest, H. G., Ko, E., Rademaker, A., Chan, P., Robaire, B. & Martin, R. H. (2009). Intra-individual and inter-individual variations in sperm aneuploidy frequencies in normal men. *Fertil.Steril.*, Vol.91, No.1, pp. 185-192

Templado, C., Vidal, F. & Estop, A. (2011). Aneuploidy in human spermatozoa. *Cytogenet.Genome Res.*, Vol.133, No.2-4, pp. 91-99

Thomas, N. S. & Hassold, T. J. (2003). Aberrant recombination and the origin of Klinefelter syndrome. *Hum.Reprod.Update*, Vol.9, No.4, pp. 309-317

Tournaye, H., Devroey, P., Liu, J., Nagy, Z., Lissens, W. & Van Steirteghem, A. (1994). Microsurgical epididymal sperm aspiration and intracytoplasmic sperm injection: a new effective approach to infertility as a result of congenital bilateral absence of the vas deferens. *Fertil.Steril.*, Vol.61, No.6, pp. 1045-1051

Ushijima1, C., Kumasako, Y., Kihaile, P. E., Hirotsuru, K. & Utsunomiya, T. (2000). Analysis of chromosomal abnormalities in human spermatozoa using multi-colour fluorescence in-situ hybridization. *Hum.Reprod.*, Vol.15, No.5, pp. 1107-1111

Vallente, R. U., Cheng, E. Y. & Hassold, T. J. (2006). The synaptonemal complex and meiotic recombination in humans: new approaches to old questions. *Chromosoma*, Vol.115, No.3, pp. 241-249

Van Opstal, D., Los, F. J., Ramlakhan, S., Van Hemel, J. O., Van Den Ouweland, A. M., Brandenburg, H., Pieters, M. H., Verhoeff, A., Vermeer, M. C., Dhont, M. & In't Veld, P. A. (1997). Determination of the parent of origin in nine cases of prenatally detected chromosome aberrations found after intracytoplasmic sperm injection. *Hum.Reprod.*, Vol.12, No.4, pp. 682-686

Van Steirteghem, A. C., Nagy, Z., Joris, H., Liu, J., Staessen, C., Smitz, J., Wisanto, A. & Devroey, P. (1993). High fertilization and implantation rates after intracytoplasmic sperm injection. *Hum.Reprod.*, Vol.8, No.7, pp. 1061-1066

Van Steirteghem, A., Bonduelle, M., Devroey, P. & Liebaers, I. (2002). Follow-up of children born after ICSI. *Hum.Reprod.Update,* Vol.8, No.2, pp. 111-116

Vegetti, W., Van Assche, E., Frias, A., Verheyen, G., Bianchi, M. M., Bonduelle, M., Liebaers, I. & Van Steirteghem, A. (2000). Correlation between semen parameters and sperm aneuploidy rates investigated by fluorescence in-situ hybridization in infertile men. *Hum.Reprod.,* Vol.15, No.2, pp. 351-365

Vendrell, J. M., Garcia, F., Veiga, A., Calderon, G., Egozcue, S., Egozcue, J. & Barri, P. N. (1999). Meiotic abnormalities and spermatogenic parameters in severe oligoasthenozoospermia. *Hum.Reprod.,* Vol.14, No.2, pp. 375-378

Viville, S., Warter, S., Meyer, J. M., Wittemer, C., Loriot, M., Mollard, R. & Jacqmin, D. (2000). Histological and genetic analysis and risk assessment for chromosomal aberration after ICSI for patients presenting with CBAVD. *Hum.Reprod.,* Vol.15, No.7, pp. 1613-1618

Yanagimachi, R., Yanagimachi, H. & Rogers, B. J. (1976). The use of zona-free animal ova as a test-system for the assessment of the fertilizing capacity of human spermatozoa. *Biol.Reprod.,* Vol.15, No.4, pp. 471-476

9

Morphology and Aneuploidy of *in vitro* Matured (IVM) Human Oocytes

Lidija Križančić Bombek[1], Borut Kovačič[2] and Veljko Vlaisavljević[2]
[1]*Institute of Physiology, Faculty of Medicine, University of Maribor*
[2]*Department of Reproductive Medicine and Gynecologic Endocrinology*
University Clinical Centre Maribor
Slovenia

1. Introduction

In vitro matured (IVM) human oocytes are very sensitive to culturing conditions. There are many external factors influencing their nuclear and cytoplasmic maturation, which can lead to morphologic or genetic abnormalities. Even oocytes themselves can possess some intrinsic abnormalities in biochemical cell cycle regulation which prevent them from reaching maturity *in vivo*. The following chapter will describe different morphological characteristics and their possible connection to aneuploidy, fertilization and embryo development. Also it will cover some aspects of oocyte IVM and describe mechanisms leading to aneuploidy. The second part of the chapter will be devoted to fluorescent *in situ* hybridization (FISH) analysis of IVM oocytes and first polar bodies (PB1) with the emphasis on aneuploidy occurrence in oocytes with prolonged cultivation.

2. Changes in the oocyte during maturation (oogenesis)

2.1 Introduction

Oogenesis includes many mechanisms that enable cytoplasmic and nuclear maturation in exact timing and succession. The first meiotic arrest occurs early in prenatal life when the oocyte proceeds through the first stages of meiosis and stops at the diplotene of the first prophase. This stage is called germinal vesicle stage (GV) and is characterized by a clearly visible large nucleus with nucleolus (Figure 1b). The maintenance of the meiotic arrest involves many complex molecular mechanisms and interactions with cumulus cells that communicate with the oocyte through cell junctions (Brower & Schultz, 1982; Gilchrist et al., 2004; Goud et al., 1998; Motta et al., 1994).

Human oocytes acquire the ability to overcome the meiotic arrest during simultaneous nuclear and cytoplasmic maturation. During nuclear maturation chromatin remodeling enables the transition of the oocyte through the succeeding meiotic phases from the first prophase to the second meiotic metaphase (M II; Figure 1d), where the second meiotic arrest occurs. On the other hand, cytoplasmic maturation involves synthesis of ribonucleic acids (RNA) and proteins, oocyte growth, rearrangement of organelles and cytoskeleton changes (Albertini et al., 2003). Research on mice has shown that nuclear and the cytoplasmic maturation can be achieved independently. Nevertheless, normal oocyte development can only take its proper course if the two modes are temporarily matched (Eppig, 1996).

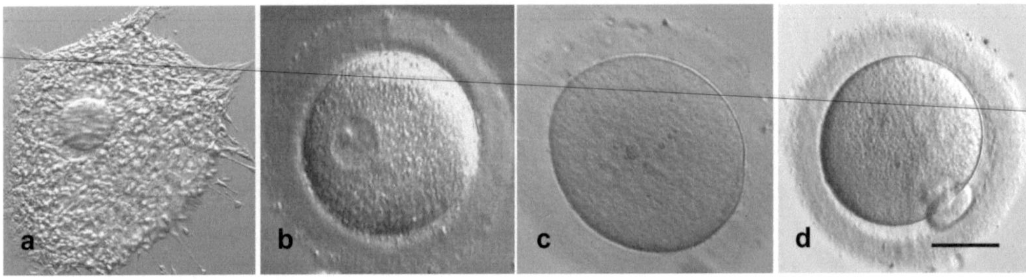

Fig. 1. Stages of oocyte maturation.
Oocyte surrounded by cumulus cells (a), Immature oocyte with visible germinal vesicle (GV) after mechanical and enzymatic removal of cumulus cells (b); immature oocyte in first metaphase (M I) (c); mature oocyte in second metaphase (M II) with clearly visible first polar body (PB1) (d). Magnification: ×100 (a), ×400 (b - d); bar: 150 µm (a), 50 µm (b - d).

2.1.1 Chromatin

Growth of a GV oocyte depends on intensive RNA synthesis which stops as the oocyte reaches its final size (Miyara et al., 2003). Studies including animal and human oocytes have shown that chromatin in GV oocytes of different final sizes is distinctly organized, which affects their maturation competence and later determines the course of embryo development (Combelles et al., 2002; Motlik & Fulka, 1976; Lefevre et al., 1989; Liu et al., 2006; Sun et al., 2004; Zuccotti et al., 1995). Chromatin remodeling includes morphologic changes such as condensation and de-condensation as well as functional changes such as transcription of particular chromatin regions. The major post-translational biochemical events during remodeling include acetylation and phosphorylation of different histones and chromatin methylation (De La Fuente, 2006; Spinaci et al., 2004).

Chromatin condensation is an indirect indicator of the cessation of gene transcription as well as RNA translation into proteins that have been taking place during the growth phase (Albertini et al., 2003). Those oocytes that have reached their final size and at the same time have the majority of chromatin configured in a circle around the nucleolus with some dense chromatin granules scattered across the nucleus, have optimum maturation capacity (Combelles et al., 2002).

The first visible sign of meiosis resumption is a gradual germinal vesicle breakdown (GVBD). The nuclear envelope disintegrates while the chromosomes remain at their position (Motlik & Fulka, 1976). *In vitro*, GVBD starts in less than 6 hours after the removal of the oocyte from the ovary (Combelles et al., 2002), presuming that the oocyte has already reached its final size before the establishment of *in vitro* conditions (Mrazek & Fulka, 2003). The GVBD phase itself lasts for approximately 12 hours (Angell, 1995).

2.1.2 Cytoskeleton

GV oocytes possess a dense sub-cortical microtubular network that is characteristic of interphase cells (Combelles et al., 2002). At the onset of GVBD, microtubules begin to assemble in the centrosomes (which contain microtubules organizing centers - MTOCs) as small star-like structures called asters, whereas there are no free microtubules in the cytoplasm. Later, the microtubules elongate and asters migrate towards opposite poles forming a barrel-like structure called meiotic spindle. The highly condensed chromosomes attach to the microtubules at their centromeric regions and align in the metaphase equatorial plane between both poles of the meiotic spindle (Battaglia et al., 1996).

In the first anaphase, chromosomes move toward the poles of the meiotic spindle located at the animal pole of the oocyte (Matsuura & Chiba, 2004). In the next phase, namely the first telophase microtubules can be observed as very dense network of threads spreading between the chromatin of the oocyte and its first polar body (PB1).

Actin filaments, also called microfilaments, regulate various dynamic processes during oocyte maturation. Although they are not directly involved in GVBD and meiotic spindle formation, they play a key role in rearrangement of cell organelles and cell polarization (Albertini et al., 2003). They are also responsible for the positioning of the meiotic spindle, movement and separation of chromosomes and extrusion of the PB1 (Kim et al., 1998; Sun & Schatten, 2006).

2.1.3 Cell organelles

Growth of an oocyte is also characterized by redistribution of cell organelles into a sub-cortical region beneath the cell membrane, whereas during the maturation phase they are distributed more centrally (Albertini et al., 2003). The only exceptions are the cortical granules which are translocated from the smooth endoplasmic reticulum towards the periphery of the oocyte by the microfilaments and are distributed immediately beneath the plasma membrane in the fully grown mature oocyte (Sun et al., 2001).

The cytoplasm of the oocyte contains many mitochondria providing energy for all cell processes (Van Blerkom, 2004). Their redistribution and gathering around the nucleus (germinal vesicle) during maturation has been attributed to the action of microtubules (Sun & Schatten, 2006).

The cytoplasm of a mature oocyte contains smooth endoplasmic reticulum and lysosomes, whereas there is almost no rough endoplasmic reticulum or ribosomes since the mature oocyte is quiescent and the protein synthesis does not take place (Sathananthan, 1997; Sathananthan et al., 2006).

2.1.4 Biochemical regulation of the cell cycle

One of the most important factors enabling the continuation of the cell cycle is the M-phase (maturation) promoting factor (MPF), consisting of cyclin B and $p34^{cdc2}$ (Gautier et al,. 1988). In the immature oocyte, it is present in its inactive phosphorylated form (Lohka et al., 1988). The amount of cyclin B and consequently the amount of MPF are changing cyclically during the oocyte growth and are highest just prior to the GVBD. Preceding the meiosis resumption, activation of MPF by dephosphorylation takes place.

A key regulator of oocyte maturation process is a product of *c-mos* proto-oncogene called $p39^{mos}$. It belongs to a family of serine/threonine-specific protein kinases and is sensitive to concentration of Ca^{2+} ions, which is involved in activation or stabilization of MPF (Gebauer

& Richter, 1997; Sagata, 1997). A direct consequence of MPF's action on a variety of different molecules in the cell is GVBD, protein phosphorylation and chromosome condensation (Chian et al., 2003; Smitz et al., 2004; Whitaker, 1996). In the first anaphase, the concentration of MPF abruptly declines due to cyclin B degradation. But in the subsequent first telophase, it increases again as the PB1 is extruded and the now mature oocyte is arrested in the second metaphase without the intervening interphase (Dekel, 1995, 2005).

The stimulatory effects of MPF are counteracted by cyclic adenosine monophosphate (cAMP). It acts so as to attain the cell in the quiescent state by activating protein kinase A (PKA) which in turn hinders $p34^{cdc2}$ dephosphorylation and consequently prevents GVBD. Sufficient cAMP concentration is achieved by purine bases such as hypoxanthine and adenosine which impede phosphodiesterase activity thereby stopping the meiosis (Downs et al., 1989). Both molecules enter the oocyte through cell junctions from cumulus cells surrounding it. When the cell junctions are interrupted in the course of maturation, the level of cAMP drops under a critical level and meiosis can resume (Schultz et al., 1983).

3. *In vitro* maturation (IVM) of human oocytes

3.1 IVM methods

The increasing frequency of infertility in women and men has facilitated the development of assisted reproduction technology (ART). Among ART methods is also the *in vitro* maturation (IVM) method, whereby oocytes are aspirated immature and grown in an incubator in a medium supplied with proper growth factors and in suitable atmosphere until they eventually reach M II stage. It has been shown that 34-82 % of the immature oocytes reach M II stage (Cha & Chian, 1998; Chian & Tan, 2002; Goud et al., 1998; Janssenswillen et al., 1995; Kim et al., 2000; Roberts et al., 2002).

Oocytes can be matured *in vitro* following two main protocols. In the first one, oocytes are acquired by aspiration of antral follicles with the diameter of up to 10 mm without any preceding ovarian hormonal stimulation. This method requires presence of cumulus-oophorus cells surrounding the oocyte during the cultivation period, since they secrete certain biochemical factors responsible for proper oocyte development and maturation (Chian et al., 2004a, 2004b; Schramm & Bavister, 1995; Tan & Child, 2002; Trounson et al., 2001). When using the alternative IVM method, oocytes are aspirated after a short hormonal stimulation, with or without the application of human chorionic gonadotropin (HCG), which increases the efficacy and the speed of their maturation (Smitz et al., 2004). In this protocol, cumulus cells are not essential for the oocyte development (Kim et al., 2000; Chian and Tan, 2002), however maturation is more synchronous in the presence of the cumulus oophorus (Kim et al., 2000) and more oocytes reach the maturity (Goud et al., 1998).

Metabolism of immature oocytes differs from that of mature oocytes or embryos. As a consequence, oocyte's maturation competence is affected by the composition of the cultivation medium (Cekleniak et al., 2001; Chian and Tan, 2002; Christopikou et al., 2010; Downs & Hudson, 2000; Herrick et al., 2006; Kovačič &Vlaisavljević, 2002; Sutton et al., 2003). Furthermore, it has been shown that FSH, which is sometimes used to speed up maturation, increases oocyte aneuploidy rate (Roberts et al., 2005; Xu et al., 2011).

In vitro matured oocytes are capable of normal fertilization and embryo development but the success rate is rather low (De Vos et al., 1999; Kim et al., 2000) and only a few children have been born after IVM (Edirisinghe et al., 1997; Friden et al., 2005; Liu et al., 1997; Liu et al., 2003; Nagy et al., 1996; Vanhoutte et al., 2005). Possible reasons include suboptimal IVM conditions as well as genetic and epigenetic characteristics of oocytes themselves. In many human and animal 6 to 8-cell IVM embryos, genome activation does not take place (Kim et al. 2004; Schramm et al., 2003). This hindered embryo development is thought to be a consequence of disturbed cytoplasmic maturation or asyncronicity between the cytoplasmic and nuclear maturation in the oocyte.

In vitro, oocytes begin their maturation earlier than *in vivo* (Motlik & Fulka, 1976) which is most probably a consequence of their premature extraction from the ovaries (Sanfins et al., 2004). Ovarian follicles contain inhibiting factors that retain the oocyte at proper meiotic phase for adequate time. If the oocyte is extracted from the follicle too soon the growth and developmental phase is shortened which can lead to nuclear and cytoplasmic anomalies (Trounson et al., 1998). Furthermore, the majority of IVM oocytes are unable to maintain M II phase until fertilization but undergo spontaneous transition into first mitotic interphase within the next 24 hours. This could be caused by impeded cell cycle regulation at the level of microtubules dynamics or chromatin phosphorylation (Combelles et al., 2002).

Following IVM many oocytes do not reach M II phase at all or they mature but are unable to develop into normal embryos. Reasons for development stagnation could be manifold, ranging from cytoplasmic immaturity and meiotic spindle formation abnormalities (Combelles et al., 2003; Eichenlaub-Ritter et al., 1988; Miyara et al., 2003; Mrazek & Fulka, 2003; Neal et al., 2002; Pickering et al., 1988) to chromatin fragmentation followed by the appearance of micronuclei (Junk et al., 2002). Also, the *in vitro* cultivation conditions can be sub-optimal (Chian and Tan, 2002; Junk et al., 2002; Trounson et al., 2001) or the intrinsic factors such as abnormal cell cycle control or affected gene regulation can impede proper oocyte development (Combelles et al., 2003; Eichenlaub-Ritter & Peschke, 2002; Kim et al., 2004). For all those reasons, the safe routine clinical use of IVM oocytes is still under debate, since the quality of such oocytes seems low. Some investigations have been done concerning structural characteristics of chromatin and meiotic spindle, however little is actually known about chromosomal abnormalities of IVM oocytes.

3.2 Morphological characteristics of IVM oocytes

The cytoplasm of a good-quality mature (M II) human oocyte is clear and homogenous, its perivitelline space containing the oval-shaped first polar body (PB1) is narrow, and the zona pellucida is colorless (Veeck, 1988). During the development of ART methods, it was observed that embryos originating from *in vivo* matured oocytes develop and implant better than those originating form IVM oocytes (Trounson et al., 1998; Mikkelsen & Lindenberg, 2001). Furthermore, an increased number of IVM embryos contain multinuclear blastomeres (Nogueira et al., 2000).

IVM oocytes show similar morphological characteristics as *in vivo* matured oocytes regarding cytoplasm, PB1 and perivitelline space. About 56 % of IVM oocytes have normal morphology, the rest having one (34 %), two (8-9 %) or all three (1-2 %) characteristics abnormal (Mikkelsen & Lindenberg, 2001).

3.2.1 Cytoplasm

The cytoplasm is normal in about 72-88 % of IVM oocytes (Figure 2a), but it can also be evenly granular (8-13 %, Figure 2b), unevenly granular (4 %, Figure 2d) or it can contain vacuoles (2–3 %, Figure 2c) (Balaban et al., 1998; De Sutter et al., 1996; Van Blerkom & Henry, 1992). The length of the cultivation period as well as hormonal stimulation, patients' age and cultivation medium somewhat change the frequency of each cytoplasmic type (Xia, 1997; Van Blerkom & Davis, 2001).

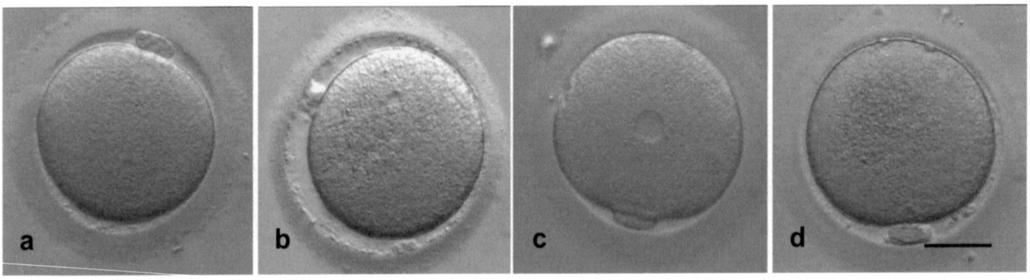

Fig. 2. Cytoplasm morphology of IVM oocytes.
Cytoplasm of a mature oocyte can be normal (a), evenly granular and darker (b), vacuolated (c) or unevenly granular resembling halo (d). Magnificaion: ×400; bar: 50 µm.

The presence of cytoplasmic inclusions is a marker of cellular irregularities which can lead to decreased fertilization as well as decreased number of good-quality embryos. Blastomere division and embryo quality is most strongly affected by cytoplasmic irregularities such as granular or dark cytoplasm and vacuoles (Mikkelsen & Lindenberg, 2001).

In mature oocytes from stimulated ART cycles, seven types of cytoplasmic irregularities were identified that were clearly associated with various fertilization and embryo development problems as well as with chromosomal abnormalities (Van Blerkom, 1990; Van Blerkom & Henry, 1992). The greatest frequency of aneuploid oocytes (32-50 %) has been observed among oocytes with dark or granular cytoplasm, and with clustered organelles such as smooth endoplasmic reticulum (Van Blerkom, 1990; Otsuki et al., 2004).

It seems that vacuoles have little influence on the aneuploidy frequency (4 % of vacuolated oocytes are aneuploid). However, increasing vacuole diameter negatively influences the fertilization rate because vacuoles interfere with cytoskeleton functioning and formation of the meiotic spindle (Ebner et al., 2005; Van Blerkom, 1990).

3.2.2 First polar body (PB1)

The most reliable indicator of nuclear maturity of the oocyte is the extruded first polar body (PB1), whose fragmentation has clearly been linked to decreased fertilization, embryo development, blastulation and implantation (Ebner et al., 1999, 2000, 2006).

PB1 of IVM oocytes shows four major morphological appearances. It can be normal - oval shaped (68-71 %, Figure 3a), fragmented (9 %, Figure 3b), invaginated (7-18 %, Figure 3c) or enlarged (3-6 %, Figure 3d). There is a clear tendency towards increasing frequency of invaginated PB1s in those oocytes that need longer time to attain maturity, suggesting that some intrinsic cellular mechanisms, which are most probably affecting proper meiotic spindle functioning, prevent normal diakinesis and PB1 extrusion. Further evidence for impaired meiotic spindle functioning in oocytes with invaginated PB1 is only 25 % fertilization rate and embryo arrest at a 2-cell stage (Xia, 1997).

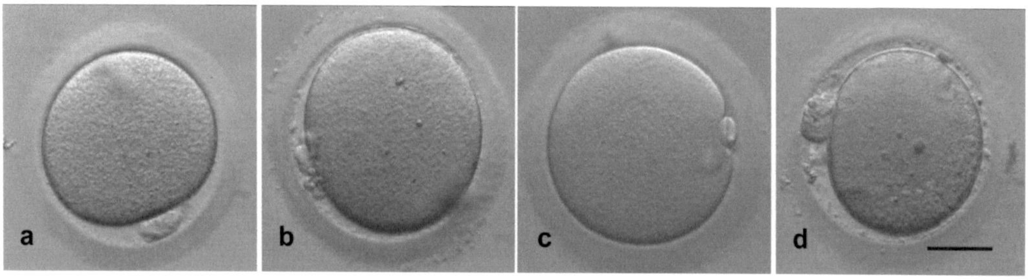

Fig. 3. First polar body (PB1) morphology of IVM oocytes.
PB1 can be normal (a), fragmented (b), invaginated (c) or enlarged (d). Magnificaion: ×400; bar: 50 μm.

Morphology of PB1 strongly depends on the age of the oocyte. Very soon after its extrusion it begins to deteriorate which changes its appearance in just a few hours. Mainly the deterioration is seen as PB1 fragmentation, which implies that attention has to be paid to morphology evaluation timing (Ciotti et al., 2004; Verlinsky et al., 2003). In IVM procedures, PB1s are usually assessed within a few hours after being extruded from the oocyte. Consequently, the frequency of fragmented PB1s (9 %) is a reflection of its actual morphology anomalies. If the incidence of fragmentation is assessed among *in vivo* matured oocytes, the frequency is usually 25-34 % (Ciotti et al., 2004; Verlinsky et al., 2003), which might be a consequence of evaluation timing after the PB1 extrusion, or an aftermath of stimulation protocols, cultivation media or even high concentrations of hormones in the follicular fluid, to which the *in vivo* matured oocytes are exposed (Xia & Younglai, 2000).

3.2.3 Perivitelline space and zona pellucida

Normally perivitelline space is narrow and contains no inclusions or debris. However, in many oocytes from ART cycles there is a substantial amount of inclusions of various sizes between the plasma membrane and zona pellucida. Their origin is not yet completely elucidated, but most probably they are the remnants of cumulus cells' extensions, through which the oocyte has been communicating with its surrounding during the growth phase. It is interesting to note that no debris is present in the GV stage, whereas its amount increases simultaneously with maturation progression, so that around 4 % of M I cells and 34 % of M II cells have some inclusions in their perivitelline space. This phenomenon is most probably completely physiological (Hassan-Ali et al., 1998).

Perivitelline space morphology is normal in 85-87 % of IVM oocytes (Figure 4a). Some have little (3-4 %) or plenty (1-2 %) of debris under zona pellucida (Figures 4b-c), whereas in 4-10 % of oocytes the perivitelline space is enlarged (Figure 4d). The later is created by a premature release of cortical granules (Okada et al., 1986) and there is a tendency of increasing percentage of oocytes with the enlarged perivitelline space in oocytes with longer duration of IVM.

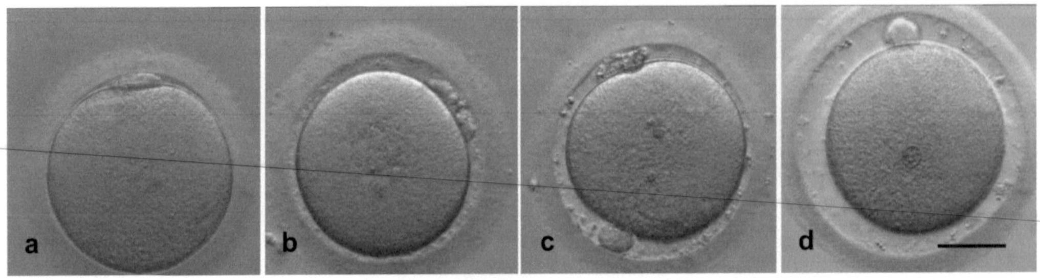

Fig. 4. Perivitelline space morphology of IVM oocytes.
Normal perivitelline space (a) can be easily distinguished from a perivitelline space with little (b) or plenty of debris (c) as well as from the enlarged one (d). Magnificaion: ×400; bar: 50 µm.

Opinions of different researchers on the correlation between oocyte morphology and aneuploidy as well as on implantation and embryo development remain divided due to large discrepancies in ovarian stimulation protocols, oocyte cultivation conditions and embryo assessment criteria (Balaban et al., 1998; Ciotti et al., 2004; De Santis et al., 2005; De Sutter et al., 1996; Ebner et al., 1999, 2000, 2006; Van Blerkom, 1990, 1996; Xia, 1997).

After the introduction of polarization microscopy to human ART methods, it has become possible not only to observe meiotic spindle characteristics and chromosome alignment in live oocytes (Wang et al., 2001) but also to evaluate the integrity of zona pellucida, the outermost barrier between the oocyte and its surrounding. When exposed to polarized light, human zona pellucida shows three-layer architecture defined by different birefringence characteristics (double refraction of light) of each layer. It has been suggested that birefringence is associated with the arrangement of proteins, polysaccharides and glycoproteins within the zona, which change during maturation. The best fertilization rate and embryo development has clearly been linked with those oocytes that possess highly birefringent zona pellucida (reviewed by Montag et al., 2011).

4. Aneuploidy mechanisms during meiosis

4.1 Introduction

Chromosome abnormalities can appear at different stages during oogenesis. Even before the entrance into meiosis, gonadal stem cells divide mitoticaly many times whereby each division represents an opportunity for emergence of gonadal mosaicism (Cozzi et al., 1999). The majority of oocyte aneuploidies originate in the first meiotic division. There are two major mechanisms causing aneuploidies, namely whole chromosome non-disjunction and premature balanced or unbalanced chromatid separation (Cupisti et al., 2003; Delhanty, 2005; Hassold et al., 1995; Kuliev et al., 2003; Kuliev & Verlinsky, 2004; Pellestor, 1991; Pellestor et al., 2002, 2006).

4.2 Chromosome non-disjunction

In case of whole chromosome non-disjunction during anaphase I, a whole tetrad (bivalent; a pair of associated homologous chromosomes, each consisting of two chromatids after

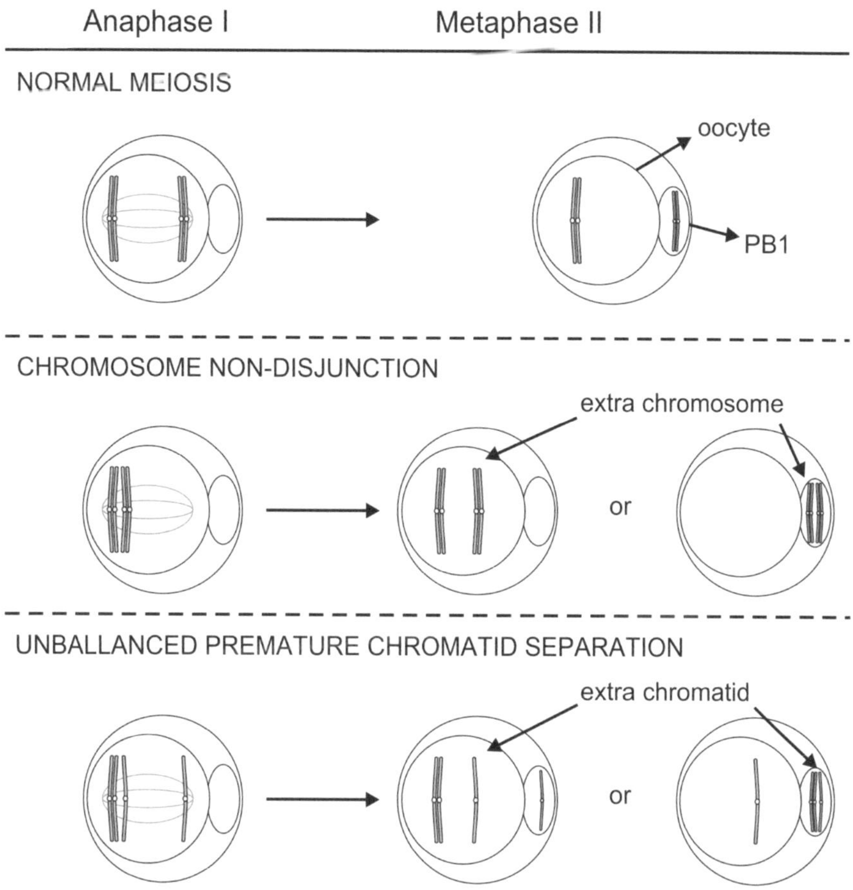

Fig. 5. Aneuploidy types.
Chromatid (FISH signals) arrangement in diakinezis I, anaphase I and metaphase II in case of normal meiosis, chromosome non-disjunction and unballanced premature chromatid separation.

chromosome replication) is moved to one pole of the meiotic spindle instead of the two homologous chromosomes moving one to each pole (Figure 5). Usually the chromatids in the two homologous chromosomes do not remain attached to each other (Angell, 1997). Non-disjunction can affect any chromosome in the cell independently or it can affect all of them at the same time. Upon analyzing an oocyte with fluorescent *in situ* hybridization (FISH) four signals in an oocyte (disomy, Figure 7b) and none in its corresponding PB1 are seen for the affected chromosome. In case of nullisomy no FISH signal for a particular chromosome are present in the oocyte, whereas there are four in its PB1 (Figure 7a).

If the chromosome non-disjunction affects all chromosomes of the oocyte in the same way, the newly formed oocyte is said to be diploid (Figure 7f). All chromosomes remain in the oocyte, whereas in its PB1 there is no genetic material. Non-disjunction is more frequent in oocytes of older women (Angell, 1997; Dailey et al., 1996; Pellestor et al., 2003) and is in cases of chromosomes 15, 16, 18 and 21 sometimes linked to decreased number of chiasmata or changes in recombination sites (Hassold et al., 2000; Lamb et al., 2005).

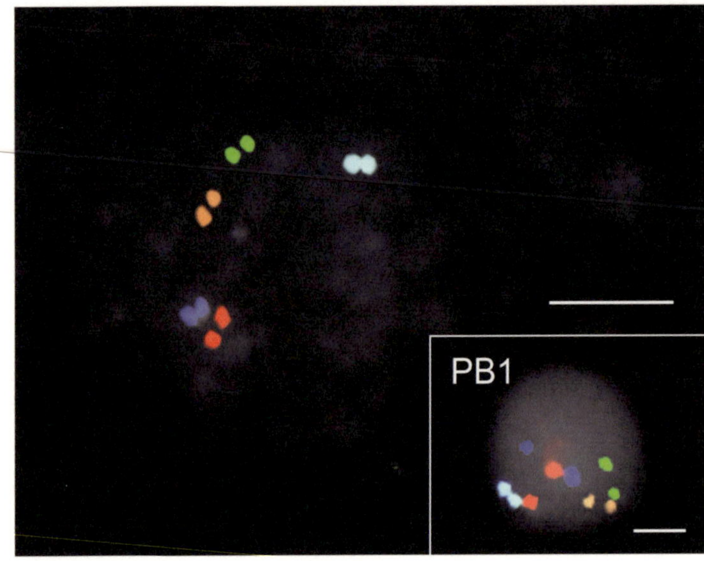

Fig. 6. Normal oocyte and PB1 in IVM oocyte.
In the oocyte and its corresponding PB1 (inset) two signals for each of the chromosomes 13 (red arrows), 16 (light blue arrows), 18 (blue arrows), 21 (green arrows) and 22 (orange arrows) are clearly seen. Each signal represents one chromatid. Magnification ×1000; bar 10 µm.

4.3 Premature chromatid separation

In meiosis I, the most frequent aneuploidy producing mechanism is premature chromatid separation in anaphase I (Fragouli et al., 2011). It is characterized by premature decomposition of cohesins which serve to establish a link between the two sister chromatids after chromosome replication (Michaelis et al., 1997). In case of premature chromatid separation, upon segregation the two free chromatids of one homologous chromosome can be pulled to the same or to different poles of the meiotic spindle. In a situation where both chromatids of one homologous chromosome travel to the same spindle pole, whereas the other homologous chrome travels to the opposite pole, a FISH analysis would show two signals for that particular chromosome in the oocyte as well as in its PB1 (balanced premature chromatid separation). Therefore, a normal chromatid count would be obtained except that in either the oocyte or PB1 the two signals will be separated (homologous chromosome with separated chromatids) whereas in the other the two signals will be close to each other (normal homologous chromosome). This type of premature chromatid separation is more common in oocytes that were exposed to *in vitro* conditions for longer time and its frequency increases from 6 to 53 % within 24-48 hours (Munne et al., 1995b).

In unbalanced premature chromatid separation, chromatids of the affected homologous chromosome travel to opposite poles of the meiotic spindle. If an oocyte contains one whole homologuous chromosome plus one extra chromatid of the other homologuous chromosome, which should normally be expelled from the oocyte into the PB1, FISH analysis would reproduce three signals for that particular chromosome in the oocyte. Such oocyte is said to be hyperhaploid (Figure 7d) for that specific chromosome, whereas its corresponding BP1 contains only one chromatid and is said to be hypohaploid. In case of one missing chromatid in the oocyte, the oocyte is said to be hypohaploid (Figure 7c) and its PB, which contains three signals is hyperhaploid.

Unbalanced premature chromatid separation can affect any chromosome, but is more frequent in chromosomes of groups D (chromosomes 13 to 15), E (chromosomes 16 to 18) and G (chromosomes 21 and 22) (Pellestor, 1991; Pellestor et al., 2002). The only factor unequivocally linked to increased aneuploidy rate is women age (Dailey et al., 1996; Kuliev et al., 2005; Sandalinas et al., 2002). In younger women (25-34 years of age) the frequency of premature chromatid separation is only 1.5 %, whereas in women aged 40-45 years it increases to more than 24 % (Dailey et al., 1996).

4.4 Aneuploidy of ART oocytes

Most research regarding oocyte aneuploidy in ART cycles has been done on oocytes that failed to be fertilized within 24-48 hours after insemination (Anachory et al., 2003; Angell et al., 1991a, Benkhalifa et al., 2003; Clyde et al., 2003; Cupisti et al., 2003; Kim et al., 2004; Pellestor et al., 2002, 2005, 2006). There are great discrepancies on the aneuploidy rate ranging from 8-54 %, which can be a consequence of different stimulation protocols (Munne et al., 1997), women age (Kuliev et al., 2003, 2005; Pellestor et al., 2003; Sandalinas et al., 2002; Vialard et al., 2006), and number of chromosomes analyzed per oocyte (Gutierrez-Mateo et al., 2004a; Pellestor et al., 2003, 2006; Sandalinas et al., 2002). Studies analyzing all 23 chromosomes revealed very high percentage of abnormal oocytes in unfertilized and *in vitro* matured oocytes (48-57 %, Gutierrez-Mateo et al., 2004a, 2004b) as well as in mature donated oocytes (29-56 % with respect to women age; Sandalinas et al., 2002).

Most frequently chromosomes 13, 15, 16, 21, 22 and X are affected in oocytes (Anahory et al., 2003; Benkhalifa et al., 2003; Clyde et al., 2003; Cupisti et al., 2003; Pellestor et al., 2002; Pujol et al., 2003; Sandalinas et al., 2002), which is similar to most affected chromosomes in embryos that include chromosomes 13, 15, 16, 17, 18, 21, 22, X and Y (Abdelhadi et al., 2003; Munne & Weier, 1996; Munne et al., 2003, 2004), supporting the idea that meiosis I is the main source of aneuploidies in human.

5. Preimplantation Genetic Diagnosis (PGD) on a single cell

Preimplantation genetic diagnosis (PGD) of aneuploidies is usually based on a biopsy of the first or both polar bodies of an oocyte (Durban et al., 1998; Kuliev et al., 2003; Verlinsky et al., 2001), or on a biopsy of 1-2 blastomeres of the created embryo (Gianaroli et al., 1999; Munne et al., 1993, 1995a, 1999). Lately, PGD has also been performed on a few trophectodermal cells of the blastocyst developed from the fertilized oocyte (de Boer et al., 2004). By analyzing oocytes and early embryos, different chromosomal abnormalities including aneuploidies, translocations and mutations can be detected (Durban et al., 2001; Munne et al., 1998a; Verlinsky & Kuliev, 2003; Verlinsky et al., 2004). Selection of chromosomally normal embryos increases implantation rate (Gianaroli et al., 1997, 1999, 2005) as well as decreases the frequency of spontaneous abortions (Munne et al., 2006).

The least invasive PGD method is the analysis of PB1, which is a byproduct of the first meiosis and does not play any significant role in further embryo development. Therefore, making a biopsy on the oocyte and taking its PB1 for aneuploidy analysis does not alter the oocyte's chromosomal status and only minimally affects the oocyte (Verlinsky et al., 1990). However, it provides a very useful indirect means for determining the oocyte's chromosomal status. Supplementing the PB1 analysis with the PB2 analysis, we get a powerful tool for uncovering the majority of aneuploidies derived from the oocyte during meiosis. In this way, ART clinicians can avoid intrauterine transfers of embryos affected by the oocyte's meiotic aneuploidies (Verlinsky et al., 1996, 1997-1998). Information about the oocyte's chromosomal status before fertilization, which we gain from the PB1 analysis, is indirect since PB1 contains exactly the complementary chromosomes / chromatids to the oocyte. Thus, a normal mature oocyte contains one copy of each of the 22 autosomal chromosomes (two chromatids each) and one copy of gonosome X (two chromatids). Exactly the same chromosomal status is found in PB1 of this oocyte. If any chromosomal abnormalities occurred during meiosis I, oocyte could carry an extra chromosome or chromatid, leaving a deficit of a specific chromosome or chromatid in the PB1, or vice versa (Verlinsky & Kuliev, 2000).

5.1 Oocyte, PB1 or blastomere fixation

The most critical step preceding chromosome analysis is PB1 or blastomere fixation. Because in PGD chromosome analysis is frequently done on a single cell, an ideal fixation method should provide as reliable spreading and fixation of chromosomes on the microscope slide as possible. Ideally, no chromosome or chromatid should be lost otherwise artificial aneuploidy would be diagnosed.

Classical fixation method, which uses a solution of methanol and acetic acid followed by air drying of the specimen (Tarkowski, 1966) produces a significant percentage of misdiagnoses due to chromosome or chromatid loss (Sugawara & Mikamo, 1986). Since its invention, it has been modified many times to ensure better reproducibility and reduce genetic material losses (Durban et al., 1998; Wramsby & Liedholm, 1984) or to be adapted for blastomere fixation (Coonen et al., 1994; Dozortsev & McGinnis, 2001). A comparative study has shown that among different fixation methods the one described by Dozortsev and McGinnis (2001) is simple to apply and returns satisfying percentage (83 %) of useful samples (Velilla et al., 2002).

When doing FISH on PB1 or blastomere it is essential to pay much attention to handling of the cell since both are very small and delicate. Therefore, they are easily damaged or even lost during fixation.

The most critical step in specimen preparation for FISH is spreading, during which the cell membrane breaks and chromosomes swim in hypotonic solution on the microscope slide. The amount of the hypotonic solution should be large enough, so that the spreading is sufficient and there is no overlap of chromosomes, enabling clear distinction between different signals (Velilla et al., 2002). At the same time, the spreading should not be too large so that all chromosomes can be clearly seen in a single visual field under large magnification of the microscope (Munne et al., 1996; Munne et al., 1998b). Despite the very precise handling, the percentage of non-applicable preparations due to PB1 loss is still around 12 % (Table 1).

	Total
Analyzed MII oocytes	**192**
Normal oocytes (%)	88 (45,8)
Aneuploid oocytes (%)	88 (45,8)
Lost oocytes during fixation (%)	7 (3,7)
FISH errors (%)	9 (4,7)
Analyzed PB1s	**129**
Oocyte diagnoses confirmed by PB1 diagnosis	102 (79,1)
Lost PB1 (%)	15 (11,6)
FISH errors (%)	8 (6,2)
Non-applicable oocyte preparations with good PB1 preparation (%)	4 (3,1)

Table 1. FISH analysis of chromosomes 13, 16, 18, 21 and 22 (MultiVysion® PB, Vysis) in oocytes and PB1s, which attained maturity after 24-36 hours of IVM in a simple embryo-cultivation medium.

The success of fixation method partially depends on the number of chromosomes tested and the analytical method used. With increasing number of tested chromosomes there is also an increasing probability of signal overlap. This is clearly demonstrated in FISH studies involving 6 to 9 chromosomes, where the percentage of analyzable slides decreased to some 61 % (Anahory et al., 2003; Gutierrez-Mateo et al., 2004a; Pujol et al., 2003). With the use of multicolor-FISH (M-FISH; Clyde et al., 2003), spectral karyotyping (SKY; Marquez et al., 1998; Sandalinas et al., 2002) or centromeric multicolor FISH (cenM-FISH; Gutierrez-Mateo et al., 2005), which enable simultaneous analysis of all 23 chromosomes, the percentage of useful specimen preparations decreases to mere 31-36 %. From the single cell analysis point of view, this low efficiency is inacceptable for clinical use.

5.2 Fluorescent *in situ* hybridization (FISH) and sources of FISH errors

Today, chromosome analysis is mostly done with FISH. It enables staining and detection of whole chromosomes or their parts on the basis of probe fluorescence after attachment to specific DNA sequences. By selecting a whole-chromosome probe, it is possible to identify aneuploidies as well as chromosome or chromatid structural malformations such as breaks, large deletions, translocations, etc. On the other hand, structural aberrations such as breaks, deletions, insertions and translocations cannot be identified with locus specific probes if they lie in the part of the genome not labeled with the probe. When there is a chance for embryo inheriting a known familiar chromosome aberration, a particular probe for a chromosome or locus of interest can be selected.

As already mentioned one of the most frequent FISH errors is a consequence of loosing genetic material during fixation or overspreading of chromosomes on the microscopic slide so that the chromosomes / chromatids cannot be seen in the same visual field. In preliminary studies of IVM oocytes, we had a chance to simultaneously analyze oocytes and their pertaining PB1s (Table 2). Whereas the analysis of the oocytes alone reported 50 % aneuploidy rate, this rate was lower (40.2 %) if pairs of oocyte-PB1 were analyzed. This is because only the diagnoses where the PB1 had exactly complementary chromosome status to the oocyte were considered accurate. The difference between the two approaches gives us an estimate of the occurrence (9.8 %) of FISH errors if only the oocyte is analyzed.

	Total
Analyzed MII oocytes	**176**
% of aneuploid oocytes	50.0
Analyzed MII oocytes with diagnoses confirmed by corresponding PB1s	**102**
% of aneuploid oocytes	40.2
% of FISH errors	**9.8**

Table 2. Estimation of the frequency of FISH errors using oocyte analysis alone compared to analysis of oocyte-PB1 pairs.

Another frequent cause of FISH errors is signal overlap, whereby we cannot discern between one signal and two or more overlapping ones for the same or for different chromosomes. Also there might appear some difficulties when using centromeric probes, since the two signals for sister chromatids may lie so close that it is hard to differentiate between one strong large signal and two weaker ones (usually they appear as two touching dots).

When analyzing chromosomes of the IVM oocytes and PB1s, special attention has to be paid to removing all cumulus oophorus cells surrounding the oocyte, since their genetic material might appear on the FISH specimens and thus cause diagnostic mistakes. Best way to eliminate the cumulus cells is to remove entire zona pellucida, and any attached cells or remnants of the cumulus, by partial enzymatic digestion followed by mechanical pipetting of the oocyte through a very thin pipette.

Because of FISH limitations, there is an increasing use of comparative genomic hybridization (CGH) for single cell analysis. In this method, polymerase chain reaction (PCR) is used to multiply the entire genome of the cell followed by identification of chromosomes or their parts with missing or excess amount of genetic material (Voullaire et al., 1999; Wells et al., 1999). The method is reliable however it does not enable the detection of genetic errors that affect all chromosomes equally (such as diploidy, triploidy, etc.) or balanced premature chromatid separation (Gutierrez-Mateo et al., 2004b). Besides, CGH takes a few days to be carried out, which is inappropriate for ART treatments since the tested embryos cannot be transferred to uterus at the right time or they have to be frozen until the results of genetic analysis are known (Wilton et al., 2003).

5.3 Aneuploidy occurrence in IVM oocytes

There were only few studies regarding chromosome analysis of IVM oocytes done so far, all of them reporting a high incidence of aneuploidy which ranges from 38 to 70 % (Clyde et al., 2003; Gutierrez-Mateo et al., 2004b; Magli et al., 2006; Pujol et al., 2003; Vlaisavljević et al., 2007). Different methods were used to elucidate the oocyte aneuploidy, among which M-FISH (multicolor-fluorescent *in situ* hybridization) and CGH (comparative genomic hybridization) were used to assess all 23 chromosomes and reported 38–48 % aneuploidy rate, that was increasing with the women's' age from 23 % in women 24 - 35 years of age up to 75 % in women older than 36 years (Clyde et al., 2003; Gutierrez-Mateo et al., 2004b). The consequences of the high aneuploidy rate are many abnormal embryos that develop from fertilized IVM oocytes. It was shown that up to 61 % of analyzed IVM embryos contain aneuploid blastomeres (Emery et al., 2005).

There is an increase in aneuploidy rate from 35 % to 49 % with increasing duration of *in vitro* maturation from 24-36 hours (Table 3A). Furthermore, multiple (complex, Figure 7e) aneuploidies are more common if the oocytes are exposed to maturation protocol for longer time (Table 3B). Also the number of affected chromosomes significantly increases with prolonged IVM (Table 3C) (Križančić Bombek L. et al., 2011). Possible reasons for these observations include exposure of oocytes to artificial milieu, lack of some unknown specific signals or growth factors in the cultivation medium, etc. On the contrary, it is also possible that oocytes already containing chromosome aberrations attain maturity later since their chromosomal abnormalities hinder the cell cycle continuation.

A	24 h	36 h
Analyzed oocyte-PB1 pairs	65	37
Normal oocytes (%)	42 (64.6)	19 (51.4)
Aneuploid oocytes (%)	23 (35.4) [a]	18 (48.6) [a]
B		
Oocytes with single aneuploidy (%)	15 (23.1)	12 (32.4)
Oocytes with double aneuploidy (%)	6 (9.2)	2 (5.4)
Oocytes with multiple aneuploidies (%)	2 (3.1) [b]	4 (10.8) [b]
C		
Analyzed chromosomes	325	185
Aneuploid chromosomes (%)	33 (10.15) [c]	32 (17.3) [c]

Table 3. Aneuploidy frequency of IVM oocytes matured for 24 or 36 hours.
FISH analysis (MultiVysion® PB, Vysis) of chromosomes 13, 16, 18, 21 and 22 in IVM oocytes.
[a] not statistically significant (chi-square test)
[b] No. too small for statistical analysis
[c] $p < 0.05$ (chi-square test)

When considering aneuploidy types, a difference between faster-maturing and slower-maturing oocytes can be observed. There is an increase in occurrence of hyperhaploid chromosomes compared to hypohaploid ones in slower-maturing oocytes (Table 4A) whereas such trend is not observed in oocytes attaining M II phase within 24 hours (Križančić Bombek L. et al., 2011). Similar results regarding oocytes were reported by other authors (Clyde et al., 2003; Gutierrez-Mateo et al., 2004a; Vialard et al., 2006) whereas the opposite situation, namely the excess of hypohaploid chromosomes, was found in studies analyzing PB1s (Kuliev et al. 2003, 2005, 2011) which is logical since the chromosomal status of PB1 is complementary to the oocyte's.

Unbalanced premature chromatid separation is approximately equally frequent in faster-maturing and slower-maturing oocytes (Table 4B) (Križančić Bombek L. et al., 2011) and is thought to be a consequence of negative influence of *in vitro* conditions (Munne et al., 1995b). However it has also been documented in fresh *in vivo* matured oocytes (Sandalinas et al., 2002) confirming the hypothesis that it is one of the mechanisms of aneuploidy emergence (Angell 1991b). On the other hand, whole chromosome non-disjunction is significantly more frequent in oocytes maturing for longer time (Table 4B) suggesting that this second mechanism of aneuploidy emergence is more prone to cultivation conditions.

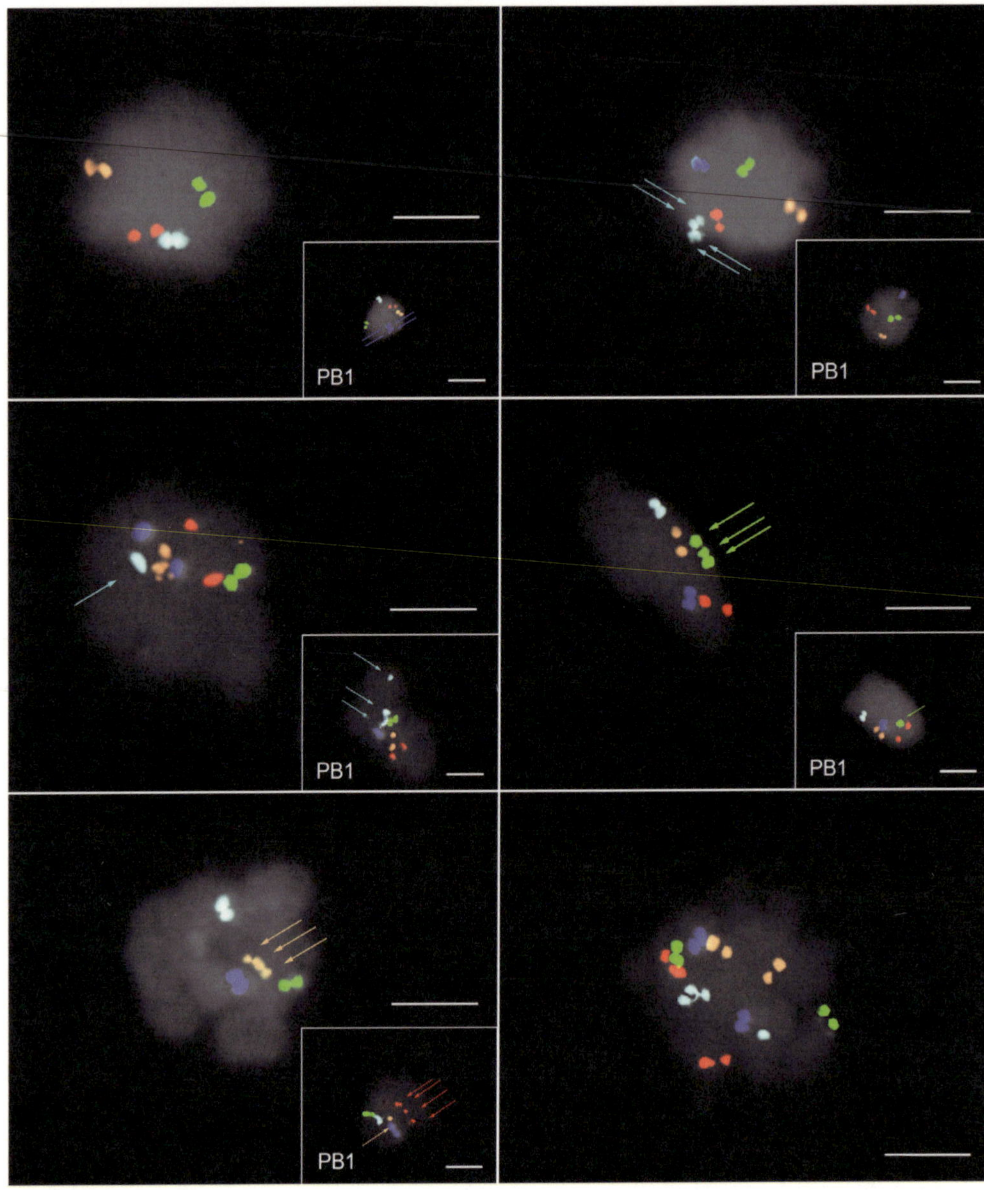

Fig. 7. Aneuploidy types obtained by FISH analysis of chromosomes 13, 16,18, 21 and 22 in IVM oocyte-PB1 pairs. During metaphase I, chromosome non-disjunction may result in nullisomy containing no signal for chromosome 18 (dark blue arrows) in the oocyte and four in its PB1 (a), or in disomy of chromosome 16 (light blue arrows), containing four signals in the oocyte and none in the PB1 (b). On the other hand, unballanced premature chromatid separation may produce hypohaploidy of chromosome 16 (light blue arrows), containing one signal in the oocyte and three in PB1 (c), or hyperhaploidy of chromosome 21 (green arrows), containing three signals in the oocyte and one in the PB1 (d). Furthermore, many IVM oocytes have complex (multiple) aneuploidies of more than just one chromosome (e) or may even be diploid with no genetic material in the PB1 (f). Magnification x1000; bar: 10 µm.

In both aneuploidy mechanisms there is a preference of the genetic material retention in the oocyte instead of its extrusion into the PB1. Consequently there is an excess of hyperhaploid and disomic oocytes over the hypohaploid and nullisomic ones (Table 4C) (Križančić Bombek L. et al., 2011). According to previous analyses of first and second polar bodies (Kuliev et al., 2003, 2005), the existence of an unknown intrinsic mechanism has been proposed that prevents genetic material to be lost from the oocyte during meiosis.

Frequencies and aneuploidy types of individual chromosomes differ, which is influenced by the women age (Benadiva et al., 1996; Petersen & Mikkelsen, 2000; Weier et al., 2005) as well as with the sensitivity of chromosomes themselves (Hassold et al., 2000; Li et al., 2006). Different studies have revealed that the most aneuploidy-sensitive are chromosomes 13 (Magli et al., 2006), 15 (Gutierrez-Mateo et al., 2004b), 16 (Pujol et al., 2003), 21 (Cupisti et al., 2003; Kuliev et al., 2005, 2011) and 22 (Clyde et al., 2003; Kuliev et al. 2003, 2011; Sandalinas et al., 2002). These chromosomes, together with chromosomes 1, 7 and 17, are also commonly diagnosed as aneuploid in early embryos (Munne & Cohen, 1998).

Similarly, in IVM oocytes some chromosomes are more frequently affected than others. Aneuploidy rate may increase with prolonged *in vitro* cultivation. This is most notable in chromosomes 18 and 22 which are 6- and 4.4-times more frequently involved in aneuploidies in oocytes with 36-hours maturation period compared to those with 24-hours maturation period, respectively (Table 4D), suggesting that these two chromosomes may be extremely sensitive to cultivation conditions (Križančić Bombek L. et al., 2011).

From the data obtained for aneuploidies of individual chromosomes and on the assumption that aneuploidies approximately equally affect all 23 chromosomes of the human genome, an average and total aneuploidy rate can be estimated (Table 4E). The later is significantly higher in IVM oocytes requiring longer time to achieve maturity (79.6 %) than in those reaching M II phase in less than 24 hours (46.7 %). However, this estimate is most probably somewhat exaggerated since the five tested chromosomes are among those most frequently found in aneuploidies.

IVM oocytes are more prone to different chromosomal aberrations since they are exposed to suboptimal maturation conditions (Chian and Tan, 2002; Chian et al., 2004a; Trounson et al., 2001) and *in vitro* aging (Warburton, 2005). Also IVM in a simple medium may not provide all necessary growth signals and factors which might influence meiotic processes, resulting in aneuploidies and other chromosomal aberrations. During IVM, oocytes undergo maturation phases from GV to MII that can be easily characterized. Usually the oocytes are considered mature, when MII phase is reached, i.e. the PB1 extruded. However, this is only an indicator of nuclear maturity. From the mare presence of PB1, nothing can be deduced about the oocyte's cytoplasmic maturity or chromosome organization. In fact, increased incidence of oocytes with non-organized meiotic-spindle microtubules (43.7) and irregularly arranged chromosomes (33.3 %) can be found among IVM oocytes from stimulated ovarian cycles compared to *in vivo* matured oocytes among which only 13.6 % of cells have non-organized microtubules and 9.1 % have irregularly arranged chromosomes (Li et al., 2006). Our data show similar results (Table 5) with 30.6 % of *in vitro* matured GV oocytes having abnormal shape of meiotic spindle (Figure 8) which is significantly higher than in donated fresh mature oocytes among which only 6.1 % of oocytes show abnormal spindle. Furthermore, in 29 % of IVM oocytes with normal meiotic spindle, chromosomes are irregularly arranged within the spindle itself (Wang & Keefe, 2002).

		24 hours	36 hours
No. of analyzed chromosomes		325	185
A			
Unbalanced premature chromatid separation	Hypohaploidy (%)	8 (2.46)	1 (0.54) [a]
	Hyperhaploidy (%)	6 (1.85)	8 (4.32) [a]
	Total	14 (4.31)	9 (4.86) [i]
Chromosome non-disjunction	Nullisomy (%)	7 (2.15)	8 (4.32)
	Disomy (%)	12 (3.69) [b]	15 (8.11) [b]
	Total	19 (5.84) [j]	23 (12.43) [i,j]
B			
Unbalanced premature chromatid separation (hypohaploidy + hyperhaploidy) (%)		14 (4,31)	9 (4,86) [c]
Chromosome non-disjunction (nullisomy + disomy) (%)		19 (5,85) [d]	23 (12,43) [c,d]
C			
Genetic material loss in oocyte (hypohaploidy + nullisomy)		15 (4.62)	9 (4.86) [f]
Genetic material excess in oocyte (hyperhaploidy + disomy)		18 (5.54) [e]	23 (12.43) [e, f]
D			
Chromosomes with aneuploidy (%)	Chromosome 13	7 (2.15)	6 (3.24)
	Chromosome 16	13 (4.00)	5 (2.70)
	Chromosome 18	2 (0.62) [g]	7 (3.78) [g]
	Chromosome 21	7 (2.15)	4 (2.16)
	Chromosome 22	4 (1.23) [h]	10 (5.41) [h]
E			
	Average aneuploidy rate*	2.03	3.46
	Total aneuploidy rate	46.7 [k]	79.6 [k]

Table 4. Occurrence of different aneuploidy types with respect to IVM duration. FISH analysis (MultiVysion® PB, Vysis) of chromosomes 13, 16, 18, 21 and 22 in IVM oocytes.
[a-d] $p < 0.05$ (chi-square test with Yates correction)
[e-j] $p < 0.01$ (chi- square test with Yates correction)
[k] $p < 0.05$ (chi- square test)
* based on the five analyzed chromosomes

		Normal spindle	Abnormal spindle
Meiotic stage before and after IVM	M I to M II (n = 31)	25 (80.6%)	6 (19.4%)
	GV to M II (n = 36)	25 (69.4%)	11 (30.6%) [a]
	M I arrest (n = 21)	12 (57.1%)	9 (42.9%) [b]
	Fresh M II (n = 33)	31 (93.9%)	2 (6.1%) [a, b]

Table 5. Configuration of meiotic spindle of *in vitro* matured prophase I (GV) and metaphase I (M I) human oocytes. [a] $p < 0.01$; [b] $p < 0.005$

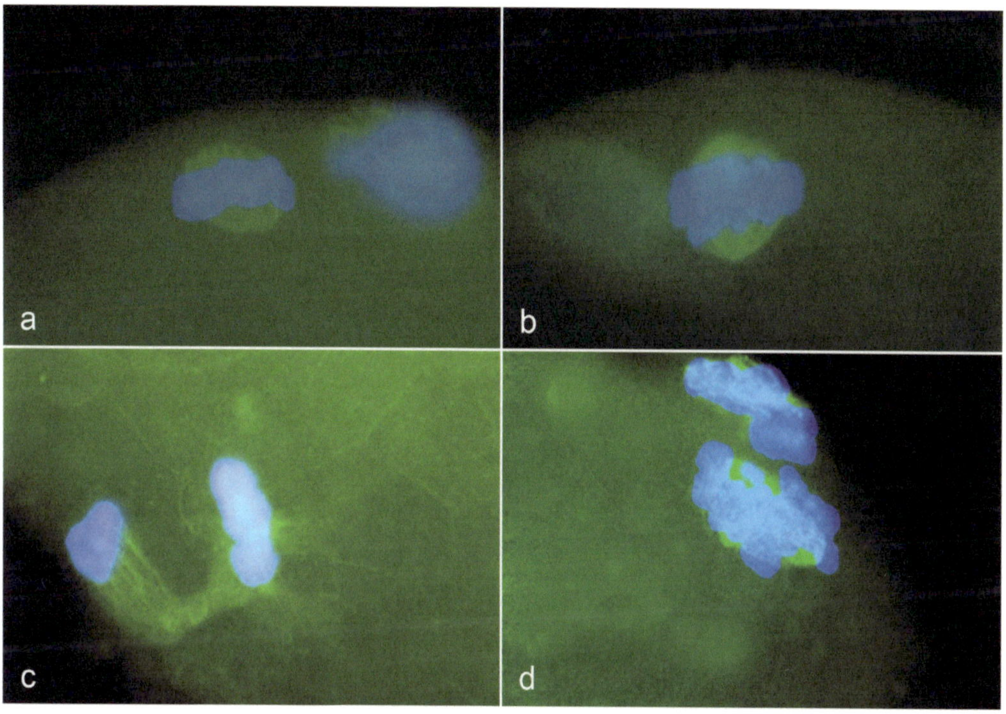

Fig. 8. Second meiotic spindles in metaphase II oocytes after IVM.
Many *in vitro* matured oocytes have normal barrel-shaped second meiotic spindles with chromosomes aligned in equatorial plane (a, b). On the right side of (a), chromosomes of PB1 are visible in a different focal plane. In IVM oocytes with abnormal spindle chromosomes can segregate between the oocyte and PB1 but microtubules remain attached to both chromosome masses instead of forming a proper meiotic spindle in the oocyte (c). It is also possible that meiotic spindles are disrupted or multipolar (d).

6. Conclusion

IVM oocytes can be used in clinical ART cycles however it has to be kept in mind that at least among those oocytes which acquire maturity later the aneuploidy incidence is very high. Therefore, for safer clinical use preimplantation genetic diagnosis and the selection of chromosomally normal embryos is recommended before embryo transfer into the uterus. Such selection significantly increases implantation rate as well as decreases the frequency of spontaneous abortions and birth of affected children.

7. References

Abdelhadi I., Colls P., Sandalinas M., Escudero T. & Munne S. (2003). Preimplantation genetic diagnosis of numerical abnormalities for 13 chromosomes. *Reprod Biomed Online* 6: 226-31

Albertini D.F., Sanfins A. & Combelles C.M.H. (2003). Origins and manifestations of oocyte maturation competencies. *Redprod Biomed Online* 6: 410-5

Anahory T., Andreo B., Regnier-Vigouroux G., Soulie J.P., Baudouin M., Demaille J. & Pellestor F. (2003). Sequential multiple probe fluorescence in-situ hybridization analysis of human oocytes and polar bodies by combining centromeric labeling and whole chromosome painting. *Mol Hum Reprod* 9: 577-85

Angell R.R., Ledger W., Yong E.L., Harkness L. & Baird D.T. (1991a). Cytogenetic analysis of unfertilized human oocytes. *Hum Reprod* 6: 568-73

Angell R.R. (1991b). Predivision in human oocytes at meiosis I: a mechanism for trisomy formation in man. *Hum Genet* 86: 383-7

Angell R.R. (1995). Meiosis I in human oocytes. Cytogenet Cell Genet 69: 266-272

Angell R. (1997). First-meiotic-division nondisjunction in human oocytes. *Am J Hum Genet* 61: 23-32

Balaban B., Urman B., Sertac A., Alatas C., Aksoy S. & Mercan R. 1998. Oocyte morphology does not affect fertilization rate, embryo quality and implantation rate after intracytoplasmic sperm injection. Hum Reprod 13: 3431-3

Barnes F.L., Crombie A., Gardner D.K., Kausche A., Lacham-Kaplan O., Suikkari A.M., Tiglias J., Wood C. & Trounson A.O. (1995). Blastocyst development and birth after in-vitro maturation of human primary oocytes, intracytoplasmic sperm injection and assisted hatching. *Hum Reprod* 10: 3243-7

Battaglia D.E., Klein N.A. & Soules M.R. (1996). Changes in centrosomal domains during meiotic maturation in the human oocyte. *Mol Hum Reprod* 2: 845-851

Benadiva C.A., Kligman I. & Munne S. (1996). Aneuploidy 16 in human embryos increases significantly with maternal age. *Fertil Steril* 66: 248-55

Benkhalifa M., Kahraman S., Caserta D., Domez E. & Qumsiyeh M.B. (2003). Morphological and cytogenetic analysis of intact oocytes and blocked zygotes. Prenat Diagn 23: 397-404

Brower P.T. & Schultz R.M. (1982). Intercellular communication between granulosa cells and mouse oocytes: Existence and possible nutritional role during oocyte growth. *Dev Biol* 90: 144-53

Cekleniak N.A., Combelles C.M.H., Ganz D.A., Jingly Fung B.A., Albertini D.F. & Racowsky C. (2001). A novel system for in vitro maturation of human oocytes. *Fertil Steril* 75: 1185-93

Cha K.Y. & Chian R.C. (1998). Maturation *in vitro* of immature human oocytes for clinical use. *Hum Reprod Update* 4: 103-20

Chian R.C. & Tan S.L. (2002). Maturational and developmental competence of cumulus-free immature human oocytes derived from stimulated and intracytoplasmic sperm injection cycles. *Reprod Biomed Online* 5: 125-32

Chian R.C., Chung J.T., Niwa T., Sirard M.A., Downey B.R. & Tan S.L. (2003). Reversible changes in protein phosphorylation during germinal vesicle breakdown and pronuclear formation in bovine oocytes *in vitro*. *Zygote* 11: 119-29

Chian R.C., Buckett W.M. & Tan S.L. (2004a). In-vitro maturation of human oocytes. *Reprod Biomed Online* 8: 148-66

Chian R.C., Buckett W.M., Abdul Jalil A.K., Son W.Y., Sylvestre C., Rao D. & Tan S.L. (2004b). Natural-cycle in vitro fertilization combined with in vitro maturation of immature oocytes is a potential approach in infertility treatment. *Fertil Steril* 82: 1675-8

Christopikou D., Karamalegos C., Doriza S., Argyrou M., Sisi P., Davies S. & Mastrominas M. (2010). Spindle and chromosome configurations of human oocytes matured in vitro in two different culture media. *Reprod Biomed Online* 20: 639- 48

Ciotti P.M., Notarangelo L., Morselli-Labate A.M., Felletti V., Porcu E. & Venturioli S. (2004). First polar body morphology before ICSI is not related to embryo quality or pregnancy rate. *Hum Reprod* 19: 1334-9

Clyde J.M., Hogg J.E., Rutherford A.J. & Picton H.M. (2003). Karyotyping of human metaphase II oocytes by multifluor fluorescence in situ hybridization. Fertil Steril 80: 1003-11

Combelles C.M.H., Cekleniak N.A., Racowsky C. & Albetrini D.F. (2002). Assessment of nuclear and cytoplasmic maturation in in-vitro matured human oocytes. *Hum Reprod* 17: 1006-16

Combelles C.M.H., Albetrini D.F. & Racowsky C. (2003). Distinct microtubule and chromatin characteristics of human oocytes after failed in-vivo and in-vitro meiotic maturation. *Hum Reprod* 18: 2124-30

Coonen E., Dumoulin J.C., Ramaekers F.C. & Hopman A.H. (1994). Optimal preparation of preimplantation embryo interphase nuclei for analysis by fluorescence in-situ hybridization. *Hum Reprod* 9: 533-7

Cozzi J., Conn C.M., Harper J.C., Winston R.M.L. & Delhanty J.D.A. (1999). A trisomic germ cell line and precocious chromatid separation leads to recurrent trisomy 21 conception. *Hum Genet* 104: 23-8

Cupisti S., Conn C.M., Fragouli E., Whalley K., Mills J.A., Faed M.J.W. & Delhanty J.D.A. (2003). Sequential FISH analysis of oocytes and polar bodies reveals anevploidy mechanisms. Prenat Diagn 23: 663-8

Dailey T., Dale B., Cohen J. & Munne S. (1996). Association between nondisjunction and maternal age in meiosis-II human oocytes. *Am J Hum Genet* 59: 176-84

De Boer K.A., Catt J.W., Jansen R.P.S., Leigh D. & McArthur S. (2004). Moving to blastocyst biopsy for preimplantation genetic diagnosis and single embryo transfer at Sydney IVF. *Fertil Steril* 82: 295-8

Dekel N. (1995). Molecular control of meiosis. *Trends Endocrinol Metab* 6: 165-9

Dekel N. (2005). Cellular, biochemical and molecular mechanisms regulating oocyte maturation. *Mol Cell Endocrinol* 234: 19-25

De La Fuente R. (2006). Chromatin modifications in the germinal vesicle (GV) of mammalian oocytes. *Dev Biol* 292: 1-12

Delhanty J.D.A. (2005). Mechanisms of aneuploidy induction in human oogenesis and early embryogenesis. *Cytogenet Genome Res* 111: 237-44

De Santis L., Cino I., Rabellotti E., Calzi F., Persico P., Borini A. & Coticchio G. (2005). Polar body morphology and spindle imaging as predictors of oocyte quality. *Reprod Biomed Online* 11: 36-42

De Sutter P., Dozortsev D., Qian C. & Dhont M. (1996). Oocyte morphology does not correlate with fertilization rate and embryo quality after intracytoplasmic sperm injection. *Hum Reprod* 11: 595-7

De Vos A., Van de Velde H., Joris H. & Van Steirteghem A. (1999). In-vitro matured metaphase-I oocytes have a lower fertilization rate but similar embryo quality as mature metaphase-II oocytes after intracytoplasmic sperm injection. *Hum Reprod* 14: 1859-63

Downs S.M., Daniel S.A.J., Bornslaeger E.A., Hoppe P.C. & Eppig J.J. (1989). Maintenance of meiotic arrest in mouse oocytes by purines: modulation of cAMP levels and cAMP phosphodiesterase activity. *Gamete Res* 23: 323-34

Downs S.M. & Hudson E.D. (2000). Energy substrates and the completion of spontaneous meiotic maturation. *Zygote* 8: 339-51

Dozortsev DI &McGinnis KT. (2001). An improved fixation technique for fluorescence in-situ hybridization for preimplantation genetic diagnosis. *Fertil Steril* 76: 186-8

Durban M., Benet J., Sarquella J., Egozcue J. & Navarro J. (1998). Chromosome studies in first polar bodies from hamster and human oocytes. *Hum Reprod* 13: 583-7

Durban M., Benet J., Boada M., Fernandez E., Calafell J.M., Lailla J.M., Sanchez-Garcia J.F., Pujol A., Egozcue J. & Navarro J. (2001). PGD in female carriers of balanced Robertsonian and reciprocal translocations by first polar body analysis. *Hum Reprod Update* 7: 591-602

Ebner T., Moser M., Yaman C., Feichtinger O., Hartl J. & Tews G. (1999). Elective transfer of embryos selected on the basis of first polar body morphology is associated with increased rates of implantation and pregnancy. *Fertil Steril* 72: 599-603

Ebner T., Yaman C., Moser M., Sommergruber M., Feichtinger O. & Tews G. (2000). Prognostic value of first polar body morphology on fertilization rate and embryo quality in intracytoplasmic sperm injection. *Hum Reprod* 15: 427-30

Ebner T., Moser M., Sommergruber M., Gaiswinkler U., Shebl O., Jesacher K. & Tews G. (2005). Occurrence and developmental consequences of vacuoles through preimplantation development. *Fertil Steril* 83: 1635-40

Ebner T., Moser M. & Tews G. (2006). Is oocyte morphology prognostic of embryo developmental potential after ICSI? *Reprod Biomed Online* 12: 507-12

Edirisinghe W.R., Junk S.M., Matson P.L. & Yovich J.L. (1997). Birth from cryopreserved embryos following in-vitro maturation of oocytes and intracytoplasmic sperm injection. *Hum Reprod*, 12: 1056-8

Edwards R.G., (1965). Maturation *in vitro* of mouse, sheep, cow, pig, rhesus monkey and human ovarian oocytes. *Nature* 208: 349-51

Eichenlaub-Ritter U., Stahl A. & Luciani J.M. (1988). The microtubular cytoskeleton and chromosomes of unfertilized human oocytes aged *in vitro*. *Hum Genet* 80: 259-264

Eichenlaub-Ritter U. & Peschke M. (2002). Expression in in-vivo and in-vitro growing and maturing oocytes: focus on regulation of expression at the translational level. *Hum Reprod Update* 8: 21-41

Emery B.R., Wilcox A.L., Aoki V.W., Peterson C.M. & Carrell C.M. (2005). In vitro oocyte maturation and subsequent delayed fertilization is associated with increased embryo aneuploidy. *Fertil Steril* 84: 1027-9

Eppig J.J. (1996). The ovary: oogenesis. in: *Scientiffic Essentials of Reproductive Medicine*. Hillier S.G., Kitshener H.C., Neilson J.P. (eds). WB Saunders Company Ltd. London, 147-59

Fragouli E., Alfarawati S., Goodall N., Sanchez-Garcıa J.F., Colls P. & Wells D. (2011). The cytogenetics of polar bodies: insights into female meiosis and the diagnosis of aneuploidy. *Mol Hum Reprod* 17, 286–95.

Friden B., Hreinsson J. & Hovata O. (2005). Birth of a healthy infant after in vitro oocyte maturation and ICSI in a woman with diminished ovarian response: case report. *Hum Reprod* 20: 2556-8

Gebauer F. & Richter J.D. (1997). Synthesis and function of Mos: the control switch of vertebrate oocyte meiosis. *Bioessays* 19: 23-28

Gianaroli L., Magli M.C., Ferraretti A.P., Fiorentino A., Garrisi J. & Munne S. (1997). Preimplantation genetic diagnosis increases the implantation rate in human in vitro fertilization by avoiding the transfer of chromosomally abnormal embryos. *Fertil Steril* 68: 1128-31

Gianaroli L., Magli M.C., Ferraretti A.P. & Munne S. (1999). Preimplantation diagnosis for aneuploidies in patients undergoing in vitro fertilization with a poor prognosis: identification of the categories for which it should be proposed. *Fertil Steril* 72: 837-44

Gianaroli L., Magli M.C., Ferraretti A.P., Tabanelli C., Trengia V., Farfalli V. & Cavallini G. (2005). The beneficial effects of preimplantation genetic diagnosis for aneuploidy support extensive clinical application. *Reprod Biomed Online* 10: 633-40

Gilchrist R.B., Ritter L.J. & Armstrong D.T. (2004). Oocyte - somatic cell interactions during follicle development in mammals. *Anim Reprod Sci* 82-83: 431-46

Goud P.T., Goud A.P., Qian C., Laverge H., Van der Elst J., De Sutter P. & Dhont M. (1998). In-vitro maturation of human germinal vesicle stage oocytes: role of cumulus cells and epidermal growth factor in the culture medium. *Hum Reprod* 13: 1638-44

Gutierrez-Mateo C., Benet J., Wells D., Colls P., Bermudez M.G., Sanchez-Garcia J.F., Egozcue J., Navarro J. & Munne S. (2004a). Aneuploidy study of human oocytes first polar body comparative genomic hybridization and metaphase II fluorescence in situ hybridization analysis. *Hum Reprod* 19: 2859-68

Gutierrez-Mateo C., Wells D., Benet J., Sanchez-Garcia J.F., Bermudez M.G., Belil I., Egozcue J., Munne S. & Navarro J. (2004b). Reliability of comparative genomic hybridization to detect chromosome abnormalities in first polar bodies and metaphase II oocytes. *Hum Reprod* 19: 2118-25

Gutierrez-Mateo C., Benet J., Starke H., Oliver-Bonet M., Munne S., Liehr T. & Navarro J. (2005). Karyotyping of human oocytes by cenM-FISH, a new 24-colour centromere-specific technique. *Hum Reprod* 20: 3395-401

Hassan-Ali H., Hisham-Saleh A., El-Gezeiry D., Baghdady I., Ismaeil I. & Mandelbaum J. (1998). Perivitelline space granularity: a sign of human menopausal gonadotrophin overdose in intracytoplasmic sperm injection. *Hum Reprod* 13: 3425-30

Hassold T., Merrel M., Adkins K., Freeman S. & Sherman S. (1995). Recombination and maternal age dependent nondisjunction: molecular studies of trisomy 16. *Am J Hum Genet* 57: 867-74

Hassold T., Sherman S. & Hunt P. (2000). Counting cross-overs: characterizing meiotic recombination in mammals. *Hum Mol Genet* 9: 2409-19

Herrick J.R., Brad A.M. & Krisher R.L. (2006). Chemical manipulation of glucose metabolism in porcine oocytes: effects on nuclear and cytoplasmic maturation in vitro. *Reproduction* 131: 289-98

Janssenswillen C., Nagy Z.P. & Van Steirteghem A. (1995). Maturation of human cumulus-free germinal vesicle-stage oocytes to metaphase II by coculture with monolayer Vero cells. *Hum Reprod* 10: 375-8

Junk S.M., Murch A.R., Dharmarajan A. & Yovich J.L. (2002). Cytogenetic analysis of embryos generated from *in vitro* matured mouse oocytes reveals an increase in micronuclei due to chromosome fragmentation. *J Assist Reprod Genet* 19: 67-71

Kim N.H., Chung H.M., Cha K.Y. & Chung K.S. (1998). Microtubule and microfilament organization in maturing human oocytes. *Hum Reprod* 13: 2217-22

Kim B.K., Lee S.C., Kim K.J., Han C.H. & Kim J.H. (2000). *In vitro* maturation, fertilization, and development of human germinal vesicle oocytes collected form stimulated cycles. Fertil Steril 74: 1153-8

Kim D.H., Ko D.S., Lee H.C., Lee H.J., Park W.I., Kim S.S., Park J.K., Yang B.C., Park S.B., Chang W.K. & Lee H.T. (2004). Comparison of maturation, fertilization, development, and gene expression of mouse oocytes grown *in vitro* and in vivo. *J Assist Reprod Genet* 21: 233-40

Kovačič B. & Vlaisavljević V. (2002). Results of in vitro maturation of meiotically immature human oocytes in a simple medium. Zdrav Vestn 71 (Suppl I): I13-7

Križančić Bombek L., Vlaisavljević V. & Kovačič B. (2011). Does the prolonged *in vitro* maturation of human oocytes influence the aneuploidy type? *Zdrav Vestn* 80: 362–9

Kuliev A., Cieslak J., Ilkevitch Y. & Verlinsky Y. (2003). Chromosomal abnormalities in a series of 6,733 human oocytes in preimplantation diagnosis for age-related aneuploidies. *Reprod Biomed Online* 6: 54-9

Kuliev A. & Verlinsky Y. (2004). Meiotic and mitotic nondisjunction: lessons from preimplantation genetic diagnosis. *Hum Reprod Update* 10: 401-7

Kuliev A., Cieslak J. & Verlinsky Y. (2005). Frequency and distribution of chromosome abnormalities in human oocytes. *Cytogenet Genome Res* 111: 193-8

Kuliev A., Zlatopolsky Z., Kirillova I, Spivakova J. & Cieslak Janzen J. (2011). Meiosis errors in over 20,000 oocytes studied in the practice of preimplantation aneuploidy testing. *Reproductive BioMedicine Online* 22, 2– 8

Lamb N.E., Sherman S.L. & Hassold T.J. (2005). Effect of meiotic recombination on the production of aneuploid hametes in humans. Cytogenet Genome Res 111: 250-5

Lefevre B., Gougeon A., Nome F. & Testart J. (1989). In vivo changes in oocyte germinal vesicle related to follicular quality and size at mid-follicular phase during stimulated cycles in the cynomolgus monkey. *Reprod Nutr Dev* 29: 523-31

Li Y., Feng H.L., Cao Y.J., Zheng G.J., Yang Y., Mullen S., Critser J.K. & Chen Z.J. (2006). Confocal microscopic analysis of the spindle and chromosome configurations of human oocytes matured *in vitro. Fertil Steril* 85: 827-32

Liu J., Katz E., Garcia J.E., Compton G. & Baramki T.A. (1997). Successful in vitro maturation of human oocytes not exposed to human chorionic gonadotrophin during ovulation induction, resulting in pregnancy. *Fertil Steril* 67: 566-8

Liu J., Lu G., Qian Y., Mao Y. & Ding W. (2003). Pregnancies and births achieved from in vitro matured oocytes retrieved from poor responders undergoing stimulation in *in vitro* fertilization cycles. *Fertil Steril* 80: 447-9

Liu Y., Sui H.S., Wang H.L., Yuan J.H., Luo M.J., Xia P. & Tan J.H. (2006). Germinal vesicle chromatin configurations of bovine oocytes. *Microsc Res Tech* 69: 799-807

Lohka M.J., Hayes M.K. & Maller J.L. (1988). Purification of maturation-promoting factor, an intracellular regulator of early mitotic events. *Proc Natl Acad Sci USA* 85: 3009-13

Magli M.C., Ferraretti A.P., Crippa A., Lappi M., Feliciani E. & Gianaroli L. (2006). First meiosis errors in immature oocytes generated by stimulated cycles. *Fertil Steril* 86: 629-35

Mahmoud K.Gh.M., Mohamed Y.M.A., Amer M.A., Noshy M.M. & Nawito M.F. (2010). Aneuploidy in in vitro matured buffalo oocytes with or without cumulus cells. *Nature and Science* 8: 46-51

Marquez C., Cohen J. & Munne S. (1998). Chromosome identification in human oocytes and polar bodies by spectral karyotyping. *Cytogenet Cell Genet* 81: 254-8

Matsuura R.K. & Chiba K. (2004). Unequal cell division regulated by the contents of germinal vesicles. *Dev Biol* 273: 76-86

Michaelis C., Ciosk R. & Nasmyth K. (1997). Cohesins: chromosomal proteins that prevent premature separation of sister chromatids. *Cell* 91: 35-45

Mikkelsen A.L. & Lindenberg S. (2001). Morphology of in-vitro matured oocytes: impact on fertility potential and embryo quality. *Hum Reprod* 16: 1714-8

Miyara F., Migne C., Dumont-Hassan M., Le Meur A., Cohen-Bacrie P., Aubriot F.X., Glissant A., Nathan C., Douard S., Stanovici A. & Debey P. (2003). Chromosome configuration and transcriptional control in human and mouse oocytes. *Mol Reprod Dev* 64: 458-70

Montag M., Köster M., van der Ven K. & van der Ven H. (2011). Gamete competence assessment by polarizing optics in assisted reproduction. *Hum Reprod Update* 17: 654-66

Motlik J. & Fulka S. (1976). Breakdovn of the germinal vesicle in pig oocytes in vivo and in vitro. *J Exp Zool* 198: 155-62

Motta P.M., Makabe S., Naguro T. & Correr S. (1994). Oocyte follicle cells association during development of human ovarian follicle. A study by high resolution scanning and treanmission electron microscopy. *Arch Histol Cytol* 57: 369-94

Mrazek M. & Fulka J.Jr. (2003). Failure of oocyte maturation: Possible mechanisms for oocyte maturation arrest. *Hum Reprod* 18: 2249-52

Munne S., Lee A., Rosenwaks Z., Grifo J. & Cohen J. (1993). Diagnosis of major chromosome aneuploidies in human preimplantation embryos. *Hum Reprod* 8: 2185-91

Munne S., Alikani M., Tomkin G., Grifo J. & Cohen J. (1995a). Embryo morphology, developmental rates, and maternal age are correlated with chromosome abnormalities. *Fertil Steril* 64: 382-91

Munne S., Dailey T., Sultan K.M., Grifo J. & Cohen J. (1995b). The use of first polar bodies for preimplantation diagnosis of aneuploidy. *Hum Reprod* 10: 1014-20

Munne S. & Weier H.U. (1996). Simultaneous enumeration of chromosomes 13, 18, 21, X, and Y in interphase cells for preimplantation genetic diagnosis of aneuploidy. *Cytogenet Cell Genet* 75: 263-70

Munne S., Dailey T., Finkelstein M. & Weier H.U. (1996). Reduction in signal overlap results in increased FISH efficiency: implications for preimplantation genetic diagnosis. *J Assist Reprod Genet* 13: 149-56

Munne S., Magli C., Adler A., Wright G., de Boer K., Mortimer D., Tucker M., Cohen J. & Gianaroli L. (1997). Treatment-related chromosome abnormalities in human embryos. *Hum Reprod* 12: 780-4

Munne S. & Cohen J. (1998). Chromosome abnormalities in human embryos. *Hum Reprod Update* 4: 842-55

Munne S., Fung J., Cassel M.J., Marquez C. & Weier H.U.G. (1998a). Preimplantation genetic analysis of translocations: case-specific probes for interphase cell analysis. *Hum Genet* 102: 663-74

Munne S., Marquez C., Magli C., Morton P. & Morrison L. (1998b). Scoring criteria for preimplantation genetic diagnosis of numerical abnormalities for chromosomes X, Y, 13, 16, 18 and 21. *Mol Hum Reprod* 4: 863-70

Munne S., Magli C., Cohen J., Morton P., Sadowy S., Gianaroli L., Tucker M., Marquez C., Sable D., Ferraretti A.P., Massey J.B. & Scott R. (1999). Positive outcome after preimplantation diagnosis of aneuploidy in human embryos. *Hum Reprod* 14: 2191-9

Munne S., Sandalinas M., Escudero T., Velilla E., Walmsley R., Sadowy S., Cohen J. & Sable D. (2003). Improved implantation after preimplantation genetic diagnosis of aneuploidy. *Reprod Biomed Online* 7: 91-7

Munne S., Bahce M., Sandalinas M., Escudero T., Marquez C., Velilla E., Colls P., Oter M., Alikani M. & Cohen J. (2004). Differences in chromosome susceptibility to aneuploidy and survival to first trimester. *Reprod Biomed Online* 8: 81-90

Munne S., Fischer J., Warner A., Chen S., Zouves C., Cohen J. & Referring Centers PGD Group. (2006). Preimplantation genetic diagnosis significantly reduces pregnancy loss in infertile couples: a multicenter study. *Fertil Steril* 85: 326-32

Nagy Z.P., Cecile J., Liu J., Loccufier A., Devroey P. & Van Steirteghem A. (1996). Pregnancy and birth after intracytoplasmic sperm injection of in vitro matured germinal-vesicle stage oocytes: case report. *Fertil Steril* 65: 1047-50

Neal M.S., Cowan L., Pierre Louis J., Hughes E., King W.A. & Basrur P.K. (2002). Cytogenetic evaluation of human oocytes that failed to complete meiotic maturation *in vitro*. *Fertil Steril* 77: 844-5

Nogueira D., Staessen C., Van de Velde H. & Van Steirteghem A. (2000). Nuclear status and cytogenetics of embryos derived from *in vitro* matured oocytes. *Fertil Steril* 74: 295-8

Okada A., Yanagimachi R. & Yanagimachi H. (1986). Development of a cortical granule-free area of cortex and the perivitelline space in the hamster oocyte during maturation and following ovulation. *J Submicrosc Cytol* 18: 233-47

Otsuki J., Okada A., Morimoto K., Nagai Y. & Kubo H. (2004). The relationship between pregnancy outcome and smooth endoplasmic reticulum clusters in M II human oocytes. *Hum Reprod* 19: 1591-7

Pellestor F. (1991). Frequency and distribution of aneuploidy in human female gametes. Hum Genet 86: 283-8

Pellestor F., Andreo B., Arnal F., Humeau C. & Demaille J. (2002). Mechanisms of non-disjunction in human female meiosis: the co-existence of two modes of malsegregation evidenced by the karyotyping of 1397 in-vitro unfertilized oocytes. *Hum Reprod* 17: 2134-45

Pellestor F., Andreo B., Arnal F., Humeau C. & Demaille J. (2003). Maternal aging and chromosomal abnormalities: new data drawn from in vitro unfertilized human oocytes. *Hum Genet* 112: 195-203

Pellestor F., Anahory T. & Hamamah S. (2005). The chromosomal analysis of human oocytes. An overview of established procedures. *Hum Reprod Update* 11: 15-32

Pellestor F., Andreo B., Anahory T. & Hamamah S. (2006). The occurence of aneuploidy in human: lessons from the cytogenetic studies of human oocytes. *Eur J Med Genet* 49: 103-16

Petersen M.B. & Mikkelsen M. (2000). Nondisjunction in trisomy 21: origin and mechanisms. *Cytogenet Cell Genet* 91: 199-203

Pickering S.J., Johnson M.H., Braude P.R. & Houliston E. (1988). Cytoskeletal organization in fresh, aged and spontaneously activated human oocytes. *Hum Reprod* 3: 978-89

Pujol A., Boiso I., Benet J., Veiga A., Durban M., Campillo M., Egozcue J. & Navarro J. (2003). Analysis of nine chromosome probes in first polar bodies and metaphase II oocytes for the detection of aneuploidies. *Eur J Hum Genet* 11: 325-36

Roberts R., Franks S. & Hardy K. (2002). Culture environment modulates maturation and metabolism of human oocytes. *Hum Reprod* 17: 2950-6

Roberts R., Iatropoulov A., Ciantar D., Stark J., Becker D.L., Franks S. & Hardy K. (2005). Follicle-stimulating hormone affects metaphase I chromosome alignment and increases aneuploidy in mouse oocytes matured *in vitro*. *Biol Reprod* 72: 107-118

Sagata N. (1997). What does Mos do in oocytes and somatic cells? *Bioessays* 19:13-21

Sandalinas M., Marquez C. & Munne S. (2002). Spectral karyotyping of fresh, non-inseminated oocytes. *Mol Hum Reprod* 8: 580-5

Sanfins A., Plancha C.E., Overstrom E. & Albertini D.F. (2004). Meiotic spindle morphogenesis in *in vivo* and *in vitro* matured mouse oocytes: insights into the relationship between nuclear and cytoplasmic quality. *Hum Reprod* 19: 2889-2899

Sathananthan A.H., (1997). Ultrastructure of the human egg. Hum Cell 10: 21-38

Sathananthan A.H., Selvaraj K., Girijashankar M.L., Ganesh V., Selvaraj P. & Trounson A.O. (2006). From oogonia to mature oocytes: inactivation of the maternal centrosome in humans. *Microsc Research and Technique* 69: 396-407

Schramm R.D. & Bavister B.D. (1995). Effects of granulosa cells and gonadotrophins on meiotic and developmental competence of oocytes *in vitro* in non-stimulated rhesus monkeys. *Hum Reprod* 10: 887-95

Schramm R.D., Paprocki A.M. & Vande Voort C.A. (2003). Causes of developmental failure of in-vitro matured rhesus monkey oocytes: impairment in embryonic genome activation. *Hum Reprod* 18: 826-33

Schultz R.M., Montgomery R.R. & Belanoff J.R. (1983). Regulation of mouse oocyte maturation: implications of a decrease in oocyte cAMP and protein dephosphorylation in commitment to resume meiosis. *Dev Biol* 97: 267-73

Smitz J., Nogueira D., Vanhoutte L., de Matos D.G. & Cortvindt R.N. (2004). Oocyte in vitro maturation. in: *Textbook of assisted reproductive techniques. Laboratory and Clinical Perspectives.* Gardner D.K., Weissman A., Howles C.M., Shoham Z. (eds). Boca Raton, Taylor & Francis Group: 125-61

Spinaci M., Seren E. & Mattioli M. (2004). Maternal chromatin remodeling during maturation and after fertilization in mouse oocytes. *Mol Reprod Dev* 69: 215-21

Sugawara S. & Mikamo K. (1986). Maternal ageing and non-disjunction: a comparative study of two chromosomal techniques on the formation of univalents in first meioticmetaphase oocytes of the mouse. *Chromosoma* 93: 321-5

Sun Q.Y., Lai L., Park K.W., Kühholzer B., Prather R.S. & Schatten H. (2001). Dynamic events are differently modulated by microfilaments, microtubules, and mitogen-activated protein kinase during porcine oocyte maturation and fertilization in vitro. *Biol Reprod* 64: 879-89

Sun X.S., Liu Y., Yue K.Z., Ma S.F. & Tan J.H. (2004). Changes in germinal vesicle (GV) chromatin configurations during growth and maturation of porcine oocytes. *Mol Reprod Dev* 69: 228-34

Sun Q.Y. & Schatten H. (2006). Regulation of dynamic events by microfilaments during oocyte maturation and fertilization. *Reproduction* 131: 193-205

Sutton M.L., Gilchrist R.B. & Thompson J.G. (2003). Effects of in-vivo and in-vitro environments on the metabolism of the cumulus-oocyte complex and its influence on oocyte developmental capacity. *Hum Reprod Update* 9: 35-48

Tan S.L. & Child T.J. (2002). In-vitro maturation of oocytes from unstimulated polycystic ovaries. *Reprod Biomed Online* 4 (Suppl 1): 18-23.

Tarkowski A.K. (1966). An air-drying method for chromosome preparation from mouse eggs. *Cytogenetics* 5: 394-400

Trounson A., Anderiesz C., Jones G.M., Kausche A., Lolatgis N. & Wood C. (1998). Oocyte maturation. *Hum Reprod* 13: 52-62

Trounson A., Anderiesz C. & Jones G. (2001). Maturation of human oocytes *in vitro* and their developmental competence. *Reproduction* 121: 51-75

Van Blerkom J. (1990). Occurrence and developmental consequences of aberrant cellular organization in meiotically mature human oocytes efter exogenous ovarian hyperstimulation. *J Electron Microsc Tech* 16: 324-46

Van Blerkom J. & Henry G. (1992). Oocyte dysmorphism and aneuploidy in meiotically mature human oocytes after ovarian stimulation. *Hum Reprod* 7: 379-90

Van Blerkom J. (1996). The influence of intrinsic and extrinsic factors on the developmental potential and chromosomal normality of the human oocyte. *J Soc Gynecol Invest* 3: 3-11

Van Blerkom J. & Davis P. (2001). Differential effects of repeated ovarian stimulation on cytoplasmic and spindle organization in metaphase II mouse oocytes matured *in vivo* and *in vitro*. *Hum Reprod* 16: 757-64

Van Blerkom J. (2004). Mitochondria in human oogenesis and preimplantation embryogenesis: engines of metabolism, ionic regulation and developmental competence. *Reproduction* 128: 269-80

Vanhoutte L., De Sutter P., Van der Elst J. & Dhont M. (2005). Clinical benefit of metaphase I oocytes. *Reprod Biol Endocrinol* 3: 71-6

Veeck L.L. (1988). Oocyte assessment and biological performance. *Ann N Y Acad Sci* 541: 259-74

Velilla E., Escudero T. & Munne S. (2002). Blastomere fixation techniques and risk of misdiagnosis for preimplantation genetic diagnosis of aneuploidy. *Reprod Biomed Online* 4: 210-7

Verlinsky Y., Ginsberg N., Lifchez A., Valle J., Moise J. & Strom C.M. (1990). Analysis of the first polar body: preconception genetic diagnosis. *Hum Reprod* 5: 826-9

Verlinsky Y., Cieslak J., Freidine M., Ivakhnenko V., Wolf G., Kovalinskaya L., White M., Lifchez A., Kaplan B., Moise J., Valle J., Ginsberg N., Strom C. & Kuliev A. (1996). Polar body diagnosis of common aneuploidies by FISH. *J Assist Reprod Genet* 13: 157-62

Verlinsky Y., Cieslak J., Ivakhnenko V., Evsikov S., Wolf G., White M., Lifchez A., Kaplan B., Moise J., Valle J., Ginsberg N., Strom C. & Kuliev A. (1997-1998). Prepregnancy genetic testing for age-related aneuploidies by polar body analysis. *Genet Test* 1: 231-5

Verlinsky Y. & Kuliev A. (2000). Normal and abnormal preimplantation development: selection of material for preimplantation genetic diagnosis. in: *An atlas of preimplantation genetic diagnosis.* Verlinsky Y. in Kuliev A. (eds.). New York, The Parthenon Publishing Group Inc: 15-8

Verlinsky Y., Cieslak J., Ivakhnenko V., Evsikov S., Wolf G., White M., Lifchez A., Kaplan B., Moise J., Valle J., Ginsberg N., Strom C. & Kuliev A. (2001). Chromosomal abnormalities in the first and second polar body. *Mol Cell Endocrinol* 183 (Suppl 1): S47-9.

Verlinsky Y. & Kuliev A. (2003). Current status of preimplantation diagnosis for single gene disorders. *Reprod Biomed Online* 7: 145-50

Verlinsky Y., Lerner S., Illkevitch N., Kuznetsov V., Kuznetsov I., Cieslak J. & Kuliev A. (2003). Is there any predictive value of first polar body morphology for embryo genotype or developmental potential? *Reprod Biomed Online* 7: 336-41

Verlinsky Y., Cohen J., Munne S., Gianaroli L., Simpson J.L., Ferraretti A.P. & Kuliev A. (2004). Over a decade of experience with preimplantation genetic diagnosis: a multicenter report. *Fertil Steril* 82: 292-4

Vialard F., Petit C., Bergere M., Molina Gomes D., Martel-Petit V., Lombroso R., Ville Y., Gerard H. & Selva J. (2006). Evidence of a high proportion of premature unbalanced separation of sister chromatids in the first polar bodies of women of advanced age. *Hum Reprod* 21: 1172-1178

Vlaisavljević V., Križančić Bombek L., Kokalj Vokač N., Kovačič B. & Čižek Sajko M. (2007). How safe is germinal vesicle stage oocyte rescue? Aneuploidy analysis of *in vitro* matured oocytes. *Eur J Obstet Gynecol Reprod Biol* 134: 213-9

Voullaire L., Wilton L., Slater H. & Williamson R. (1999). Detection of aneuploidy in single cells using comparative genomic hybridization. *Prenat Diagn* 19: 846-51

Xia P. (1997). Intracytoplasmic sperm injection: correlation of oocyte grade based on polar body, periviteline space and cytoplasmic inclusions with fertilization rate and embryo quality. *Hum Reprod* 12: 1750-5

Xia P. & Younglai E.V. (2000). Relationship between steroid concentrations in ovarian follicular fluid and oocyte morphology in patients undergoing intracytoplasmic sperm injection (ICSI) treatment. *J Reprod Fertil* 118: 229-33

Xu Y-W., Peng Y-T., Wang B., Zeng Y-H., Zhuang G-Lun & Zhou C-Q. (2011). High follicle-stimulating hormone increases aneuploidy in human oocytes matured in vitro *Fertil Steril* 95: 99-104

Yun Q., Ting F., Chen J., Cai L.B., Liu J.Y., Mao Y.D., Ding W. & Sha J.H. (2005). Pregnancies and births resulting from in vitro matured oocytes fertilized with testicular spermatozoa. *J Assist Reprod Genet* 22: 133-6

Wang W.H., Meng L., Hackett R.J. & Keefe D.L. (2001) Developmental ability of human eggs with or without birefringent spindles imaged by PolScope before insemination. *Hum Reprod* 16: 1464-8

Wang W.H. & Keefe D.L. (2002). Prediction of chromosome misalignment among *in vitro* matured human oocytes by spindle imaging with the PolScope. *Fertil Steril* 78: 1077-81

Warburton D. (2005). Biological aging and the etiology of aneuploidy. *Cytogenet Genome Res* 111: 266-72

Weier H.U., Weier J.F., Renom M.O., Zheng X., Colls P., Nureddin A., Pham C.D., Chu L.W., Racowsky C. & Munne S. (2005). Fluorescence in situ hybridization and spectral imaging analysis of human oocytes and first polar bodies. *J Histochem Cytochem* 53: 269-72

Wells D., Sherlock J.K., Handyside A.H. & Delhanty J.D.A. (1999). Detailed chromosomal and molecular genetic analysis of single cells by whole genome amplification and comparative genomic hybridization. *Nucleic Acids Res* 27: 1214-8

Whitaker M. (1996). Control of meiotic arrest. *Reviews of Reproduction* 1: 127-35

Wilton L., Voullaire L., Sargeant P., Williamson R. & McBain J. (2003). Preimplantation aneuploidy screaning using comparative genomic hybridization or fluorescence in situ hybridization of embryos from patients with recurrent implantation failure. *Fertil Steril* 80: 860-8

Wramsby H. & Liedholm P. (1984). A gradual fixation method for chromosomal preparations of human oocytes. *Fertil Steril* 41: 736-738

Zuccotti M., Piccinelli A., Giorgi Rossi P., Garagna S. & Redi C.A. (1995). Chromatin organization during mouse oocyte growth. *Mol Reprod Dev* 41: 479-85

10

Comparing Pig and Amphibian Oocytes: Methodologies for Aneuploidy Detection and Complementary Lessons for MAPK Involvement in Meiotic Spindle Morphogenesis

Michal Ješeta[1] and Jean-François L. Bodart[2]
[1]Veterinary Research Institute, Department of Genetics and Reproduction, Brno
[2]University of Lille 1, Laboratoire de Régulation des Signaux de Division
[1]Czech Republic
[2]France

1. Introduction

Maintenance of ploidy is crucial to the fate of daughter cells in any reproduction process. Improper genetic material segregation leads in general to mitotic catastrophe and subsequent cell death, but may also lead to the formation of aneuploid cells. Chromosomal unbalance, or aneuploidy, has been one of the main concerns in human reproduction for decades. About 20 % of all human oocytes are aneuploid and this percentage is believed to increase with ovarian aging, which is one of the major detrimental factors in pregnancy achievement (Battaglia *et al.*, 1996; Younis, 2011). Besides age, oocyte-related aneuploidy is linked to spindle morphology abnormalities, non-disjunction of chromosomes in meiosis I and II, and related to toxic compounds exposure (Hassold and Hunt, 2001; Wang and Sun, 2006). Most embryos, that are formed from aneuploid oocytes, are non-viable and do not result in pregnancy. However, viable aneuploidic embryos can be produced but in many cases carry genetic disorders, such as monosomies for chromosomes X and 21, autosomal trisomies [for instance, Patau syndrome (trisomy 13), Down syndrome (trisomy 21)] and triploidy. The latter is associated with tumor development (Hitzler and Zipursky, 2005).

Imbalance in chromosome number is thought to result in the failure of the organization/assembly or disassembly of the mitotic or meiotic spindle, which is in charge of the correct segregation of the genetic material to the daughter cells (oocytes and polar bodies in the case of female gametogenesis). Indeed, chromosomes that are not organized correctly on the microtubule spindle apparatus may be lost or inappropriately segregated during cell division, which results in aneuploidy. Abnormalities in spindle organization and chromosomal dynamics are predominant in aging oocytes and are regarded as the major factors responsible for infertility, miscarriage and to some extent, birth defects. For these reasons the cell cycle is considered to be tightly controlled through many checkpoints, in a manner to avoid "madness" at the helm, which would drive to genomic instability. Then, any failure in cell cycle regulation is called to promote accumulation alteration in genomic material and in some cases, may lead to aneuploidy.

Studies of human aneuploidy have been hampered by the lack of a suitable animal model. Most studies so far have been performed using the mouse model, which in many aspects does not allow direct comparison with humans (Alvarez Sedo *et al.*, 2011; Neuber and Powers, 2000; Schatten and Sun, 2011). It may be underlined that mouse model is a poor one regarding the methods of centrosome inheritance (due to the fact that mouse follows a maternal method for centrosome inheritance, in contrast to human where fertilization restores centrosome). As well, differences may be observed in the failure of fertilization between the two models. In human oocytes, the failure results from cytoplasm inability to support pronuclear formation while in mouse oocytes, the failure is rather due to inability of spermatozoa to penetrate the oocyte (Neuber and Powers, 2000). Other differences may also be reported between mouse and human oocytes, in contrast to non-rodent oocytes, mouse oocytes depend not upon protein synthesis for meiosis resumption and metaphase II spindle organization depends upon the assembly of cytoplasmic asters, including gamma-tubulin (see Table1). Still, the mouse model could promote strategies to sustain oocyte quality in mammals and provide evidences on the effects of environmental factors that may negatively impact oogenesis (Alvarez Sedo *et al.*, 2011; Combelles *et al.*, 2005; Farin and Yang, 1994; Gordo *et al.*, 2001; Hunter and Moor, 1987; Liang *et al.*, 2007; Lu *et al.*, 2002; Meinecke and Krischek, 2003; Memili and First, 1998; Schatten and Sun, 2011; Sun *et al.*, 1999; Sun *et al.*, 2002). Nevertheless, further efforts have to be performed to promote other mammalian non-rodent models, whose meiotic regulation, cytoskeletal organization and fertilization are more closely related to human system (Schatten and Sun, 2011).

	Xenopus oocytes	Mouse oocytes	Pig oocytes	Bovine oocytes	Human oocytes
Does maturation depends upon protein synthesis?	Yes	No	Yes	Yes	n.d.
Does initiation of meiosis depends upon transcription?	No	Yes	No (DO) Yes (COC)	No (DO) Yes (COC)	n.d.
Do maturation and spindle morphogenesis rely on MPF activation?	Yes	Yes	Yes	Yes	n.d.*
Does initiation of meiosis depends upon MAPK network activation?	No	No	No	No	n.d.*
Does spindle morphogenesis depends upon MAPK network activation?	Yes	Yes	Yes	Yes	n.d.*
Does metaphase II spindle formation depends upon cytoplasmic asters assembly?	No	Yes	No	No	No

Table 1. Meiosis characteristics in *Xenopus*, mouse, porcine, bovine and human oocytes. (DO: denuded oocyte; COC: Cumulus Oocyte Complexes ; n.d.: not determined; * Dynamical observations have been solely gathered for these kinases) (Alvarez Sedo *et al.*, 2011; Combelles *et al.*, 2005; Farin and Yang, 1994; Gordo *et al.*, 2001; Hunter and Moor, 1987; Liang *et al.*, 2007; Lu *et al.*, 2002; Meinecke and Krischek, 2003; Memili and First, 1998; Schatten and Sun, 2011; Sun *et al.*, 1999; Sun *et al.*, 2002).

Organisms enabling studies of spindle morphogenesis and aneuploidy might be divided into two classes: (1) meiotic models from non-mammalian species, which offer opportunities to unravel the fundamental mechanisms of meiotic spindle morphogenesis, and (2) meiotic models that correspond closely to human oocytes, taking into account both morphology and timing of meiotic maturation. Among the non-mammalian models, *Xenopus* has appeared as a model of choice since it shared similarities regarding mechanisms controlling meiotic progression with many mammalian species (see Table 1). In most vertebrates, oocytes are arrested at the first meiotic prophase until meiotic resumption is induced by hormonal stimulation. In both amphibian and pig models, resumption of meiosis and completion of oocytes maturation depend on protein translation, and are independent upon transcription. The factor promoting entry into M-phase, or division, was first reported in amphibians (Masui and Markert, 1971) and isolated almost two decades later in amphibian oocytes, based on genetic analysis performed in yeast (Gautier *et al.*, 1988; Lohka *et al.*, 1988). Named M-phase or Meiosis Promoting Factor (MPF), this factor is comprised of a catalytic subunit $p34^{Cdc2/Cdk1}$, and a regulatory subunit Cyclin B, whose association is crucial for the kinase activity of the complex. Together with the Mitogen Activated Protein Kinase (MAPK) pathway, MPF rules the coordination of the cellular reorganization during M-phase (Bodart *et al.*, 2005; Haccard and Jessus, 2006; Kotani and Yamashita, 2002). The maintenance of low levels of MPF activity is a prerequisite for the maintenance of meiotic arrest at prophase, while high levels of MPF activity are required for arrest at metaphase II (Bodart *et al.*, 2002a).

This chapter aims at comparing pig and *Xenopus* oocytes regarding their respective advantages and inconveniences, in comparison to other animal models. Standard methodologies for spindle morphogenesis analysis and aneuploidy detection in both models will be described. The role of the MAPK network in spindle morphogenesis and in ploidy maintenance will also be largely discussed, since female gametes have offered case studies to emphasize the potential role of MAPK's deregulation in aneuploidy.

2. Comparing advantages and inconveniences of pig and amphibian oocytes as models for spindle morphogenesis and aneuploidy studies

Xenopus has mainly been used in an aneuploidy context for cancer study purposes and has been less regarded as a valuable source for reproductive studies. Although it may appear as an attractive model, enabling structural approaches of spindle morphogenesis, it is not appropriate for accurate studies of genetic imbalance. To study the unbalance, porcine oocytes have appeared as a valuable and suitable model.

2.1 Strengths and disadvantages of amphibian oocyte model

The current understanding of meiosis regulation in vertebrate oocytes has benefited from studies performed in amphibian models such as *Xenopus laevis*. Fully-grown oocytes, blocked in prophase I resume meiosis upon hormonal stimulation and arrest in metaphase II as mature oocytes, or eggs, in anticipation of fertilization. Neither somatic cells nor *in vitro* systems offer a similar amenability for *in vivo* studies of the mechanisms that control cell cycle and orchestrate the cellular reorganization that occurs during mitosis or meiosis (Liu and Liu, 2006). This model could be advantageous to analyze the role of molecular networks involved in the morphological events of cell division. Indeed, *Xenopus* oocytes offer impressive opportunities for studies at the biochemical level: oocytes contain high levels of proteins (each oocyte contains for example 50 to 70 ng of the catalytic subunit of Protein Kinase A (PKA), 1 oocyte is equivalent to 50 000 somatic cells) and makes it possible to perform anti-MAPK immunoblotting on one-tenth of a single cell, allowing to study feed-back regulation mechanisms within one cell. Thus, extracts of either oocytes or eggs from amphibian are an abundant source for cytoskeletal and cell cycle proteins. In addition to their physiological synchronization in G2-like state or metaphase block, *Xenopus* oocytes are also known and used for their high capacity of protein synthesis (200-400 ng per day, per oocyte) and their size (1.2 to 1.4 mm), which facilitates micromanipulations, exploration of signaling network or electrophysiological properties. Finally, the use of this model of lower vertebrate fits into the ethical policy of the 3R (Replace, Refine, Reduce) on animal experimentation, which aims at promoting non mammalian alternative models in order to noticeably reduce and refine the use of upper vertebrates in experimental studies.

In addition, for several decades *Xenopus* oocytes have appeared to be one of the best cellular model to study *in vivo* enzymatic activities, assembly of cell division spindle, aneuploidy and characterization of parthenogenetic events. Nevertheless, this model suffers from several disadvantages: (1) amphibians are not oviparous models and oocytes maturation, as well as fertilization, is independent of any cumulus cells; (2) oocytes contain yolk, which does not facilitate structural analysis, and exhibit autofluorescence; (3) *Xenopus laevis* is a allotetraploid species, making it less/not suitable for genetic studies and careful analysis of genetic imbalances.

2.2 Strengths and disadvantages of porcine oocyte model

As mentioned above, mouse models may be optimal for studying molecular mechanisms underlying the maturation of mammalian oocytes, but several differences may been outlined when comparing to the maturation of non-rodent oocytes (Table 1). Porcine oocytes are closely related to human oocytes, in term of morphology and timing of meiotic maturation. Nuclear envelope breakdown, also called germinal vesicle breakdown (GVBD) in oocytes, occurs after 20 hours (2-5 hours in mice). Oocytes are reaching the second meiotic metaphase block approximately 40 hours after the lutheinizing hormone (LH) peak (*in vivo*) or after isolation from follicles (*in vitro* condition) (9-13 hours in mouse). It is known that pig oocytes rely on *de novo* protein synthesis for GVBD, whereas this occurs independently of protein synthesis in murine oocytes.

Several studies have reported that fertilization of pig oocytes resembles more that of lower vertebrates than mice (Long *et al.*, 1993; Sun *et al.*, 2001a). In sea urchin, starfish, porcine or bovine oocytes, sperm interaction with the oocyte or their penetration is impaired by microfilament inhibitors (Schatten *et al.*, 1982). In murine oocytes, however, microfilament inhibitor Latrunculin A did not block sperm penetration (Schatten *et al.*, 1986). Similarly, it was reported that the microfilament modulator JAS inhibited sperm incorporation and prevented cortical granules (CG) exocytosis in murine oocytes (Terada *et al.*, 2000). In murine oocytes, pronucleus migration is blocked upon inhibition of microfilament assembly (Schatten *et al.*, 1989; Terada *et al.*, 2000), while in pigs (Sun *et al.*, 2001a) or urchins (Schatten *et al.*, 1992), microtubule assembly is not required for pronucleus formation. During fertilization in sea urchins, pigs, cattle and humans, sperm introduces the centrosome into the egg. Microtubules nucleated by centrosomes cause the syngamy between male and female pronuclei (Kim *et al.*, 1997; Sun *et al.*, 2001a; Sutovsky *et al.*, 1996; Van Blerkom *et al.*, 1995). In mice, the situation is quite different because centrosomes are maternally inherited. Microtubules are organised by numerous cytoplasmic sites and microtubules and microfilament activity are required for pronuclear migration. For the above-mentioned reasons, porcine egg may be a more appropriate model for studies with the aim to make a comparison with human reproduction.

The access to porcine ovaries is straightforward since they can be obtained as "bioproducts" from local slaughterhouses. Nevertheless, working with pig oocytes may be hampered because of the heterogeneity of the isolated oocytes and the heterogeneity of the donor animals. Two types of ovaries may be obtained from slaughterhouses, depending whether killed animals are monitored or not. When performed, monitoring includes exact reproduction phase, age and farming conditions (including composition of feeding rations). Monitoring is expensive, but often necessary to obtain better standard conditions. For any work using porcine oocytes isolated from ovaries obtained from a slaughterhouse, it is necessary to perform a rigorous and strict selection of the ovaries and oocytes. Apart from ovaries collected at slaughterhouses, oocytes might be obtained by endoscopic ovum pick-up (OPU) from living animals. Antral follicles are punctured and cumulus oocyte complexes (COCs) are aspirated with the follicular fluid into an aspiration cannula using vacuum pressure. In contrast to the previous method, oocytes obtained in this way are homogenous and of high quality. Unfortunately, this method is expensive and labor-intensive and results in a low recovery of oocytes compared to the previous method.

Porcine and murine oocytes are different in their *in vitro* requirements during maturation. In contrast to mouse oocytes, porcine oocytes require cumulus cells for successful maturation, and they are very sensitive to maturation conditions and manipulation. For instance, culture conditions of cumulus cells may alter the meiotic spindle morphology (Ueno *et al.*, 2005), may impair successful micro-injection and subsequent scanning by confocal microscopy during maturation. Thus, live imaging experiments in this model are time-consuming and may appear as "complex".

3. Chromatin configuration, spindle morphogenesis and aneuploidy detection

3.1 *Xenopus laevis* oocytes

3.1.1 Morphological signs of maturation by external observation

In *Xenopus* oocytes, spindle formation is associated with migration of nucleoplasm and chromosomes to the apex of the cells. Upon hormonal stimulation, the germinal vesicle breaks down at its basis and migrates towards the apex of the oocyte, creating a large white area without pigment. This area is called white spot or maturation spot (Figure 1). The chromosomes are condensed and the first metaphase spindle is formed at the cortical area, located near the plasma membrane. After extrusion of the first polar body, the metaphase II spindle will be anchored at the plasma membrane. A dot may be detected within the white spot, corresponding to the anchored metaphase II spindle at the plasma membrane.

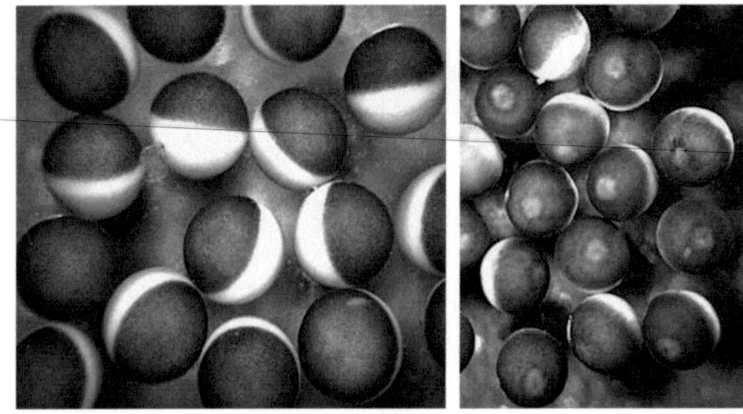

Fig. 1. External morphology of *Xenopus* oocytes. Immature oocytes (left panel) exhibit a dark pigmented hemisphere where the nucleus, or germinal vesicle, is found. Upon stimulation by progesterone, a small white spot appears at the apex of the cell, which is correlated with GV migration and its breakdown (right panel).

3.1.2 Spindle morphogenesis and aneuploidy detection

Classically, oocytes are fixed overnight in Smith's fixative, embedded in paraffin and sectioned (7µm thickness). Sections are then stained with Nuclear Red to detect nuclei and chromosomes, and with picroindigocarmine, which reveals cytoplasmic structures (Bodart *et al.*, 1999). This method enables the detection of spindle and condensed chromosomes, even if not located near the plasma membrane. Atypical structures can be detected in depth of the oocytes, such as tripolar spindle or nuclear envelope reformation around chromosomes in deep cytoplasm (Figure 2, 3). These methods can be coupled with electrophysiological procedures or calcium measurements to perform oocyte-by-oocyte analysis (Bodart *et al.*, 2001).

To perform immunocytological studies, oocytes are fixed in cold methanol, which is gradually replaced by butanol before embedding in paraffin. 7 µm-thin sections are subsequently incubated with antibodies directed towards spindle structures (e.g. towards alpha-tubulin). Structures are revealed with second antibodies conjugated with a fluorescent marker such as Oregon Green or Fluorescein Isothiocyanate. To detect structures located near the plasma membrane, section and embedding should be avoided. In this case, oocytes are fixed in cold methanol, which is gradually replaced by PBS (phosphate buffered saline). Next the oocytes are incubated in a low percentage of detergent for permeabilization purposes together with diluted antibodies and revealed as previously mentioned. Treated oocytes are bisected and animal halves are placed on standard slides with mounting medium including glycerol and Hoechst 33342, which reveals chromosomes, and observed under an epifluorescent microscope (Figure 4) (Baert *et al.*, 2003; Bodart *et al.*, 2005; Bodart and Duesbery, 2006).

To overcome autofluorescence and to increase the number of observed structures, many studies have been undertaken using egg extract together with sperm nuclei (Cross and Powers, 2009; Garner and Costanzo, 2009; Maresca and Heald, 2006). Though these methods are of interest, they have to be performed in a cell-membrane-free context and only focus on mitotic spindle formation. Indeed differences remain, albeit meiosis and mitosis share quite a lot of similarities: (1) centrosomes are absent in oocytes, (2) kinetochores appear later in MI and (3) the Ran GTPase might be dispensable for MI but requested for MII and mitosis (Brunet *et al.*, 1999; Dumont *et al.*, 2007).

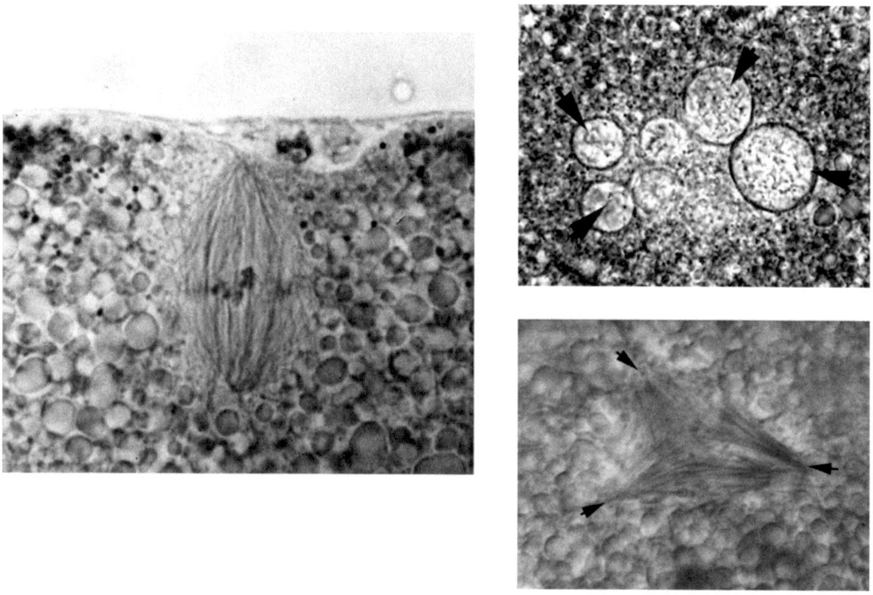

Fig. 2. Bipolar spindle and first polar body (left panel), abnormal tripolar spindle (right panel, bottom), and multiple envelope reformation around chromosomes in deep cytoplasm (right panel, top). Metaphase II spindle has, like seen in most species, a typical barrel shape.

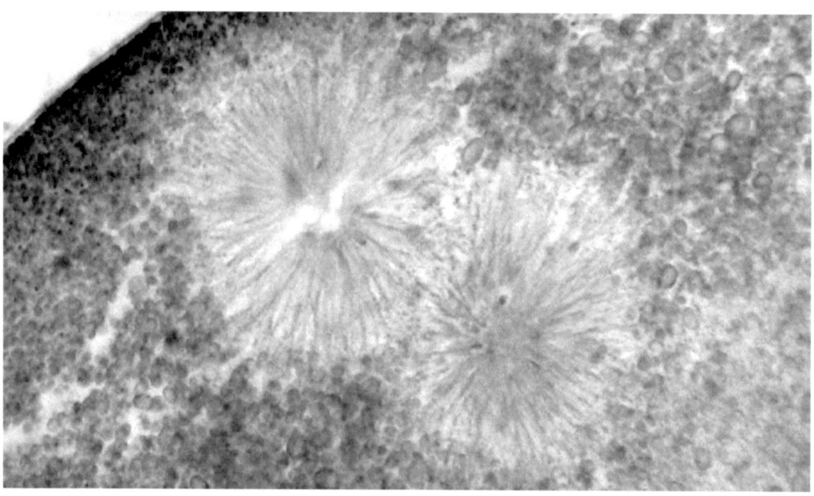

Fig. 3. Double aster formation in *Xenopus* oocyte where MAPK activity has been impaired. Structures are located in the subcortical layer but are not associated with the plasma membrane.

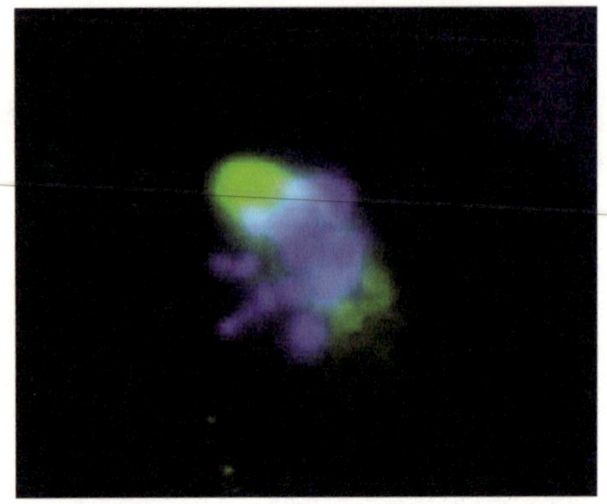

Fig. 4. Bipolar spindle in metaphase-II arrested *Xenopus* oocyte; DNA (blue), beta-Tubulin (green).

3.2 Porcine oocytes

3.2.1 Germinal vesicle stages

Full meiotic competence of pig oocytes is reached in ovarian follicles of 2 mm or more in diameter. Germinal vesicle breakdown is initiated *in vivo* by either preovulatory surge of gonadotropins or atretic degeneration of the follicle. Spontaneous (gonadotropin-independent) maturation occurs upon removal of the oocyte, or the oocyte-cumulus cell complex, from antral follicles when cultured in an appropriate supportive medium. Several protein kinases have been shown to regulate meiotic resumption. MPF is a key regulator of the meiotic resumption. Its inhibition totally blocks GVBD in pig oocytes. Nevertheless, MAPK, Protein Kinase C and Calmodulin-dependent Kinase (CAMKII) also play crucial roles during meiotic resumption in pig oocytes. In pigs, like in other domestic species and amphibians, protein synthesis is a prerequisite for oocyte meiotic resumption. In porcine oocytes, four GV chromatin configurations (GV1-GV4) were described, based on chromatin stages, nucleolus and nuclear chromatin disappearance (Motlik and Fulka, 1976). Stages GV1 (Figure 5), GV2 and GV3 exhibit a typical perinucleolar ring. At stage GV4 chromatin makes clumps and strands, nuclear membrane is less distinct, and nucleolus disappears completely. In oocytes undergoing GVBD, GV membrane disappears completely and chromatin condenses into clumps. Growing oocytes (diameter ≤90 μm) are unable to resume meiosis *in vitro*. Acquisition of meiotic competence in growing pig oocyte rather correlates with its ability to activate both MPF and MAPK pathways (Kanayama *et al.*, 2002).

3.2.2 Spindle morphogenesis

Metaphase II spindle is a crucial structure for genetic material segregation within oocytes and eggs; this structure is maintained in a highly dynamic status from ovulation to fertilization. The spindle morphogenesis during maturation begins after GVBD, when microtubule-organizing centres (MTOCs) are recruited in the vicinity of chromosomes: small microtubule asters are observed near the condensed chromatin. During the prometaphase stage, microtubule asters are found in association with each chromatin mass. Randomly growing microtubules are then stabilized and organized into a bipolar spindle. Next, asters elongate and encompass the chromatin at the metaphase-I stage. At this step,

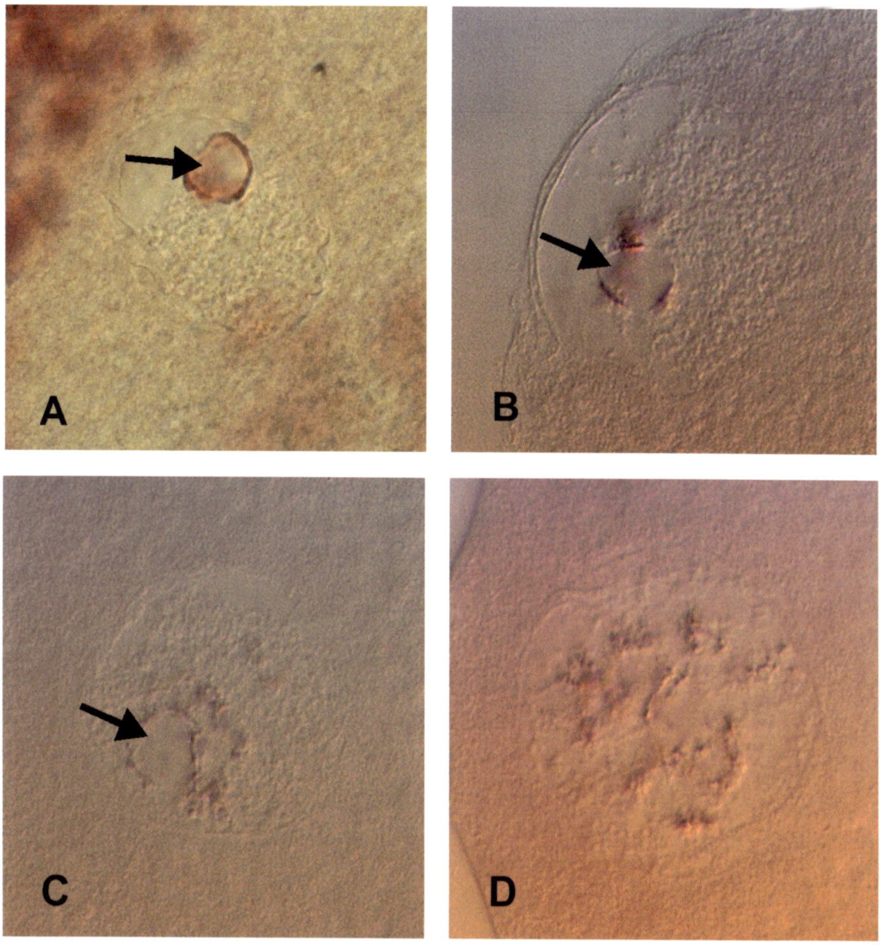

Fig. 5. Morphology of porcine oocyte nucleus exhibiting different GV configurations. (A) GV1: nucleolus surrounded by condensed chromatin, (B) GV2: condensed chromatin are not only around the nucleolus, (C) GV3: chromatin is condensed in many clumps or strands, (D) GV4: nucleolus disappears completely and condensed chromatin is in clumps (black arrows indicate nucleolus).

microtubules are seen only in the spindle (Figure 6, left). During anaphase-I and telophase-I, microtubules are detected around the chromatin (Figure 6, right). At the metaphase-II stage, microtubules are only observed in the second meiotic spindle. The meiotic spindle has a symmetric barrel-shaped structure containing anastral broad poles peripherally located and radially oriented (Kim *et al.*, 1996).

3.2.3 Aneuploidy detection

To detect aneuploidy there are applicable methods such as fluorescence *in situ* hybridization (FISH) or karyotyping from chromosomal spreads. These methods require spreading the metaphase II oocyte on a slide, risking the loss of chromosomal material. Modern cytogenetic method of comparative genomic hybridization is also suitable for aneuploidy

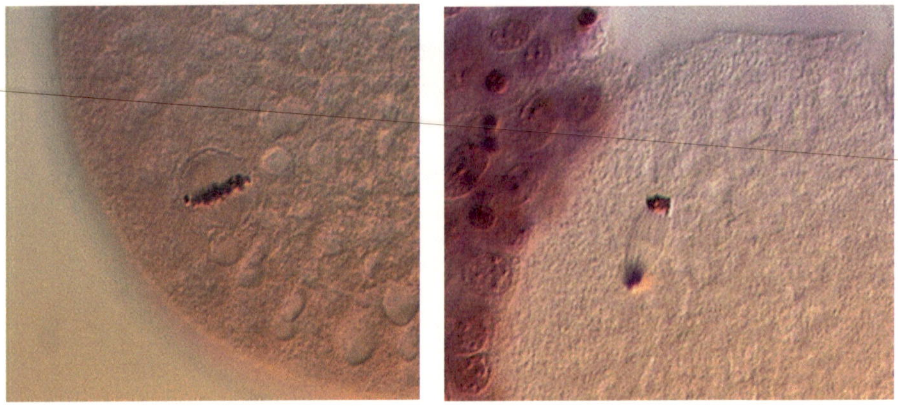

Fig. 6. Spindle detection in pig oocyte; (left) spindle at metaphase-I stage; (right) spindle at telophase-I stage.

detection in oocyte or polar body. The comparative genomic hybridization (CGH) method relies on whole oocyte DNA amplification in a single reaction, preventing artificial changes of chromosome content. These methods are suitable for detection of numeric aberrations, chromosomal non-disjunction and frequency of premature segregation of sister chromatids (an extra or a missing copy of a single chromatid).

3.2.3.1 Karyotyping from spreads

Giemsa staining is suitable only for hyperhaploid spreads. Hypohaploidy is rather considered as an artifact, because air-drying step used in slide preparation can account for chromosome loss during rapid evaporation of alcohol containing fixative. For karyotype analysis, only cells in metaphase can be analyzed because they present identifiable individual chromosomes (Figure 7). Furthermore, poor chromosome morphology and artefactual loss of chromosomes can compromise cytogenetic results.

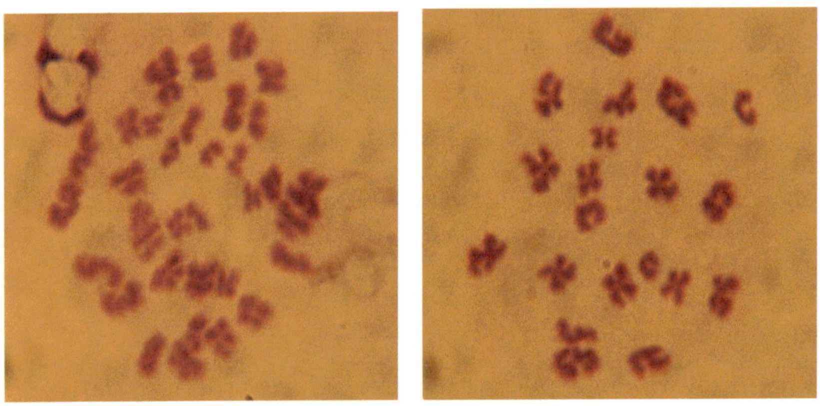

Fig. 7. Chromosomal analysis of porcine oocytes (Giemsa staining); (right) haploid chromosome set (n=19), (left) diploid chromosome set (2n=38) (Lechniak *et al.*, 2007)

3.2.3.2 Fluorescence *in situ* hybridization (FISH)

Fluorescence *in situ* hybridization (FISH, Figure 8) is a well-established technique for chromosome analysis and aneuploidy screening (Foster *et al.*, 2010; Lechniak *et al.*, 2007). In contrast to previously described methods, FISH data can be obtained from interphase nuclei or at least in cases where not all chromosomes are separated during spreading. Concerning oocyte, analysis of the corresponding polar bodies can be performed in parallel to strength the observations. Unfortunately, the diagnostics of targeted aneuploidies in pig with fluorescence *in-situ* hybridization is limited to chromosome-specific DNA probes. Current protocols have used probes for up to 13 chromosomes in human samples but in pigs, they are suitable for usually two probes (specific for centromeric region of Chromosomes 1 and 10) (Lechniak *et al.*, 2007). Results are thus extrapolated for all chromosomes solely based on these 2 probes. Furthermore, premature segregation of sister chromatids is not detectable *via* this method.

3.2.3.3 Comparative genomic hybridization (CGH)

Comparative genomic hybridization (CGH, Figure 9) is a more comprehensive method than karyotyping or FISH techniques. This cytogenetic technique allows the analysis of the full set of chromosomes and it has been applied to detect aneuploidy at the single cell level in interphase or M-phase cells. The CGH protocol requires only 0,5-1 μg of genomic DNA (from oocyte or polar body). By comparison with other farm animals, pigs have a small number of chromosomes (2n=38), which ease up chromosome identification and analysis. This method also enables analysis of the whole chromosomal set and relative contribution of individual chromosomes to resulting aneuploidy. This approach was recently applied in a study looking to detect chromosome abnormalities in first polar bodies and metaphase II-arrested oocytes in pig. CGH method is also suitable for detection of chromosome non-disjunction or premature segregation of sister chromatids (an extra or a missing copy of a single chromatid).

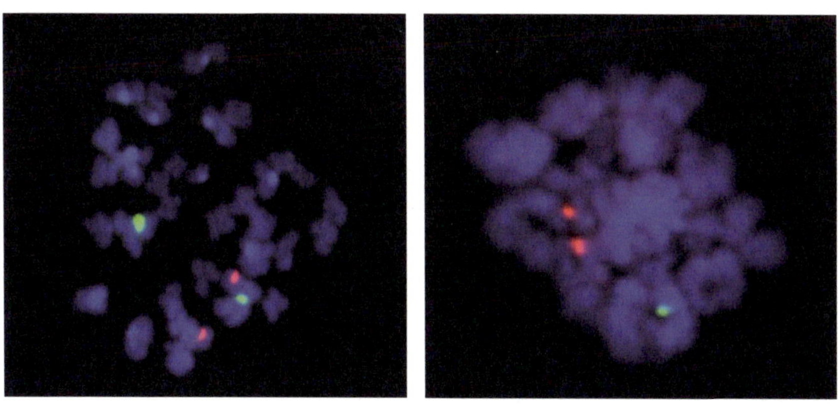

Fig. 8. Chromosomal analysis of porcine oocytes (FISH); (left) diploid oocytes (green signal - chromosome 1, red signal - chromosome 10), (right) aneuploid oocyte (disomy of chromosome 10) (Lechniak *et al.*, 2007)

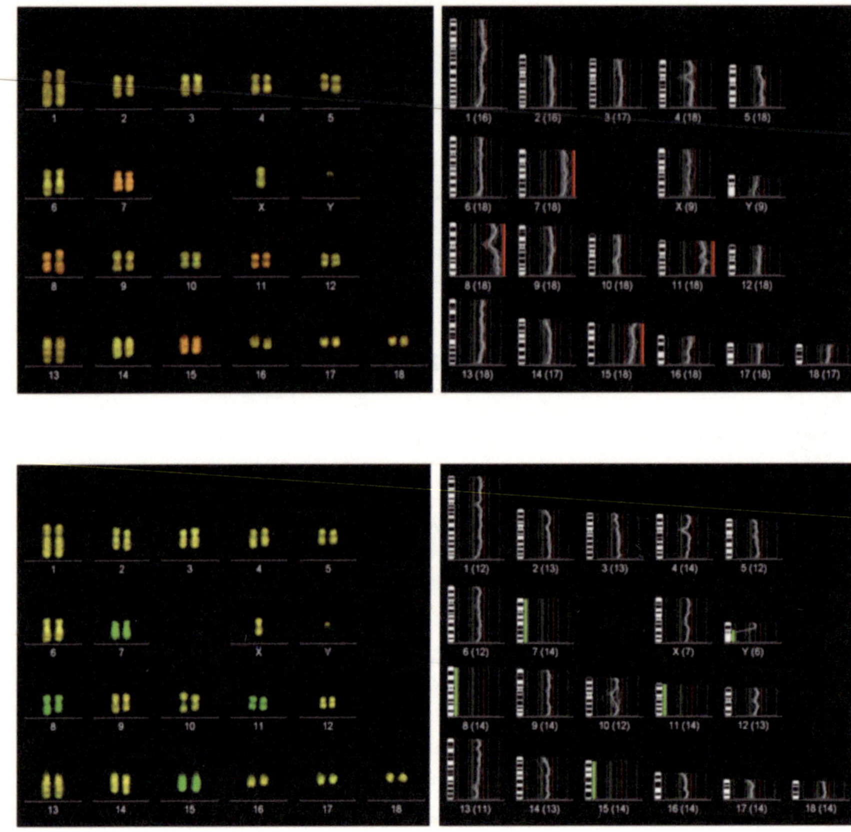

Fig. 9. Comparative genomic hybridization (CGH) in MII porcine oocytes; (upper panel) aneuploid oocyte with trisomy of chromosomes 7, 8, 11 and 15; (lower panel) corresponding polar body with nulisomy of chromosomes 7, 8, 11 and 15 (red signal - DNA from oocyte or polar body, green signal - reference DNA) (Hornak *et al.*, 2011).

3.2.3.4 Abnormalities during meiotic spindle morphogenesis in pig oocytes

Abnormalities during meiotic spindle morphogenesis are a hallmark of maternal aging. Spindle aberrations are not found so often in oocytes of animals with shorter reproductive periods like mice. In porcine oocytes, abnormal spindle morphologies include poorly shaped spindle morphologies, grossly disorganized microtubules, sometimes with thick bundles of cytoplasmic microtubules (Figure 10). These morphologies may result from the failure to organize two opposite metaphase spindle poles, either in metaphase I or metaphase II, or from the loss of attachment between microtubules and chromosomes. In oocytes coming from old pigs, one might observe various forms of abnormal spindles like multipolar spindle, large rounded spindle with microtubules emanating from most of its surface, elongated spindle, highly disorganized spindle with scattered microtubules, tripolar spindle or large irregular spindle (Miao *et al.*, 2009). In contrast to amphibians, aster formations are rare in mammals. In pigs, they were solely observed after taxol (Sun *et al.*, 2001b).

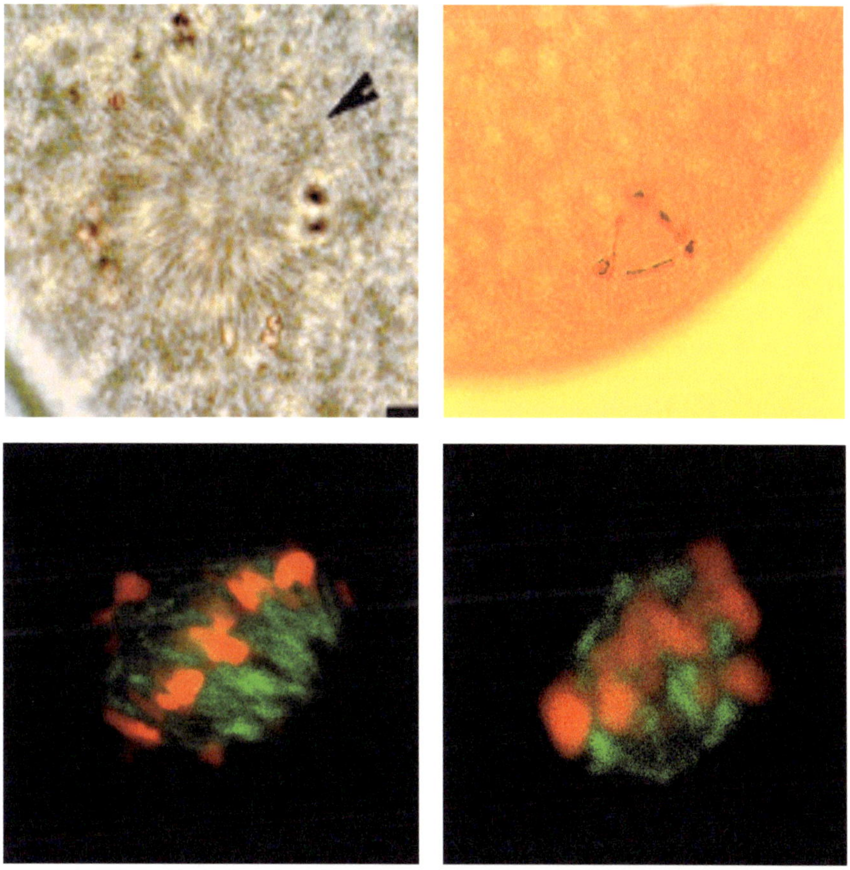

Fig. 10. Typical abnormal spindle morphologies observed in porcine oocytes: aster formation (upper panel, left) (Sun *et al.*, 2001b), tripolar spindles (upper panel, right), disorganized spindle with scattered chromosomes (lower panel, left) and irregular spindle (lower panel, right).

4. Aneuploidy case study: Unraveling the role of MAPK pathway in the cellular reorganization during meiosis

In many species, MAPK from the Extracellular regulated kinase (Erk) family has appeared as major player in the network regulating meiosis. The completion of the two meiotic metaphase offer windows of vulnerability towards aneuploidy, where MAPK are playing a crucial role. Nevertheless, the involvement of this pathway has been underestimated in its role for genome integrity. At least, the involvement of MAPK deregulation in aneuploidy remains difficult to untangle and female gametes have offered case studies to unravel MAPK's role in spindle morphogenesis. Here is outlined the involvement of the MAPK network in aneuploidy throughout different models.

4.1 Physical properties of MAPK pathway in amphibian

In many species, MAPK from the Extracellular regulated kinase (Erk) family is a crucial component in the network regulating meiosis. In vertebrate oocytes, the oncoprotein Mos acts as the upstream activator of mitogen-activated protein kinase kinase (MEK) and MAPK/Erk levels. This oocyte-expressed kinase appeared early during animal evolution and was in charge of regulating female meiosis specializations (Amiel *et al.*, 2009). Once accumulated, Mos phosphorylates MEK, which in turn activates MAPK/Erk by dual phosphorylation of a TEY motif (Ferrell and Bhatt, 1997). In amphibian oocytes, Mos-activated cascade prevents DNA synthesis during meiosis and promotes spindle morphogenesis as well as cytostatic activity present in metaphase-II arrested oocytes (Baert *et al.*, 2003; Bodart *et al.*, 2005; Dupre *et al.*, 2002; Sagata, 1997). In this model, physiological role of MAPKKK Raf, has been minored and Mos is thought to literally hijack the control of the MAPK cascade. A specific all-or-none response for MAPK/Erk activation is characteristic in these oocytes, in contrast to the gradual response of MAPK/Erk to external stimuli observed in mammalian somatic cells. The cascade arrangement of the signaling network generates the steepness of MAPK/Erk response in *Xenopus* oocytes. The physical properties of the cascade, which includes ultrasensitivity, bistability and irreversibility (Angeli *et al.*, 2004; Ferrell and Machleder, 1998; Huang and Ferrell, 1996; Russo *et al.*, 2009), are thought to mainly arise for bistability and ultrasensitivity from the existence of a feed-back loop motif. Indeed, the Mos-MEK-MAPK/Erk network has been found to be embedded in a positive feed-back loop, driven by MAPK/Erk itself (Ferrell and Machleder, 1998; Howard *et al.*, 1999; Matten *et al.*, 1996) and / or through MPF action (Castro *et al.*, 2001; Nebreda *et al.*, 1995; Paris *et al.*, 1991), which promotes Mos accumulation.

4.2 Role of MAPK/Erk network in spindle morphogenesis

4.2.1 Amphibian oocytes

MAPK/Erk activity was suggested to be required for functional spindle assembly checkpoint in amphibian oocyte extracts (Chung and Chen, 2003; Minshull *et al.*, 1994; Takenaka *et al.*, 1997). Although presence of MAPK/Erk on kinetochores has been suspected in somatic cells (Willard and Crouch, 2001), proteomic studies failed to find MAPK/Erk associated to isolated human metaphase chromosomes (Uchiyama *et al.*, 2005). Thus, whether MAPK/Erk in its active form is a component of kinetochore, and whether it is required for spindle assembly checkpoint function, remains somehow controversial.

From observations made in many species like starfish, jellyfish, urochordates, amphibians and mice, it is thought that control of meiotic spindle morphogenesis and positioning and chromatin organization are conserved functions for Mos and MAPK/Erk network. First observations were made in nullizygous mice for Mos, where MEK activation is impaired and interphase-like structure of microtubules and chromosomes are found between meiotic division, as well as formation of monopolar half-spindle (Araki *et al.*, 1996; Tong *et al.*, 2003; Verlhac *et al.*, 1996). Similar observations were made in other biological systems. MAPK/Erk cascade regulates spindle bipolarity through its direct or indirect effects on microtubule dynamics in amphibian oocytes (Bodart *et al.*, 2005; Gotoh *et al.*, 1995). No bipolar spindle anchored at the plasma membrane is observed when MAPK/Erk activity is inhibited by chemical inhibitors of MEK such as U0126 (Bodart *et al.*, 2002b; Gross *et al.*, 2000; Horne and Guadagno, 2003). *Rana japonica* oocytes treated with U0126 also fail to organize a Microtubule Organizing Center (MTOC) at the bottom of the germinal vesicle and chromosomes are partially condensed (Kotani and Yamashita, 2002). Both *in vitro* (Horne and Guadagno, 2003) and *in vivo* (Bodart *et al.*, 2005), MAPK activity inhibition leads to the formation of monopolar spindle or aster-like structures, attesting the failure to establish a bipolar organization (Figure 3). Similarly, when Mos accumulation is prevented *in vivo*, *Xenopus* oocytes exhibit aster-like structures. Such structures remain to be fully characterized but do not enable oocytes to properly segregate their genomic content (Bodart *et al.*, 2005). Finally, by inhibiting the network at different levels, it has been shown that Mos and MAPK/Erk play distinct but complementary roles in spindle morphogenesis (Bodart *et al.*, 2005). The latter observations suggested that MAPK/Erk is composed of functional modules, which may exert distinct actions at different levels of spindle organization. Then deregulation in any of this model may drive different type of aneuploidy, depending on the deregulated module.

4.2.2 Porcine oocytes

MAPK is found under an inactive form in pig oocytes at the GV stage, while its level of activity is significantly increased at GVBD time. Microinjection of c-mos RNA into porcine oocytes induces GVBD to occur earlier. But, antisense RNA towards pig c-mos protein does not affect GVBD in denuded oocytes, although MAPK phosphorylation and activation were completely inhibited (Ohashi *et al.*, 2003). Other reports show that the presence of MEK inhibitors, PD98059 or U0126 in the maturation medium blocks MAPK activation in both cumulus-enclosed and denuded oocytes, but prevents GVBD only in cumulus-enclosed oocytes (CEOs) (Meinecke and Krischek, 2003). Similarly to other models, MAPK activation is dispensable for meiotic resumption *per se*, but activation of this cascade in cumulus cells is indispensable for the gonadotropin-induced meiotic resumption of porcine cumulus-enclosed oocytes. These observations suggest that MAPK activation is not required for GVBD induction in denuded oocytes but is necessary for GVBD induction in CEOs. MPF activation correlates with GVBD occurrence, even though the activation of MAPK has been completely prevented, indicating that MPF is sufficient to induce GVBD.

Nevertheless, the activity of MAPK in porcine oocytes may be involved in the organization of chromosomes at the metaphase spindle plate (Ye *et al.*, 2003). Phosphorylated MAPK is detected at the spindle during the post-GVBD maturation period (Sugiura *et al.*, 2001). After GVBD, phosphorylated MAPK and its downstream effector p90rsk distribute to the area around the condensed chromosomes, in the meiotic spindle at the MI stage, in the midzone of the elongated spindle at anaphase I to telophase I transition, and in the spindle at MII stage (Goto *et al.*, 2002; Lee *et al.*, 2000). MAPK is kept highly phosphorylated from the MI to MII stages, when microtubules are assembled in the spindle (Sun et al., 2001a). Thus, it can be suggested that the MAPK cascade is required not to initiate resumption of maturation but for microtubule dynamics in the meiotic spindle in pig oocytes (Meinecke and Krischek, 2003). Inhibition of MAPK activation during MI-to-MII transition results in the failure of first polar body emission and MII spindle formation (Lee *et al.*, 2000). After fertilization, MAPK is kept highly active while the second meiosis resumes and the second polar body extrudes. Finally, MAPK is dephosphorylated during pronucleus formation (Sun *et al.*, 2001a). High level of MAPK is important for the oocyte to remain arrested at MII stage and is also necessary for the chromosomes to orderly align at the spindle equator. Low level of MAPK activity may cause instability of chromosomes in the spindles and may alter the precious relationship between microtubules and chromosomes (Ma *et al.*, 2005).

4.3 Mos-MAPK in human oocytes

p42Erk2 is the main form of MAPK in human oocytes (Sun *et al.*, 1999). Its pattern of activation by phosphorylation is reminiscent of other mammalian species including mice and pigs. MAPKKK Mos has also been detected in human oocytes and its expression was like in other models restricted to oocytes (Heikinheimo *et al.*, 1995; Heikinheimo *et al.*, 1996; Pal *et al.*, 1994). MAPK is inactive in immature oocyte while its activity increases during maturation and drops after fertilization. Thus, the functional role of MAPK in human oocytes remains an opened question since dynamical observations have been solely gathered (Combelles *et al.*, 2005; Sun *et al.*, 1999; Trounson *et al.*, 2001). MAPK and Mos have been then assumed to exert similar functions to those of other species.

4.4 A role for Mos in the limitation of M-phase rounds?

Mitotic exit is irreversible and irremediably followed by interphase, based on the degradation mechanisms of Cyclin B (Potapova *et al.*, 2006). This is not the case during meiosis, where exit from the first meiotic division is not followed by interphase and replication but is immediately followed by the onset of the second division. This lack of irreversibility has raised the following question: how oocytes limit the number of M-phases to just two during maternal meiosis? Switching off the activity of Mos - MAPK/Erk network appeared as an attractive hypothesis for ruling the number of M-phases, though it was clear from studies in jellyfish, starfish and amphibians that this mechanism could not be a universal one. First evidence supporting this hypothesis was recorded in mice oocytes where maintaining MAPK activity inhibits pronucleus formation (Moos *et al.*, 1995; Moos *et al.*, 1996) and where entry to meiosis III is observed in the presence of high level of MAPK/Erk activity (Verlhac *et al.*, 1996). The hypothesis that Mos-MAPK/Erk network could be the determining factor limiting the number of meiosis to two was recently formally tested in urochordates, which are at the crossroad between invertebrates and vertebrates (Dumollard *et al.*, 2011). In ascidian eggs, prolonging MAPK activity by expressing murine Mos leads to entry into supernumerary rounds of M-phases, which was attested by the increased number of polar bodies (Dumollard *et al.*, 2011). Then, urochordates offer an attractive model to unravel new observations on a conserved role of MAPK/Erk in spindle morphogenesis and to decipher the mechanisms leading to uncontrolled division and polyploidy since the successive rounds of M-phases observed in these cases occur without intervening replication.

5. Concluding remarks

Intensive fundamental research has generated a large amount of experimental data. However, it is crucial to validate this knowledge on animal models closer to humans. For analysis of aneuploidy degree and mechanism of occurrence in mammalian oocytes, pig has appeared as an attractive model. Comparing to non-human primates, pigs are cheaper and easier to maintain in controlled conditions. Porcine physiology assures a high relevance of the data obtained in this species for human-related research. Effective application of special breeds like minipigs, together with new methods for aneuploidy detection like CGH, brings new possibilities for aneuploidy research in mammalians. Usage of porcine oocytes for research on regulation pathways is still limited by the volume of oocytes collected and their sensitivity to manipulation in *in vitro* conditions. Development of *in vitro* cultivation methods and more effective live-cell imaging systems open new perspectives for aneuploidy research on porcine oocytes. To this extent, the molecular toolkits developed for kinase activity reporter will offer advantages to understand how kinases integrate and achieve cellular functions (Riquet *et al.*, 2011). Also, these methods, which aim at developing new sensors, will gain in sensitivity, kinetic properties and in spatial resolution, providing new tools for precise subcellular localization of dynamic structures such as meiotic spindles.

Nowadays pigs are used in several fields of biomedical research and its importance, as biomedical model, will increase in the near future. Last reports detecting aneuploidies in porcine oocytes bring interesting results and indicate significance of the porcine model for the study of aneuploidy in human. Nevertheless, taking advantages of the above-mentioned advantages of *Xenopus* oocytes, this amphibian might be considered as an "old dog", from which one might learn new tricks. It might also provide new insights to the scientific community interested in the field of reproduction. Proteomic approaches of the meiotic microtubule proteome are promising, since they will enable us to build a network of a microtubule-associated interactome: such approach was successfully adopted and began to validate novel spindle components like the human orthologue Mgc81475 (Smu1), which depletion drives mitotic arrest (Gache *et al.*, 2010). Further works are requested to validate this observation in other meiotic or mitotic models and to fully elucidate the role of the member of the MAPK/Erk network in spindle morphogenesis and aneuploidy. Nevertheless, approaches driven either in oocytes, eggs or extracts have generated an abundant literature, which has been attractive for modeling purposes. Computational models have been proposed to understand the self-organization of meiotic spindle (Loughlin *et al.*, 2010; Schaffner and Jose, 2006; Schaffner and Jose, 2008). These models offer a coherent picture of how microtubule dynamic instability, flux, and nucleation contribute to self-organization of a structure in a steady state.

Understanding of aneuploidy occurrence during meiosis in humans will benefit from experiments performed in various models, such as pigs and amphibians, and from the development of new tools, like sensors, and new approaches, like modeling. Further efforts will be necessary to collect and compare data obtained from these models.

6. Acknowledgments

Our work are supported by a grant from GACR 523/08/H064, MZe 0002716202, by the 'Ligue Régionale contre le Cancer" and the University Lille1, Sciences and Technologies. We thank our colleagues, Drahomira Knitlova, Franck Riquet, Brigitta Brinkman and Corentin Spriet, for helpful discussions and comments.

7. List of abbrevations

Calmodulin-dependent kinase (CAMKII); cumulus-enclosed oocytes (CEOs); cumulus oocytes complexes (COCs); cortical granule (CG); comparative genomic hybridization (CGH); denuded oocyte (DO) ; extracellular regulated kinase (Erk); fluorescence *in situ* hybridization (FISH); Germinal Vesicle (GV); germinal vesicle breakdown (GVBD); lutheinizing hormone (LH); metaphase I (MI); metaphase II (MII); mitogen activated protein kinase (MAPK); mitogen-activated protein kinase kinase (MEK); M-phase or meiosis promoting factor (MPF); microtubule organizing center (MTOC); ovum pick-up (OPU); polar body (PB); phosphate buffered saline (PBS); protein kinase A (PKA);

8. References

Alvarez Sedo, C., Schatten, H., Combelles, C. M., and Rawe, V. Y. (2011). The nuclear mitotic apparatus (NuMA) protein: localization and dynamics in human oocytes, fertilization and early embryos. *Mol Hum Reprod* 17, 392-398.

Amiel, A., Leclere, L., Robert, L., Chevalier, S., and Houliston, E. (2009). Conserved functions for Mos in eumetazoan oocyte maturation revealed by studies in a cnidarian. *Curr Biol* 19, 305-311.

Angeli, D., Ferrell, J. E., Jr., and Sontag, E. D. (2004). Detection of multistability, bifurcations, and hysteresis in a large class of biological positive-feedback systems. *Proc Natl Acad Sci U S A* 101, 1822-1827.

Araki, K., Naito, K., Haraguchi, S., Suzuki, R., Yokoyama, M., Inoue, M., Aizawa, S., Toyoda, Y., and Sato, E. (1996). Meiotic abnormalities of c-mos knockout mouse oocytes: activation after first meiosis or entrance into third meiotic metaphase. *Biol Reprod* 55, 1315-1324.

Baert, F., Bodart, J. F., Bocquet-Muchembled, B., Lescuyer-Rousseau, A., and Vilain, J. P. (2003). Xp42(Mpk1) activation is not required for germinal vesicle breakdown but for Raf complete phosphorylation in insulin-stimulated Xenopus oocytes. *J Biol Chem* 278, 49714-49720.

Battaglia, D. E., Goodwin, P., Klein, N. A., and Soules, M. R. (1996). Influence of maternal age on meiotic spindle assembly in oocytes from naturally cycling women. *Hum Reprod* 11, 2217-2222.

Bodart, J. F., Baert, F. Y., Sellier, C., Duesbery, N. S., Flament, S., and Vilain, J. P. (2005). Differential roles of p39Mos-Xp42Mpk1 cascade proteins on Raf1 phosphorylation and spindle morphogenesis in Xenopus oocytes. *Dev Biol* 283, 373-383.

Bodart, J. F., Bechard, D., Bertout, M., Gannon, J., Rousseau, A., Vilain, J. P., and Flament, S. (1999). Activation of Xenopus eggs by the kinase inhibitor 6-DMAP suggests a differential regulation of cyclin B and p39(mos) proteolysis. *Exp Cell Res* 253, 413-421.

Bodart, J. F., and Duesbery, N. S. (2006). Xenopus tropicalis oocytes: more than just a beautiful genome. *Methods Mol Biol* 322, 43-53.

Bodart, J. F., Flament, S., and Vilain, J. P. (2002a). Metaphase arrest in amphibian oocytes: interaction between CSF and MPF sets the equilibrium. Mol Reprod Dev *61*, 570-574.

Bodart, J. F., Gutierrez, D. V., Nebreda, A. R., Buckner, B. D., Resau, J. R., and Duesbery, N. S. (2002b). Characterization of MPF and MAPK activities during meiotic maturation of Xenopus tropicalis oocytes. *Dev Biol* 245, 348-361.

Bodart, J. F., Rodeau, J. L., Vilain, J. P., and Flament, S. (2001). c-Mos proteolysis is independent of the CA(2+) rise induced by 6-DMAP in *Xenopus* oocytes. *Exp Cell Res* 266, 187-192.

Brunet, S., Maria, A. S., Guillaud, P., Dujardin, D., Kubiak, J. Z., and Maro, B. (1999). Kinetochore fibers are not involved in the formation of the first meiotic spindle in mouse oocytes, but control the exit from the first meiotic M phase. *J Cell Biol* 146, 1-12.

Castro, A., Peter, M., Magnaghi-Jaulin, L., Vigneron, S., Galas, S., Lorca, T., and Labbe, J. C. (2001). Cyclin B/cdc2 induces c-Mos stability by direct phosphorylation in Xenopus oocytes. *Mol Biol Cell* 12, 2660-2671.

Chung, E., and Chen, R. H. (2003). Phosphorylation of Cdc20 is required for its inhibition by the spindle checkpoint. *Nat Cell Biol* 5, 748-753.

Combelles, C. M., Fissore, R. A., Albertini, D. F., and Racowsky, C. (2005). In vitro maturation of human oocytes and cumulus cells using a co-culture three-dimensional collagen gel system. *Hum Reprod* 20, 1349-1358.

Cross, M. K., and Powers, M. A. (2009). Learning about cancer from frogs: analysis of mitotic spindles in Xenopus egg extracts. *Dis Model Mech* 2, 541-547.

Dumollard, R., Levasseur, M., Hebras, C., Huitorel, P., Carroll, M., Chambon, J. P., and McDougall, A. (2011). Mos limits the number of meiotic divisions in urochordate eggs. *Development* 138, 885-895.

Dumont, J., Petri, S., Pellegrin, F., Terret, M. E., Bohnsack, M. T., Rassinier, P., Georget, V., Kalab, P., Gruss, O. J., and Verlhac, M. H. (2007). A centriole- and RanGTP-independent spindle assembly pathway in meiosis I of vertebrate oocytes. *J Cell Biol* 176, 295-305.

Dupre, A., Jessus, C., Ozon, R., and Haccard, O. (2002). Mos is not required for the initiation of meiotic maturation in Xenopus oocytes. *EMBO J* 21, 4026-4036.

Farin, C. E., and Yang, L. (1994). Inhibition of germinal vesicle breakdown in bovine oocytes by 5,6-dichloro-1-beta-D-ribofuranosylbenzimidazole (DRB). *Mol Reprod Dev* 37, 284-292.

Ferrell, J. E., Jr., and Bhatt, R. R. (1997). Mechanistic studies of the dual phosphorylation of mitogen-activated protein kinase. *J Biol Chem* 272, 19008-19016.

Ferrell, J. E., Jr., and Machleder, E. M. (1998). The biochemical basis of an all-or-none cell fate switch in Xenopus oocytes. *Science* 280, 895-898.

Foster, H. A., Sturmey, R. G., Stokes, P. J., Leese, H. J., Bridger, J. M., and Griffin, D. K. (2010). Fluorescence in situ hybridization on early porcine embryos. *Methods Mol Biol* 659, 427-436.

Gache, V., Waridel, P., Winter, C., Juhem, A., Schroeder, M., Shevchenko, A., and Popov, A. V. (2010). Xenopus meiotic microtubule-associated interactome. *PLoS One* 5, e9248.

Garner, E., and Costanzo, V. (2009). Studying the DNA damage response using in vitro model systems. *DNA Repair (Amst)* 8, 1025-1037.

Gautier, J., Norbury, C., Lohka, M., Nurse, P., and Maller, J. (1988). Purified maturation-promoting factor contains the product of a Xenopus homolog of the fission yeast cell cycle control gene cdc2+. *Cell* 54, 433-439.

Gordo, A. C., He, C. L., Smith, S., and Fissore, R. A. (2001). Mitogen activated protein kinase plays a significant role in metaphase II arrest, spindle morphology, and maintenance of maturation promoting factor activity in bovine oocytes. *Mol Reprod Dev* 59, 106-114.

Goto, S., Naito, K., Ohashi, S., Sugiura, K., Naruoka, H., Iwamori, N., and Tojo, H. (2002). Effects of spindle removal on MPF and MAP kinase activities in porcine matured oocytes. *Mol Reprod Dev* 63, 388-393.

Gotoh, Y., Masuyama, N., Dell, K., Shirakabe, K., and Nishida, E. (1995). Initiation of Xenopus oocyte maturation by activation of the mitogen-activated protein kinase cascade. *J Biol Chem* 270, 25898-25904.

Gross, S. D., Schwab, M. S., Taieb, F. E., Lewellyn, A. L., Qian, Y. W., and Maller, J. L. (2000). The critical role of the MAP kinase pathway in meiosis II in Xenopus oocytes is mediated by p90(Rsk). *Curr Biol* 10, 430-438.

Haccard, O., and Jessus, C. (2006). Oocyte maturation, Mos and cyclins--a matter of synthesis: two functionally redundant ways to induce meiotic maturation. *Cell Cycle* 5, 1152-1159.

Hassold, T., and Hunt, P. (2001). To err (meiotically) is human: the genesis of human aneuploidy. *Nat Rev Genet* 2, 280-291.

Heikinheimo, O., Lanzendorf, S. E., Baka, S. G., and Gibbons, W. E. (1995). Cell cycle genes c-mos and cyclin-B1 are expressed in a specific pattern in human oocytes and preimplantation embryos. *Hum Reprod* 10, 699-707.

Heikinheimo, O., Toner, J. P., Lanzendorf, S. E., Billeter, M., Veeck, L. L., and Gibbons, W. E. (1996). Messenger ribonucleic acid kinetics in human oocytes--effects of in vitro culture and nuclear maturational status. *Fertil Steril* 65, 1003-1008.

Hitzler, J. K., and Zipursky, A. (2005). Origins of leukaemia in children with Down syndrome. *Nat Rev Cancer* 5, 11-20.

Hornak, M., Jeseta, M., Musilova, P., Pavlok, A., Kubelka, M., Motlik, J., Rubes, J., and Anger, M. (2011). Frequency of aneuploidy related to age in porcine oocytes. *PLoS One* 6, e18892.

Horne, M. M., and Guadagno, T. M. (2003). A requirement for MAP kinase in the assembly and maintenance of the mitotic spindle. *J Cell Biol* 161, 1021-1028.

Howard, E. L., Charlesworth, A., Welk, J., and MacNicol, A. M. (1999). The mitogen-activated protein kinase signaling pathway stimulates mos mRNA cytoplasmic polyadenylation during Xenopus oocyte maturation. *Mol Cell Biol* 19, 1990-1999.

Huang, C. Y., and Ferrell, J. E., Jr. (1996). Ultrasensitivity in the mitogen-activated protein kinase cascade. *Proc Natl Acad Sci U S A* 93, 10078-10083.

Hunter, A. G., and Moor, R. M. (1987). Stage-dependent effects of inhibiting ribonucleic acids and protein synthesis on meiotic maturation of bovine oocytes in vitro. *J Dairy Sci* 70, 1646-1651.

Kanayama, N., Miyano, T., and Lee, J. (2002). Acquisition of meiotic competence in growing pig oocytes correlates with their ability to activate Cdc2 kinase and MAP kinase. *Zygote* 10, 261-270.

Kim, N. H., Chung, K. S., and Day, B. N. (1997). The distribution and requirements of microtubules and microfilaments during fertilization and parthenogenesis in pig oocytes. *J Reprod Fertil* 111, 143-149.

Kim, N. H., Funahashi, H., Prather, R. S., Schatten, G., and Day, B. N. (1996). Microtubule and microfilament dynamics in porcine oocytes during meiotic maturation. *Mol Reprod Dev* 43, 248-255.

Kotani, T., and Yamashita, M. (2002). Discrimination of the roles of MPF and MAP kinase in morphological changes that occur during oocyte maturation. *Dev Biol* 252, 271-286.

Lechniak, D., Warzych, E., Pers-Kamczyc, E., Sosnowski, J., Antosik, P., and Rubes, J. (2007). Gilts and sows produce similar rate of diploid oocytes in vitro whereas the incidence of aneuploidy differs significantly. *Theriogenology* 68, 755-762.

Lee, J., Miyano, T., and Moor, R. M. (2000). Localisation of phosphorylated MAP kinase during the transition from meiosis I to meiosis II in pig oocytes. *Zygote* 8, 119-125.

Liang, C. G., Su, Y. Q., Fan, H. Y., Schatten, H., and Sun, Q. Y. (2007). Mechanisms regulating oocyte meiotic resumption: roles of mitogen-activated protein kinase. *Mol Endocrinol* 21, 2037-2055.

Liu, X. S., and Liu, X. J. (2006). Oocyte isolation and enucleation. *Methods Mol Biol* 322, 31-41.

Lohka, M. J., Hayes, M. K., and Maller, J. L. (1988). Purification of maturation-promoting factor, an intracellular regulator of early mitotic events. *Proc Natl Acad Sci U S A* 85, 3009-3013.

Long, C. R., Pinto-Correia, C., Duby, R. T., Ponce de Leon, F. A., Boland, M. P., Roche, J. F., and Robl, J. M. (1993). Chromatin and microtubule morphology during the first cell cycle in bovine zygotes. *Mol Reprod Dev* 36, 23-32.

Loughlin, R., Heald, R., and Nedelec, F. (2010). A computational model predicts Xenopus meiotic spindle organization. *J Cell Biol* 191, 1239-1249.

Lu, Q., Dunn, R. L., Angeles, R., and Smith, G. D. (2002). Regulation of spindle formation by active mitogen-activated protein kinase and protein phosphatase 2A during mouse oocyte meiosis. *Biol Reprod* 66, 29-37.

Ma, W., Zhang, D., Hou, Y., Li, Y. H., Sun, Q. Y., Sun, X. F., and Wang, W. H. (2005). Reduced expression of MAD2, BCL2, and MAP kinase activity in pig oocytes after in vitro aging are associated with defects in sister chromatid segregation during meiosis II and embryo fragmentation after activation. *Biol Reprod* 72, 373-383.

Maresca, T. J., and Heald, R. (2006). Methods for studying spindle assembly and chromosome condensation in Xenopus egg extracts. *Methods Mol Biol* 322, 459-474.

Masui, Y., and Markert, C. L. (1971). Cytoplasmic control of nuclear behavior during meiotic maturation of frog oocytes. *J Exp Zool* 177, 129-145.

Matten, W. T., Copeland, T. D., Ahn, N. G., and Vande Woude, G. F. (1996). Positive feedback between MAP kinase and Mos during Xenopus oocyte maturation. *Dev Biol* 179, 485-492.

Meinecke, B., and Krischek, C. (2003). MAPK/ERK kinase (MEK) signalling is required for resumption of meiosis in cultured cumulus-enclosed pig oocytes. *Zygote* 11, 7-16.

Memili, E., and First, N. L. (1998). Developmental changes in RNA polymerase II in bovine oocytes, early embryos, and effect of alpha-amanitin on embryo development. *Mol Reprod Dev* 51, 381-389.

Miao, Y. L., Sun, Q. Y., Zhang, X., Zhao, J. G., Zhao, M. T., Spate, L., Prather, R. S., and Schatten, H. (2009). Centrosome abnormalities during porcine oocyte aging. *Environ Mol Mutagen* 50, 666-671.

Minshull, J., Sun, H., Tonks, N. K., and Murray, A. W. (1994). A MAP kinase-dependent spindle assembly checkpoint in Xenopus egg extracts. *Cell* 79, 475-486.

Moos, J., Visconti, P. E., Moore, G. D., Schultz, R. M., and Kopf, G. S. (1995). Potential role of mitogen-activated protein kinase in pronuclear envelope assembly and disassembly following fertilization of mouse eggs. *Biol Reprod* 53, 692-699.

Moos, J., Xu, Z., Schultz, R. M., and Kopf, G. S. (1996). Regulation of nuclear envelope assembly/disassembly by MAP kinase. *Dev Biol* 175, 358-361.

Motlik, J., and Fulka, J. (1976). Breakdown of the germinal vesicle in pig oocytes in vivo and in vitro. *J Exp Zool* 198, 155-162.

Nebreda, A. R., Gannon, J. V., and Hunt, T. (1995). Newly synthesized protein(s) must associate with p34cdc2 to activate MAP kinase and MPF during progesterone-induced maturation of Xenopus oocytes. *EMBO J* 14, 5597-5607.

Neuber, E., and Powers, R. D. (2000). Is the mouse a clinically relevant model for human fertilization failures? *Hum Reprod* 15, 171-174.

Ohashi, S., Naito, K., Sugiura, K., Iwamori, N., Goto, S., Naruoka, H., and Tojo, H. (2003). Analyses of mitogen-activated protein kinase function in the maturation of porcine oocytes. *Biol Reprod* 68, 604-609.

Pal, S. K., Torry, D., Serta, R., Crowell, R. C., Seibel, M. M., Cooper, G. M., and Kiessling, A. A. (1994). Expression and potential function of the c-mos proto-oncogene in human eggs. *Fertil Steril* 61, 496-503.

Paris, J., Swenson, K., Piwnica-Worms, H., and Richter, J. D. (1991). Maturation-specific polyadenylation: in vitro activation by p34cdc2 and phosphorylation of a 58-kD CPE-binding protein. *Genes Dev* 5, 1697-1708.

Potapova, T. A., Daum, J. R., Pittman, B. D., Hudson, J. R., Jones, T. N., Satinover, D. L., Stukenberg, P. T., and Gorbsky, G. J. (2006). The reversibility of mitotic exit in vertebrate cells. *Nature* 440, 954-958.

Riquet, F., Vandame, P., Sipieter, F., Cailliau-Maggio, K., Spriet, C., Héliot, L. and Bodart, J.F. (2011). Reporting Kinase activities: paradigms, tools and perspectives. *Journal of Biological Medicine* 1, 10-18.

Russo, C., Beaujois, R., Bodart, J. F., and Blossey, R. (2009). Kicked by Mos and tuned by MPF-the initiation of the MAPK cascade in Xenopus oocytes. *HFSP J* 3, 428-440.

Sagata, N. (1997). What does Mos do in oocytes and somatic cells? *Bioessays* 19, 13-21.

Schaffner, S. C., and Jose, J. V. (2006). Biophysical model of self-organized spindle formation patterns without centrosomes and kinetochores. *Proc Natl Acad Sci U S A* 103, 11166-11171.

Schaffner, S. C., and Jose, J. V. (2008). Chapter 24: Computational modeling of self-organized spindle formation. *Methods Cell Biol* 89, 623-652.

Schatten, G., Schatten, H., Bestor, T. H., and Balczon, R. (1982). Taxol inhibits the nuclear movements during fertilization and induces asters in unfertilized sea urchin eggs. *J Cell Biol* 94, 455-465.

Schatten, G., Schatten, H., Spector, I., Cline, C., Paweletz, N., Simerly, C., and Petzelt, C. (1986). Latrunculin inhibits the microfilament-mediated processes during fertilization, cleavage and early development in sea urchins and mice. *Exp Cell Res* 166, 191-208.

Schatten, H., Simerly, C., Maul, G., and Schatten, G. (1989). Microtubule assembly is required for the formation of the pronuclei, nuclear lamin acquisition, and DNA synthesis during mouse, but not sea urchin, fertilization. *Gamete Res* 23, 309-322.

Schatten, H., and Sun, Q. Y. (2011). Centrosome dynamics during mammalian oocyte maturation with a focus on meiotic spindle formation. *Mol Reprod Dev* 78, 757-768.

Schatten, H., Walter, M., Biessmann, H., and Schatten, G. (1992). Activation of maternal centrosomes in unfertilized sea urchin eggs. *Cell Motil Cytoskeleton* 23, 61-70.

Sugiura, K., Naito, K., Iwamori, N., Kagii, H., Goto, S., Ohashi, S., Yamanouchi, K., and Tojo, H. (2001). Germinal vesicle materials are not required for the activation of MAP kinase in porcine oocyte maturation. *Mol Reprod Dev* 59, 215-220.

Sun, Q. Y., Blumenfeld, Z., Rubinstein, S., Goldman, S., Gonen, Y., and Breitbart, H. (1999). Mitogen-activated protein kinase in human eggs. *Zygote* 7, 181-185.

Sun, Q. Y., Lai, L., Park, K. W., Kuhholzer, B., Prather, R. S., and Schatten, H. (2001a). Dynamic events are differently mediated by microfilaments, microtubules, and mitogen-activated protein kinase during porcine oocyte maturation and fertilization in vitro. *Biol Reprod* 64, 879-889.

Sun, Q. Y., Lai, L., Wu, G. M., Park, K. W., Day, B. N., Prather, R. S., and Schatten, H. (2001b). Microtubule assembly after treatment of pig oocytes with taxol: correlation with chromosomes, gamma-tubulin, and MAP kinase. *Mol Reprod Dev* 60, 481-490.

Sun, Q. Y., Wu, G. M., Lai, L., Bonk, A., Cabot, R., Park, K. W., Day, B. N., Prather, R. S., and Schatten, H. (2002). Regulation of mitogen-activated protein kinase phosphorylation, microtubule organization, chromatin behavior, and cell cycle progression by protein phosphatases during pig oocyte maturation and fertilization in vitro. *Biol Reprod* 66, 580-588.

Sutovsky, P., Navara, C. S., and Schatten, G. (1996). Fate of the sperm mitochondria, and the incorporation, conversion, and disassembly of the sperm tail structures during bovine fertilization. *Biol Reprod* 55, 1195-1205.

Takenaka, K., Gotoh, Y., and Nishida, E. (1997). MAP kinase is required for the spindle assembly checkpoint but is dispensable for the normal M phase entry and exit in Xenopus egg cell cycle extracts. *J Cell Biol* 136, 1091-1097.

Terada, Y., Simerly, C., and Schatten, G. (2000). Microfilament stabilization by jasplakinolide arrests oocyte maturation, cortical granule exocytosis, sperm incorporation cone resorption, and cell-cycle progression, but not DNA replication, during fertilization in mice. *Mol Reprod Dev* 56, 89-98.

Tong, C., Fan, H. Y., Chen, D. Y., Song, X. F., Schatten, H., and Sun, Q. Y. (2003). Effects of MEK inhibitor U0126 on meiotic progression in mouse oocytes: microtuble organization, asymmetric division and metaphase II arrest. *Cell Res* 13, 375-383.

Trounson, A., Anderiesz, C., and Jones, G. (2001). Maturation of human oocytes in vitro and their developmental competence. *Reproduction* 121, 51-75.

Uchiyama, S., Kobayashi, S., Takata, H., Ishihara, T., Hori, N., Higashi, T., Hayashihara, K., Sone, T., Higo, D., Nirasawa, T., *et al.* (2005). Proteome analysis of human metaphase chromosomes. *J Biol Chem* 280, 16994-17004.

Ueno, S., Kurome, M., Ueda, H., Tomii, R., Hiruma, K., and Nagashima, H. (2005). Effects of maturation conditions on spindle morphology in porcine MII oocytes. *J Reprod Dev* 51, 405-410.

Van Blerkom, J., Davis, P., Merriam, J., and Sinclair, J. (1995). Nuclear and cytoplasmic dynamics of sperm penetration, pronuclear formation and microtubule organization during fertilization and early preimplantation development in the human. *Hum Reprod Update* 1, 429-461.

Verlhac, M. H., Kubiak, J. Z., Weber, M., Geraud, G., Colledge, W. H., Evans, M. J., and Maro, B. (1996). Mos is required for MAP kinase activation and is involved in microtubule organization during meiotic maturation in the mouse. *Development* 122, 815-822.

Wang, W. H., and Sun, Q. Y. (2006). Meiotic spindle, spindle checkpoint and embryonic aneuploidy. *Front Biosci* 11, 620-636.

Willard, F. S., and Crouch, M. F. (2001). MEK, ERK, and p90RSK are present on mitotic tubulin in Swiss 3T3 cells: a role for the MAP kinase pathway in regulating mitotic exit. *Cell Signal* 13, 653-664.

Ye, J., Flint, A. P., Luck, M. R., and Campbell, K. H. (2003). Independent activation of MAP kinase and MPF during the initiation of meiotic maturation in pig oocytes. *Reproduction* 125, 645-656.

Younis, J. S. (2011). Ovarian aging: latest thoughts on assessment and management. *Curr Opin Obstet Gynecol.* 6, 427-434.

11

The Role of Aneuploidy Screening in Human Preimplantation Embryos

Christian S. Ottolini[1,2], Darren K. Griffin[2] and Alan R. Thornhill[1,2]
[1]*The London Bridge Fertility, Gynaecology and Genetics Centre, London Bridge*
[2]*School of Biosciences, University of Kent, Canterbury*
United Kingdom

1. Introduction

Aneuploidy can be defined as extra or missing whole chromosomes in the nucleus of a cell and occurs during cell division when chromosomes do not separate equally between the two new daughter cells (Hassold & Hunt 2001). Chromosome imbalance typically results in non-viability, manifesting as developmental arrest prior to implantation, miscarriage or stillbirth. Depending on the chromosomes involved, aneuploidy can also result in viable but developmentally abnormal pregnancies e.g. Down or Klinefelter Syndrome. In all cases, aneuploidy results in a non-favourable outcome for the family in question and is undoubtedly a major contributing factor to the relatively low fecundity of humans when compared with other species.

Aneuploidy is a particularly frequent event during both human gametogenesis and early embryogenesis in humans and arises due to mal-segregation of the chromosomes. The most cited mechanism is classical "non-disjunction" however this has been challenged in recent years and alternative mechanisms have been proposed (see subsequent sections). It is estimated that at least 20% of human oocytes are aneuploid, a number that increases dramatically with advancing maternal age over the age of 35 years (Dailey *et al.* 1996a; Hassold & Hunt 2001). Conversely, the incidence of aneuploidy in sperm cells from a normal fertile male is estimated to be as low as 4-7% (Martin *et al.* 1991; Shi & Martin 2000). However, this can significantly increase in some cases of severe male factor infertility.

The idea of screening pre-implantation embryos to eliminate the aneuploid ones is not new, but the ability to do this effectively has required rapid evolution of diagnostic technologies to combine speed, accuracy and reliability. To date, only direct analysis of chromosomes from cells in gametes and pre-implantation embryos (rather than indirect methods such as metabolic analysis) has proved successful in accurately detecting aneuploidy. Performing Preimplantation Genetic Screening (PGS) in this way involves the biopsy of cellular material from the embryo or oocyte at different stages of development. Since embryo biopsy is too invasive a procedure for routine embryo selection, PGS remains a test for high-risk patient groups only rather than for routine universal application. Worldwide, the test is only offered routinely to patients presenting with advanced maternal age, recurrent miscarriage, recurrent implantation failure and in some cases of severe male factor infertility. Due to the invasive nature of embryo biopsy and the complexity of human aneuploidy in the human IVF embryo, cost benefit analysis is crucial to achieve positive outcomes. It could be argued that, in the past, the practice of PGS has not given proper concern to these issues and thus, going forward, patient selection and understanding the mechanisms of aneuploidy should be central to an effective PGS strategy. This chapter explores the premise underpinning the use of PGS in human embryos, its clinical applications, current methodologies and future applications.

2. Origin of aneuploidy

Aneuploidy in pre-implantation IVF embryos (and presumably also those naturally conceived) primarily arises during three developmental stages: (i) pre-meiotic divisions of gametogenesis; (ii) meiotic divisions of gametogenesis and (iii) early mitotic divisions of embryogenesis. Understanding the mechanism behind the mal-segregation of chromosomes at these stages gives insight into the limitations of PGS when applied clinically.

2.1 Gonadal mosaicism

Errors in germ cell proliferation or errors inherited in an otherwise somatically normal individual resulting in germ cell aneuploidy (gonadal mosaicism) can also contribute to aneuploidy of the gametes. This is perhaps the least studied of the three stages. In any event, the outcome is a hyper- or hypo- gamete and thus can be considered in the same way as a meiotic error.

2.2 Meiosis

Meiosis is the production of a haploid gamete by two specialised cell divisions in which the diploid chromosome complement of normal somatic cells is reduced (a requisite for sexual reproduction). Errors in chromosome segregation during these divisions typically result in gamete aneuploidy and subsequent 'uniform' aneuploidy in any resulting embryo. Although the basic principle of chromosome mal-segregation holds for both male and female meiosis in humans, the processes and resulting gametes are vastly different. Female meiosis, the process by which a single diploid germ cell develops into a single haploid ovum, involves two unequal meiotic divisions producing a mature ovum and two non-functional products containing mirror images of the chromosomes present in the ovum. These are known as polar bodies (PB) and, once extruded, take no further part in development thus making them a useful sample for inferring chromosome constitution of the oocyte itself. Failures in female meiosis make, by far, the biggest contribution to aneuploidy in human pre-implantation embryos. Cytogenetic studies on oocytes and first polar bodies (PB1) from assisted conception cycles have shown more than 20% of oocytes from patients with an average age under 35 to be aneuploid (Selva *et al.* 1991; Fragouli *et al.* 2006). The percentage of aneuploid oocytes increases significantly with age and has been shown to affect an average of around 70% of oocytes for patients of advanced maternal age (Van Blerkom 1989; Angell *et al.* 1993; Kuliev *et al.* 2003; Gutierrez-Mateo *et al.* 2004; Kuliev *et al.* 2005).

There is conflicting evidence on the frequency of errors in both the first and second meiotic division with groups showing errors in both the first meiotic division-MI (Kuliev *et al.* 2003) and more recently in the second meiotic division-MII (Fragouli *et al.* 2011; Handyside *et al.* 2012) occurring more frequently. This discrepancy may be due in part to differences in patient maternal age of the study groups and the difference in resolution of the cytogenetic techniques used. Either way, it is clear that chromosome segregation errors occur at significant rates during both the first and second meiotic divisions of oogenesis.

Based on studies of yeast, drosophila and mouse models it was generally believed that aneuploidy arose as a result of classic nondisjunction and involved the segregation of a whole chromosome to the same pole as its homologue during meiosis. Studies of human oocytes led to an alternative model for the origin of aneuploidy (Angell 1991) suggesting that errors in meiosis can result in extra or missing chromatids (known as premature or precocious separation of sister chromatids - PS), as well as whole chromosomes in the daughter cells (See figure 1). Early studies of human oocytes supporting the hypothesis that precocious separation was the predominant mechanism leading to human aneuploidy were subject to recurring criticism (Angell 1991; Angell *et al.* 1993; Angell *et al.* 1994; Pellestor *et al.* 2002; Kuliev *et al.* 2003). It was argued that use of 'failed IVF' oocytes' prolonged time in culture, sub-optimal metaphase preparation technique, and lack of rigour in the analysis may have led to interpretation errors (Dailey *et al.* 1996b; Lamb *et al.* 1996; Lamb *et al.* 1997; Mahmood *et al.* 2000). Recently several groups, including our own, performed analyses using methodology less prone to these confounding criticisms - the results of which support the hypothesis. Quantitative analysis of loss or gain of all 24 chromosomes on PB1 (Gabriel *et al.* 2011b) and sequential 24 chromosome analysis of PB1, PB2 and zygote performed on freshly harvested oocytes used in IVF treatments (Geraedts et al. 2011) have shown PS to be the predominant mechanism of chromosome mal-segregation in assisted reproduction derived oocytes. This is consistent with recent data exploring the decline of adhesion molecules holding sister chromatids together during anaphase arrest leading to increased PS events (Chiang *et al.* 2010; Lister *et al.* 2010).

In contrast to oogenesis, male meiosis results in four equivalent functional spermatozoa from a single progenitor germ cell. The presence of typically millions of sperm per ejaculate make them easy to study *en masse* however it is impossible, with current technology, to screen a sperm head for aneuploidy then subsequently use it for PGS. This is because aneuploidy assessment of a sperm cell inevitably results in its destruction, and unlike in the ovum, there are no by-products available from which a determination of chromosome complement can be inferred.

The overall incidence of aneuploidy in sperm is estimated to be around 4-7% (Martin *et al.* 1991; Shi & Martin 2000) although some studies suggest it is as high as 14% in some infertile men (Johnson 1998; Shi & Martin 2001). Spermatogenesis can theoretically continue unchanged throughout the life of a man however several studies have shown there to be a correlation between increased sperm aneuploidy and advanced paternal age (Griffin *et al.* 1995; Robbins *et al.* 1995) albeit not as dramatic as in the female. Other factors such as male factor infertility, smoking and chemotherapy can however increase sperm aneuploidy levels, making individual couples in which these risk factors are present possible candidates for PGS.

2.3 Mitosis

Mitosis is the process by which a diploid cell usually divides into two chromosomally identical daughter cells. It is the primary mechanism by which a multicellular individual

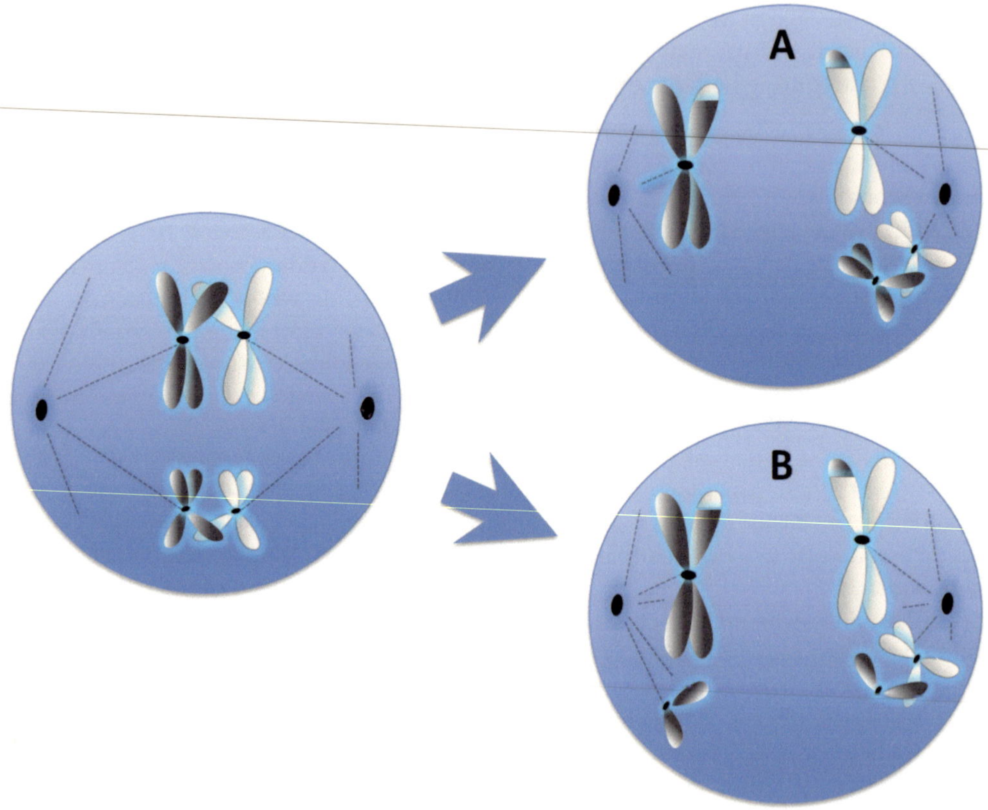

Fig. 1. Diagrammatic representation of classic nondisjunction (A) and premature separation of the sister chromatids (B), the two predominant mechanisms by which aneuploidy can arise in the first meiotic division in humans.

develops from a single fertilised oocyte (zygote). Human mitotic divisions are generally not prone to chromosome segregation errors to any great extent, except in the case of early embryo cleavage stages where cells are thought to be exquisitely prone to segregation errors (Bean *et al.* 2001). Indeed, recent studies using a variety of cytogenetic techniques on early IVF human embryos have demonstrated that over 50% are subject to some form of mitotic error (Bielanska *et al.* 2002; Munne *et al.* 2004; Delhanty 2005; Munne 2006).

Most mitotic errors in early embryo development will lead to chromosomal mosaicism which is defined as the presence of two or more chromosome complements within an embryo developed from a single zygote. There are three hypothesised mechanisms by which mitotic aneuploidy can arise: (i) chromosome loss (presumably from anaphase lag resulting in chromosome loss in one cell line), (ii) chromosome duplication (the underlying mechanisms of which are not well understood) or (iii) reciprocal chromosome loss and gain (resulting mainly from a mitotic nondisjunction event or potentially anaphase lag creating one cell line with chromosome loss and one with a reciprocal gain) (see figure 2). Following observations of increased incidence of chromosome loss in pre-implantation embryos compared to gains and the relative paucity of reciprocal events -which would indicate non-disjunction (Daphnis *et al.* 2005; Delhanty 2005) the predominant mechanism leading to post-zygotic errors in human embryos is likely to be chromosome loss resulting from anaphase lag (Coonen *et al.* 2004). Anaphase lag is described as the delayed movement during mitotic anaphase of a homologous chromosome resulting in it not being incorporated into the nucleus of the daughter cell. Often the lagging chromosome is lost creating one euploid daughter cell and a daughter cell with a monosomy for the chromosome in question.

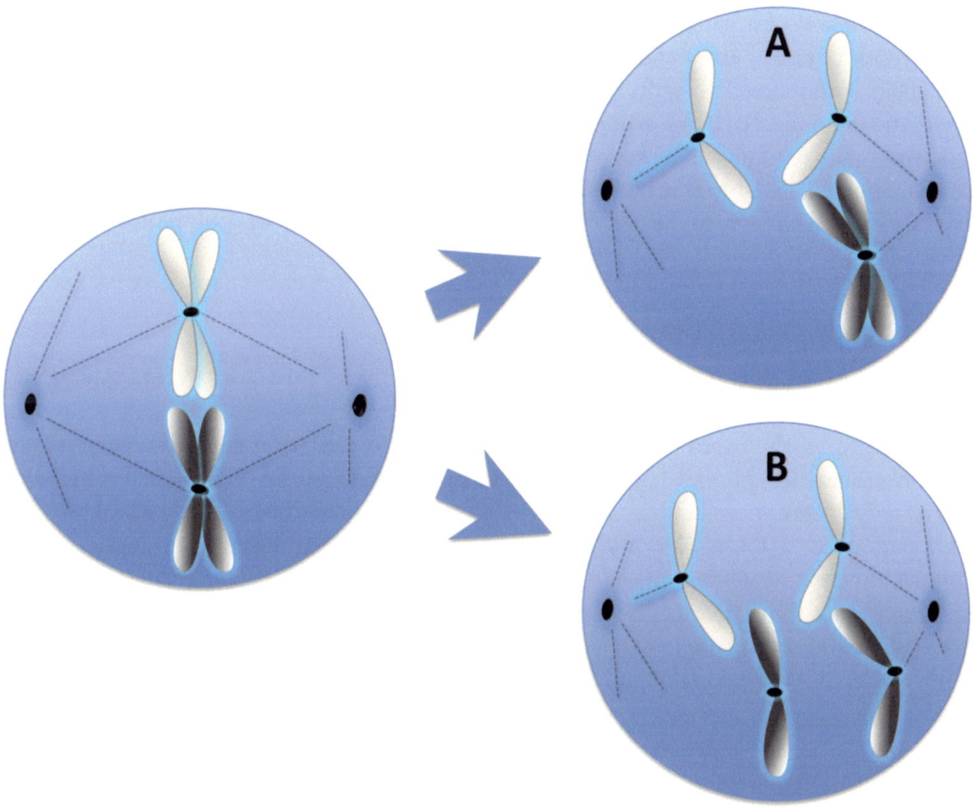

Fig. 2. Diagrammatic representation of anaphase lag (A) and mitotic nondisjunction (B), the two predominant types of mitotic errors in humans resulting in embryo mosaicism.

Mosaicism is considered to be largely independent of age (Delhanty 2005). However, it has been shown that mosaicism originating by the mechanism of mitotic non-disjunction could perhaps be related to advanced maternal age (Munne *et al.* 2002). Results also suggest that mosaicism involving multiple chromosomes and a high proportion of cells (chaotic embryos) appear to impair early embryo development considerably.

The general consensus for the viability of mosaic embryos is that, if more than half of the cells at day 3 post fertilization are aneuploid, the embryo is unlikely to be viable. Conversely, if a small proportion of cells are aneuploid in an otherwise healthy and euploid background, it is likely to be viable (Delhanty 2005).

Clearly mosaicism affects embryo development making it a key element in the selection of embryos in clinical IVF cases (Bielanska *et al.* 2002; Delhanty 2005).

2.4 Abnormal fertilisation

Abnormal fertilisation can also contribute to chromosome errors in pre-implantation embryos. Approximately 1% of conceptions contain more than two paired homologous sets of chromosomes-referred to as polyploidy rather than aneuploidy (Hassold 1986). There are two ways in which a polyploid embryo can arise: Firstly, if a diploid (2n) sperm or oocyte is involved in the fertilisation event and secondly, if two or more haploid sperm are involved in the fertilisation of a haploid oocyte (polyspermy). The majority of all polyploid embryos are the result of polyspermy and account for around 60% of polyploid conceptions (Egozcue *et al.* 2002). Following IVF with ICSI in which only a single sperm is inserted into each oocyte, the main mechanism leading to polyploidy in the embryo is the failure of the oocyte to extrude the second polar body (Grossmann *et al.* 1997). This results in a triploid embryo when fertilisation is achieved with a haploid sperm. Non-reduced or diploid sperm have also been shown to be involved in as many as 8.3% of polyploid conceptions (Egozcue *et al.* 2002).

3. Aneuploidy and IVF development

Since the first human IVF success in 1978 (Steptoe & Edwards 1978), advances in morphologic embryo grading and technologies aiding morphologic embryo selection have contributed to vastly improved IVF outcomes (Figure 3). Unfortunately, the morphological selection criteria for human gametes and embryos across all developmental stages have shown only weak correlations with aneuploidy (Munne 2006; Gianaroli *et al.* 2007; Alfarawati *et al.* 2011a). Karyotypic analysis indicates that there is a higher rate of chromosome abnormalities in morphologically abnormal monospermic embryos than morphologically normal embryos (Pellestor 1995; Almeida & Bolton 1996). However, clear distinctions cannot be made between chromosomally normal and abnormal human embryos by morphological assessment alone (Zenzes & Casper 1992). This may be because chromosome abnormalities detected at the early stages of embryogenesis cannot induce dysmorphism, since embryonic gene expression has not yet commenced (Braude *et al.* 1988; Tesarik *et al.* 1988). There is evidence from 24 chromosome copy number analysis that morphology and aneuploidy are linked at the later stages of pre-implantation embryo development (blastocyst stage). However, again the association is weak, and consequently, morphologic analysis can still not be relied upon to ensure transfer of chromosomally normal embryos. A significant proportion of aneuploid embryos are capable of achieving the highest morphologic scores even at the later stages of pre-implantation development, and, conversely, some euploid embryos achieve only poor morphological scores or even fail to develop (Alfarawati *et al.* 2011a).

Other indirect aneuploidy screening methods have been trialled in the past with limited success. More recently, proteomic studies have shown to be a potentially useful tool in prenatal aneuploidy screening (Cho & Diamandis 2011; Kolialexi *et al.* 2011). By applying the same principle to pre-implantation embryos, one study has identified the first protein secreted by human blastocysts that is associated with generic chromosome aneuploidy (McReynolds *et al.* 2011). Although promising, this technology is still some way from becoming a routine aneuploidy screening test and oocyte or embryo biopsy with molecular cytogenetic analysis is still the preferred technique for PGS.

All molecular cytogenetic techniques involving gametes and embryos require direct access to the nuclear material of the gametes or blastomeres themselves. This process is achieved by cell biopsy and inevitably results in the destruction of the cells involved. With this in mind, it is important that fertilisation or embryogenesis is not compromised and the biopsy procedure impacts minimally on developmental potential.

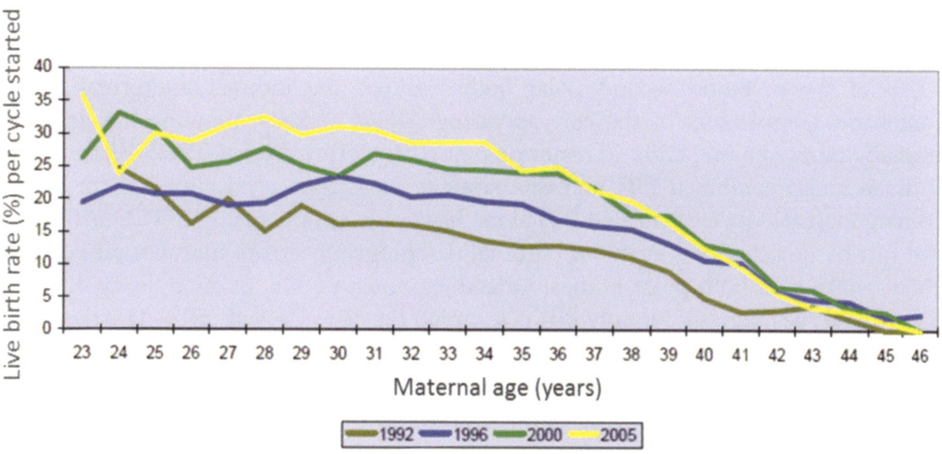

Fig. 3. Overall IVF and IVF/ICSI success rates by maternal age in the UK from 1992 - 2005. Figure adapted from Human Fertilisation and Embryology Authority website [HFEA] (2008a)

Recent clinical trials and meta-analyses of cases have suggested no benefit, and in some cases worse IVF pregnancy outcomes following PGS- presumably the result of discard of normal embryos (diagnosed as abnormal - false positives), detrimental effects of the biopsy including reduction of cellular mass and excessive micromanipulation outside of the incubator (Mastenbroek *et al.* 2007; Twisk *et al.* 2008). These results have however been dismissed by many PGS practitioners due to questionable experimental design (Munne *et al.* 1999; Handyside & Thornhill 2007). Nevertheless, at the very least, these trials have reinforced the idea that embryo biopsy can only be justifiable when the benefit of the testing outweighs the cost to the embryo, since the ultimate aim of PGS is to identify chromosomally competent embryos without compromising embryo viability.

4. Oocyte/embryo biopsy

Biopsy for PGS is currently a two-step micromanipulation process involving the penetration of the zona pellucida followed by the removal of one or more cells for chromosome analysis. Breaching the zona is generally performed by laser ablation as it has been shown, when used appropriately, to have no detrimental effects on embryo development in both animal and human studies (Montag *et al.* 1998; Park *et al.* 1999; Han *et al.* 2003). Specialised micromanipulation pipettes are then used to separate the required cells from the oocyte or embryo. Theoretically, PGS can be accomplished at any developmental stage from the mature (MII) oocyte to the blastocyst stage. To date only three discrete stages have been proposed for clinical use: (i) polar body (oocyte and/or zygote), (ii) cleavage stage (day 3 embryo) and (iii) blastocyst (day 5 or 6 embryo). Each of these stages is biologically different thus having different diagnostic limitations in terms of information to be gained and impact on embryo viability.

4.1 Polar body biopsy

The removal of PB1 and/or PB2 from a human oocyte should have no deleterious effect on subsequent embryo, foetal and infant development as neither is required for successful fertilisation or embryogenesis (Gianaroli 2000; Strom *et al.* 2000). Biopsy and subsequent analysis of the first and second polar bodies allows the indirect interpretation of the chromosome complement of the corresponding oocyte thereby allowing the detection of maternally derived aneuploidy in resulting embryos (Verlinsky *et al.* 1996). While biopsy of PB1 alone and a combined PB1 and PB2 strategy have been used clinically for PGS, it is becoming increasingly evident that PB1 alone has limited applicability to PGS as only errors in MI can be detected and even MI chromatid segregation errors may not all be detected without analysis of both polar bodies. Indeed, as much as 30% of aneuploidy of maternal origin will not be diagnosed if only PB1 is sampled (Handyside *et al.* 2012). It is therefore the authors opinion that biopsy of both first and second polar body is essential for optimal detection of oocyte aneuploidy if used as an embryo selection tool. A further limitation is that cytogenetic analysis of either polar body does not allow the detection of aneuploidies of paternal origin nor aneuploidies arising after fertilisation in the embryo.

The process of polar body biopsy is relatively labour intensive and may involve the micromanipulation of oocytes that ultimately do not develop into therapeutic quality embryos. Sometimes up to four manipulations - ICSI, PB1, PB2 and blastomere biopsy (as a reflexive test following test failure or an ambiguous PB result) may be required. However, in experienced hands, even 3 independent biopsy manipulations appear to have no deleterious effect on development (Magli *et al.* 2004; Cieslak-Janzen *et al.* 2006). Although simultaneous removal of PB1 and PB2 is possible on day 1 of embryo development (Magli *et al.* 2011) there may be advantages to sequential biopsy where PB1 is removed on day 0 (day of insemination) followed by the removal of PB2 on day 1. This is to avoid any degeneration of PB1 leading to possible diagnostic failure and also to allow for the distinction between polar bodies, thereby allowing accurate identification of errors in the first and second meiotic divisions.

4.2 Cleavage stage embryo biopsy

Historically cleavage stage biopsy was the most widely practiced form of embryo biopsy for PGS worldwide. This biopsy strategy is now becoming less popular however due to its potential detrimental effect on embryo viability and the problem of mosaicism in human cleavage stage embryos. A typical procedure for cleavage stage biopsy involves the removal of one or two blastomeres from an embryo on day 3 post-fertilization - usually those of suitable quality with at least 5 cells having entered the third cleavage division. Although cleavage stage biopsy allows the detection of maternally and paternally derived aneuploidy as well as post-zygotic errors, they are not always distinguishable. The main problem affecting cleavage stage biopsy is chromosomal mosaicism resulting in an increased rate of false positive and negative results from single cell (or two cell) analysis (Figure 4).

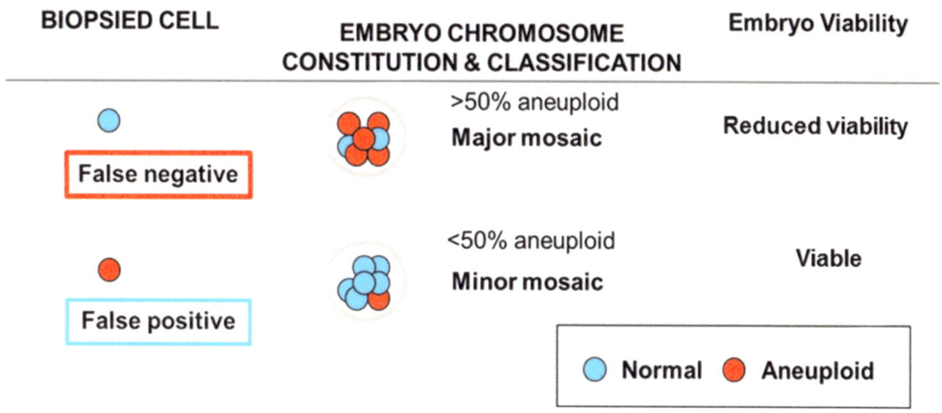

Fig. 4. Schematic representation of possible misdiagnosis following cleavage stage biopsy of a single cell

Data from studies comparing undiagnosed biopsied embryos and non-biopsied control embryos showed a detrimental effect of biopsy on implantation (Cohen & Grifo 2007; Mastenbroek *et al.* 2007), most evident in embryos of suboptimal quality. Animal models have shown that the potential for the embryo to continue to develop and implant is progressively compromised the greater the proportion of the embryo is removed (Liu *et al.* 1993). While such evidence provides fuel for the argument against performing biopsy at early cleavage stages at all, evidence from frozen-thawed embryo transfers (as a proxy for biopsied embryos) in which successful implantations and live births can be achieved even following embryonic cell death demonstrates that a certain degree of cell loss is tolerated (Cohen *et al.* 2007). However, just as in the animal models, success is inversely correlated with the amount of cellular mass lost.

The successful application of cleavage stage biopsy minimising cell removal from good quality embryos shows it is compatible with normal embryo metabolism, blastocyst development and foetal growth (Hardy *et al.* 1990). Moreover, studies of pregnancies and children born after cleavage stage biopsy have identified no significant increase in abnormalities above the rate seen in routine IVF (Harper *et al.* 2006; Banerjee *et al.* 2008; Nekkebroeck *et al.* 2008).

A general estimate therefore is that cleavage stage biopsy of 1 cell may reduce the implantation potential of an IVF embryo of around 10% although this figure would inevitably increase in less experienced hands (Cohen & Grifo 2007). The challenge for any future application of cleavage stage biopsy PGS therefore is to ensure that any benefits outweigh these costs and it remains a question whether this will be possible even with more accurate and reliable tests given the high levels of mosaicism.

4.3 Blastocyst stage biopsy

Blastocyst biopsy involves the sampling of trophectoderm (TE) cells, the spherical outer epithelial monolayer of the blastocyst stage embryo. Just as at cleavage stage, TE biopsy is able to detect aneuploidy arising in either gamete or post-fertilisation. It is more akin to early prenatal diagnosis when compared to the other biopsy stages as it involves the removal of up to 10 cells without depleting the inner cell mass (ICM) from which the foetus is derived. TE biopsy is most commonly achieved by partial zona dissection followed by a period of culture in which time the expansion of the blastocyst will cause herniation of several cells through the artificial breach. The herniating cells (~4-10 cells) are then easily removed by excision or aspiration using micromanipulation tools with or without the aid of a laser. Sampling of several cells at this stage lessens the likelihood that mosaicism will produce false positive results also overcoming the limitations of extreme sensitivity apparent with conventional single cell diagnosis.

As with cleavage stage biopsy, it has been suggested that the removal of cells may negatively impact on the embryo's developmental potential. However, skilled biopsy practitioners are able to remove TE cells and achieve comparable implantation rates to non-biopsied blastocyst stage embryos (Kokkali *et al.* 2007). It has also been proposed that sampling of the TE may not reflect the genetic composition of the ICM (Kalousek & Vekemans 1996). Recent data however comparing TE to ICM suggests 100% concordance with the exception of structural abnormalities (Johnson *et al.* 2010a).

Currently the main limitation of blastocyst biopsy is the low number of embryos that reach the blastocyst stage; a number that significantly decreases with advanced maternal age (Pantos *et al.* 1999). If very few blastocysts are available, particularly in older patients, biopsy for selection purposes may be of no benefit. Also, time constraints at the blastocyst stage dictate, in many cases, the need to cryopreserve biopsied blastocysts awaiting diagnosis. Thus, the effect of cryopreservation and subsequent thawing on embryo viability must be taken into account. Nonetheless, improved culture techniques, possible vitrification and rapid molecular analysis regimes are making blastocyst biopsy an increasingly attractive option (Schoolcraft *et al.* 2010).

5. Molecular cytogenetics – The rise and fall of fluorescence *in situ* hybridization (FISH) in PGS

Following embryo or oocyte biopsy, PGS requires cytogenetic techniques with high sensitivity and specificity to establish the chromosome composition of the embryo via the analysis of one or very few cells. Classic karyotyping techniques are not suitable for pre-implantation testing due to the difficulty of achieving good metaphase spreads with the limited cells available for testing (Angell *et al.* 1986; Papadopoulos *et al.* 1989). In 1993 the application of Fluorescent In-situ Hybridisation (FISH) for the single cell detection of the sex chromosomes in pre-implantation embryos provided a springboard for aneuploidy detection and clinical application of PGS soon followed (Griffin *et al.* 1992). FISH is a highly sensitive, relatively inexpensive molecular cytogenetic tool enabling the determination of chromosome copy number at the single cell level. Its successful application rapidly led to the implementation of PGS as a clinical adjunct to IVF globally. To date tens of thousands of PGS cases have been performed globally, attesting to its popularity. Nonetheless, advances in technology are making FISH for PGS in oocytes and embryos a less attractive option due to a range of technical and biological considerations that are becoming increasingly apparent (Table 1).

Test	Chromosomes detected	Resolution	Parental DNA required	Polyploidy	Recombination mapping	Origin of aneuploidy	
						parent of origin	MI or MII
Fluorescence in situ hybridization (FISH)	5 to 12	low	no	yes	no	no	no
Array comparative genomic hybridisation (aCGH)	24	high	no	no	no	no	no
Single nucleotide polymorphism (SNP) array	24	highest	yes	yes	yes	yes	limited to hyperploidy

Table 1. Scope and limitations of different molecular cytogenetic techniques after embryo biopsy

5.1 Fluorescent *In-situ* Hybridisation (FISH)

FISH requires the fixation of biopsied cells to a glass slide before visual analysis of hybridised fluorescent chromosome specific DNA probes. The advantage to the observer of being able to view the presence of chromosome copy number directly is considerable. Technical issues however include the fact that FISH signals can overlap (making two signals appear as one, or three as two) or "split" according to the stage of the cell cycle making a single signal appear as two (Cohen *et al.* 2009). Initially only five different fluorescent probes attached to different chromosomes (typically 13, 16, 18, 21, 22 or 13, 18, 21 X and Y) were used, however a recent study analysing twelve chromosomes (X, Y, 2, 4, 13, 15, 16, 18, 19, 20, 21, 21) at the cleavage stage described detection of 91% of chromosomally abnormal embryos reaching the blastocyst stage. In this case, if the misdiagnosis rate of each probe averaged 1%, over the two rounds of hybridisation required, an accuracy of only 88% per embryo could be achieved. The test's ability to diagnose only 91% of aneuploid embryos compounded by the 12% misdiagnosis rate per embryo would result in only 80% efficiency of the test in its ability to diagnose aneuploidy per embryo. This would inevitably result in the transfer of aneuploid embryos (false negative) or the discarding of euploid embryos (false positive). It has been widely accepted that the efficiency of each probe is reduced in subsequent hybridisation rounds (Harrison *et al.* 2000) however a 24 chromosome FISH assay has recently been applied to preimplantation human embryos with no apparent loss of signal, even after four rounds of hybridization (Ioannou *et al.* 2011).

The importance of low error rates on the diagnostic efficiency of PGS is strongly argued (Summers & Foland 2009; Munne *et al.* 2010), as is the need to detect all chromosomes simultaneously for aneuploidy. Notwithstanding the ability now to detect all 24 chromosomes by FISH, the issues of mosaicism, signal interpretation, clinical trial data and the development of microarray based methods for detecting 24 chromosome copy number are now signalling the demise of FISH based PGS approaches. Microarray based tests are now becoming the standard and these have been made possible through the advancement of whole genome amplification (WGA) technology.

5.2 Whole genome amplification (WGA)

The introduction of whole genome amplification (WGA) techniques has led to new more efficient 24 chromosome molecular karyotyping tests. WGA brought with it the potential to increase the amount of cytogenetic information that can be obtained from a single nuclear genome contained in one cell. A single cell contains 6pg of DNA, far less than the 0.2-1.0μg usually required for microarray analysis and thus the need for amplification is paramount (Wells & Delhanty 2000). The process simply involves the transfer of the cell(s) to a microfuge tube followed by cell lysis prior to genome amplification either by polymerase chain reaction based methods or, more recently, multiple displacement amplification (MDA) to yield quantities of DNA in excess of 20 μg from a single cell. These products can in turn be used for genome wide analysis studies to establish chromosome copy number with impressive accuracy. One of the biggest drawbacks of single cell DNA amplification is a phenomenon known as allele dropout (ADO) where only one of the two alleles at a locus successfully amplifies (Walsh *et al.* 1992; Findlay *et al.* 1995; Piyamongkol *et al.* 2003). This proved a limiting factor on the resolution and reliability of PGD for single gene disorders where individual gene sequences are analysed but is less of an issue for array based PGS where many probes along each chromosome are used (Ling *et al.* 2009). Further problems involving the extreme sensitivity of single cell analysis still exist in the form of failed or poor amplification. However, these failure rates can be maintained at under 3% in experienced laboratories (Gutierrez-Mateo *et al.* 2011).

5.3 Comparative genomic hybridisation (CGH)

Originally designed for molecular karyotyping of tumour cells (Kallioniemi *et al.* 1992; Kallioniemi *et al.* 1993), comparative genomic hybridisation (CGH) has been successfully adapted for the analysis of human polar bodies and pre-implantation embryonic cells (Voullaire *et al.* 2000; Wells *et al.* 2002). Originally a labour intensive and time consuming procedure involving hybridization to and analysis of standard cytogenetic metaphase chromosome preparations, CGH was adapted for use in microarray technology, which allowed streamlining of the process. Recent successful applications of the technology have enabled array CGH (aCGH) to become the current platform of choice for PGS at all biopsy stages in the majority of laboratories around the world (Hellani *et al.* 2008; Alfarawati *et al.* 2011b).

The process involves the separate labeling of the amplified DNA and normal reference sample using different fluorescent dyes followed by co-hybridization to several thousand probes derived from known regions of the genome printed on a glass slide. Using quantitative image analysis, differences in the fluorescence ratio are interpreted to identify gained or lost regions along all chromosomes simultaneously with an error rate of less than 2% (Gutierrez-Mateo *et al.* 2011). The main technical limitations of this process are (i) that it does not supply information about chromosomal ploidy *per se*, only deviations from the most frequent level of the combined fluorescence signal and (ii) the origin of the error is not determined. Thus haploid and polyploid embryos will appear diploid or 'normal' and meiotic errors are not distinguished from post-zygotic ones. Despite these limitations, aCGH is rapidly establishing itself as the "gold standard" for PGS, replacing FISH based approaches in most laboratories.

5.4 Single Nucleotide Polymorphism (SNP) arrays

Single Nucleotide Polymorphisms (SNPs) are the most frequent form of DNA variation in the genome. To date over 6 million SNPs have been identified in the human genome (Javed & Mukesh 2010). SNPs are bi-allelic genetic markers that can be used in a variety of ways to detect chromosome copy number. SNP micro-arrays are used to detect the specific alleles present in polar bodies or embryos at up to 500,000 SNP loci. This information can, in turn, be interpreted in several ways to obtain massive amounts of genetic information. Simple quantification of the SNP alleles and analysis of heterozygosity enables diagnosis of aneuploidy including uniparental isodisomy (Northrop *et al.* 2010; Brezina *et al.* 2011; Treff *et al.* 2011). Using this method, results can be difficult to interpret above the level of background 'noise' due to the problem of amplification from a single template. For this reason, methods involving comparison with parental DNA are under development (Handyside *et al.* 2010; Johnson *et al.* 2010b). Since all embryonic chromosomes are derived from parental chromosomes, predicted genotypes based on known parental data can be used to "clean" noisy single cell data resulting in a comprehensive and highly reliable molecular cytogenetic test for chromosome copy number (Johnson *et al.* 2010b). In addition to this, again with the aid of the known parental genotypes, our group has developed a test involving Mendelian inheritance analysis of SNPs known as 'Karyomapping'. By establishing the four parental haplotypes, only informative 'key' SNPs are analysed to establish chromosome copy number, parental origin and points of meiotic recombination of the tested cells can be 'Karyomapped'(Handyside *et al.* 2010). Karyomapping has the added advantage of being able to detect not only meiotic aneuploidy but also the presence of the chromosomes carrying the mutant allele for cases involving the risk of transmission of specific known inherited disorders.

SNP genotyping has the potential to be the most comprehensive platform for PGS. The interpretation of a SNP genotype allows diagnosis of all possible chromosome copy number aberrations. It has the capacity to perform as a high resolution molecular cytogenetic test at higher resolution than aCGH for all types of chromosomal gains and losses and with the added ability of linkage based analysis allowing diagnosis of inherited genetic disease (Handyside *et al.* 2010). Although largely clinically un-validated, comparative data with other platforms suggest better efficiency than both FISH and aCGH for aneuploidy screening (Johnson *et al.* 2010b; Treff *et al.* 2010a; Treff *et al.* 2010b). Recently presented clinical data of SNP array based PGS on cleavage stage embryos suggests significant improvement of pregnancy rates following embryo transfer (Rabinowitz *et al.* 2010).We anticipate that with further clinical validation, SNP genotyping will become the gold standard for PGS in the near future.

6. What we have learnt from PGS thus far?

The rationale for PGS is of course that if embryo ploidy could be determined and euploid embryos selected for embryo transfer, IVF pregnancy rates would increase and poor outcomes such as implantation failure and miscarriage would decrease. Few disagree with this premise underpinning PGS as scientifically and clinically sound.

Since its inception in the mid-90s, PGS has primarily involved the biopsy of one or two cells on the third day of embryo development followed by targeted chromosome analysis using FISH. Subsequently, diagnosed euploid embryos (for the limited number of chromosomes analysed) were transferred or cryopreserved with the remaining embryos diagnosed as aneuploid being discarded (with or without follow-up confirmation analysis). This work was based on the theoretical premise of PGS without the support of randomised controlled trials (RCTs). All recent RCTs using cleavage stage biopsy followed by FISH analysis showed no improvement in delivery rates after PGS with some even suggesting adverse outcomes (Staessen *et al.* 2004; Mastenbroek *et al.* 2007; Blockeel *et al.* 2008; Hardarson *et al.* 2008; Mersereau *et al.* 2008; Debrock *et al.* 2010). The largest of these trials included over 200 patients in each of the experimental arms (control and treatment groups) and concluded that PGS resulted in a reduced delivery rate following IVF (Mastenbroek *et al.* 2007). These results, contrary to the original premise of PGS, sparked much debate with several institutions including the practice committees of the Society of Assisted Reproductive Technology and the American Society of Reproductive Medicine [SART & ASRM] (2008b) and the British Fertility Society (Anderson & Pickering 2008) issuing statements that PGS should no longer be performed. Meanwhile, several groups criticised the trials for their poor diagnostic efficiency, practical skill levels, inappropriate patient selection and generally low pregnancy rates. They claimed that the trials were performed by inexperienced practitioners thereby generating invalid or questionable results (Cohen & Grifo 2007; Simpson 2008).

What is not in question is that these trials have ultimately highlighted the complexity of considerations PGS requires when applied clinically. FISH of cleavage stage biopsies has clearly outlined that both technical and practical limitations exist when performing PGS to improve pregnancy outcomes. Furthermore, there is great importance and careful consideration needed in patient selection as well as effective test selection and implementation on a case-by-case basis (Handyside & Thornhill 2007).

The success of aneuploidy screening as a selection tool for IVF to improve pregnancy rates is dependent on the efficacy of the entire testing process. It is now clear that FISH, especially for cleavage stage biopsy, is not the optimal tool for PGS. The process is subject to the following technical limitations: (i) the efficacy of the cell preparation technique, (ii) the accuracy of the FISH test itself and its reliable interpretation. Biologically, we are constrained by the products we have to work with (embryo quality, mosaicism and nucleation) and the time in which to work with them. We believe that there is scope for PGS to improve pregnancy rates in ART but the test used must be optimised and tailored to suit the biological and technical limitations that exist to maximise benefit at the lowest possible cost to the embryo.

7. Clinical applications and decision making

Aneuploidy screening using 24 chromosome micro-array analyses should improve IVF outcomes with the implementation of case-by-case cost-benefit analysis. For best results, PGS should be performed with the most comprehensive cytogenetic platform available. PGS is considered too invasive to be employed as a routine embryo selection tool for IVF thus, at present, it should be offered only to patients at high risk of aneuploidy. The cost of the biopsy on embryo development is only justifiable if the information gained will outweigh the cost to the cohort of embryos as a whole. For this reason, false positive results due to mosaicism and the number of testable embryos in a cohort are important in the decision making process. Advanced maternal age (AMA) is the single largest indication for PGS as an adjunct to embryo selection to improve IVF success. Careful patient selection is still required within this group of patients to achieve the best results (see figure 5). There are a number of other indications for which PGS is likely to be of most benefit, all of which are associated with a potential increased risk of aneuploidy including patients with Repeated

Implantation Failure (RIF) and Recurrent Miscarriage (RM). Patients with diagnosed high levels of sperm aneuploidy or severe male factor infertility may also benefit.

PB biopsy theoretically has the lowest cost to embryo development but only gives information about maternally derived aneuploidy. PB biopsy is therefore of most benefit to patients of AMA with no other suspected aneuploidy input. Both PB1 and PB2 should be sampled to ensure that the majority of maternally aneuploidy is detected (Geraedts *et al.* 2011).

Theoretically, blastocyst stage biopsy is the optimal stage as it partially negates the problem of mosaicism and gives maximum aneuploidy information from maternal, paternal and post-zygotic events. In addition, the biopsy of 10 or more cells virtually eliminates the problem of ADO following WGA (Ling *et al.* 2009). However, the logistical downside is that embryos may need cryopreservation whist awaiting genetics results, a potential additional 'cost' to embryos. Furthermore, *in- vitro* blastocyst development may be limited in some patients leading to a limited cohort of blastocysts that can be biopsied simultaneously reducing the chance of a live birth and genetic information from the cohort (Janny & Menezo 1996). Thus it should only be considered for patients with RIF and RM, including male factor, with evidence of good blastocyst formation or proven fertility.

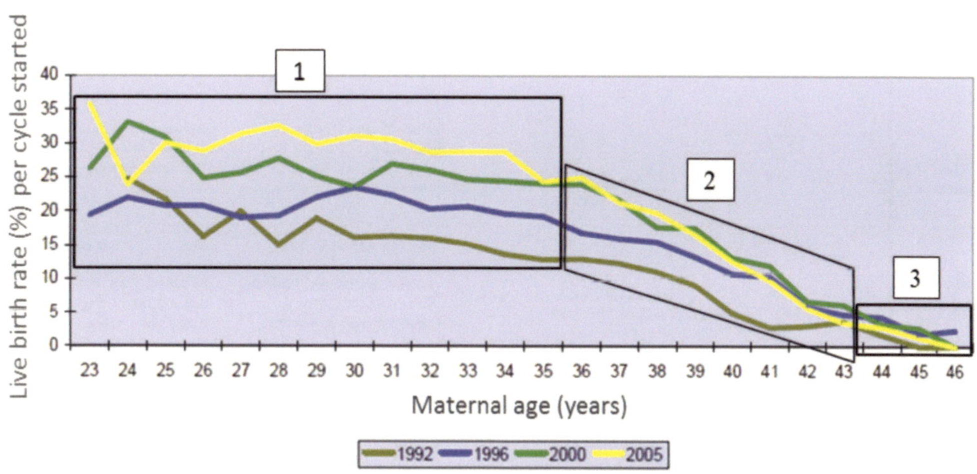

Fig. 5. Three distinct patient groups in relation to age and IVF success rates. Note the drop in success rates beyond maternal age 35 across all years (consistent with increasing rates of aneuploidy). High number of embryos and low rate of aneuploidy are expected in patient group under 35 years of age (1) thus PGS is not recommended - Cost outweighs benefit of PGS. Moderate embryo numbers and increased rate of aneuploidy consistent with reduced IVF success rates of patients above 35 years (2) indicate a target group for PGS - Benefit of PGS outweighs its cost. PGS is suggested to be of no benefit for embryo selection in patients of severe AMA due to low number of embryos and high rate of aneuploidy (3) - Cost outweighs benefit of PGS.
Figure adapted from Human Fertilisation and Embryology Authority website [HFEA] (2008a)

The inherent problem of mosaicism and false positive results is a major problem for biopsy at the cleavage stage. This, paired with the cost of removing a significant amount of the cell mass (up to 25%), suggests that use of cleavage stage biopsy should be limited to cases of male factor aneuploidy with known poor ability for blastocyst development. Removal of only a single cell is recommended to minimize cost to the embryo and prevent the dilemma of discordant results due to mosaicism (Cohen *et al.* 2007). Cleavage stage biopsy may also be considered as follow-up for equivocal results from PB biopsy (Magli *et al.* 2004; Cieslak-Janzen *et al.* 2006). The relative pros and cons of all biopsy stages are summarised in table 2.

Biopsy, irrespective of stage, should only be performed if there are a sufficient number of oocytes or embryos to be tested. If there is limited or no embryo selection to be achieved by PGS then it (PGS) should be avoided as there will be no benefit to IVF success rates and may even be a detrimental effect (Summers & Foland 2009). An exception to this is when PGS is used not as an embryo selection tool but as a diagnostic tool to avoid or diagnose aneuploidy.

	origin of aneuploidy							Associated costs and benefits	
	Maternal		Paternal			Detection of mosaicism	Day of biopsy - days post fertilisation		
Biopsy stage	MI	MII	MI	MII	Post Zygotic			Benefit	Cost
PB1	yes	no	no	no	no	no	Day 0 (day of fertilisation)	Minimal manpulations. No removal of viable cells. Maximum time for analysis prior to embryo transfer.	Only information from maternal MI.
PB1 & PB2	yes	yes	no	no	no	no	Day 0 and 1	No removal of viable cells. Maximum time for analysis prior to embryo transfer.	Only information for maternal meiotic errors.
Cleavage stage (blastomere)	yes	yes	yes	yes	yes	no (Yes with limited sensitivity if>1 cell analysed)	Day 3	Information for all origin of aneuploidy. Maximise number of embryos tested. Paternal aneuploidy detected.	Mosaicism resulting in false positive and negative results. Removal of significant proportion of cell mass.
Blastocyst stage (trophectoderm)	yes	yes	yes	yes	yes	yes (only with limitation on sensitivity)	Days 5 and 6	Information for all origin of aneuploidy. Biopsy of several cells (~10 cells). No harm to ICM. Paternal aneuploidy detected.	Reduced number of embryos for testing (requires good blastocyst formation). Reduced time for diagnosis (embryo cryopreservation potentially necessary).

Table 2. Technical limitations, costs and benefits of the established biopsy stages for PGS

Some patients may require elimination of the possibility of aneuploidy resulting in poor outcomes such as miscarriage or birth of a child with a genetic defect. These 'must screen' patients for PGS should be considered more like diagnosis of inherited genetic disease and all embryos, irrespective of the number and quality, should be tested.

8. Research and future developments

It is now well documented when and how extra or missing chromosomes arise but the big question remains 'why'. Clearly, research into the origin of human aneuploidy will continue to provide new and exciting insights in the field of reproductive medicine. The introduction of new array technology, including SNP genotyping of embryos, will further improve PGS strategies. For example, recent evidence demonstrating that errors are equally likely during the two maternal meiotic divisions (Handyside *et al.* 2012) is rapidly leading to a shift in the strategy for approaching polar body analysis for PGS with PB1 considered inadequate if embryo selection is the ultimate goal.

Continued efforts should be employed to use new technologies to correlate the rate and origin of aneuploidy with external factors in an effort to identify markers for aneuploidy risk. Patient assessment of these risk factors will lead to better personalisation of PGS treatment plans and provide an understanding of the underlying mechanisms behind chromosome segregation and the cause of aneuploidy.

Along with AMA, altered recombination in meiosis is the most important known aetiology related to aneuploidy and gives clues to the overall mechanism (Hassold *et al.* 2007). Algorithms applied to SNP genotyping data, including Karyomapping can be applied for high resolution pinpointing of recombination points (Handyside *et al.* 2010; Gabriel *et al.* 2011a). Patterns of recombination across the genome can then be correlated with chromosome mal-segregation in meiosis in an attempt to find aberrant patterns that predispose to aneuploidy. Similar strategies can be employed to different patient profiles to ascertain further aetiologies associated with aneuploidies of different origin. Further understanding of the predisposition to human aneuploidy will lead to specific patient treatment and more importantly guide the direction of studies on the molecular basis of aneuploidy. Once the mechanisms leading to aneuploidy are understood and there is an understanding of why it occurs, interventions to prevent aneuploidy could be usefully investigated.

It has been hypothesised that the high rates of aneuploidy and mosaicism following IVF procedures may in fact be an iatrogenic artefact of the procedure itself. Ovarian hyperstimulation (Baart *et al.* 2007), fertilisation in vitro (Bean *et al.* 2002) and in vitro culture environments (IVC) (Carrell *et al.* 2005; Sabhnani *et al.* 2011; Xu *et al.* 2011) appear to affect embryo aneuploidy. A recent RCT of ovarian stimulation protocols revealed that minimal stimulation, although associated with a reduced number of oocytes, results in higher proportions of chromosomally 'normal' embryos. It was hypothesised that conventional stimulation protocols result mainly in an increase of post zygotic chromosome segregation errors. Altered ovarian function (recruitment of follicles), gonadotrophin dose and GnRH analogue have been offered as potential correlates for further investigation. Furthermore, mouse studies have shown increased meiotic and post zygotic error rates following IVF and IVC respectively (Bean *et al.* 2002; Sabhnani *et al.* 2011). The sensitivity of mouse oocytes to different culture regimens resulting in differing aneuploidy rates corroborate the hypothesis that IVF affects aneuploidy (Carrell *et al.* 2005). In humans, FSH levels associated with in-vitro maturation correlate with chromosome mal-segregation in the first meiotic division (Xu *et al.* 2011). Animal models could be further employed for manipulation of IVF parameters in an effort to induce or suppress aneuploidy, although clinical IVF itself may provide the best 'experiment' to gain a better understanding of the mechanisms involved in human aneuploidy.

Full genetic sequencing seems the logical next technological advance for PGS and appears technically possible following successful genomic sequencing of microbial single cells (Zhang *et al.* 2006; Lasken 2007). Additional data at the highest possible resolution should inevitably prove more reliable for chromosome copy number analysis and, as with SNP genotyping, points of recombination as well as points of partial aneuploidy along chromosomes could be analysed with more precision. Currently, increased resolution of PGS is limited by the WGA step (Ling *et al.* 2009). Achieving the highest possible resolution is directly restricted by the phenomenon of ADO when amplifying single or very few cells. Thus it necessary to invest effort in improving WGA technology before the full benefits of genomic sequencing could be realised.

With the increasing amount of data obtained from PGS technologies comes the issue of an increasing amount of 'incidental' findings of unknown pathological significance. Careful considerations of the social, ethical and legal aspects of these findings are required to combat potential problems prior to implementing higher resolution technologies.

The ultimate goal of PGS is to provide maximum benefit (in terms of information to the parent/healthcare provider) with minimal cost to the embryo. The possibility of gaining chromosome copy number information with no cost to the embryo would enable PGS to be used routinely as an embryo selection tool for IVF. An indirect aneuploidy screening test was first explored by associations with conventional embryo morphology scoring. However, morphological embryo grading is apparently at its limits to improve IVF success rates and has only shown very limited correlation with aneuploidy (Munne 2006; Gianaroli *et al.* 2007; Alfarawati *et al.* 2011a). The implementation of time-lapse imaging to embryo culture has facilitated high resolution morphokinetic analysis of embryo development in an attempt to improve IVF success rates and eliminate potentially abnormally developing embryos. Morphokinetic analysis involves continual analysis of the morphological state and rates of change during oocyte and embryo development and provides evidence of developmental milestones that can predict embryo implantation (Meseguer *et al.* 2011). Since, cells of different genotypes are known to have slightly different cell cycle times (Varrela *et al.* 1989), it follows that algorithms involving multiple developmental time points could be used to predict embryo aneuploidy at no cost to the embryo. Embryos with an abnormal karyotype (particularly those with multiple abnormalities) may have aberrant cell cycles, detectable by morphokinetic analysis, compared with normal embryos. New studies into the morphological rates of change including such developmental markers as PB extrusion, syngamy and early mitotic divisions could find more significant correlations with chromosome mal-segregation than embryo morphology alone.

Other approaches to non-invasive assessment of embryo viability include the measurement of what is used by or what is secreted by the oocyte or embryo. All culture media contain substances that are required for embryo development. Culture media will also contain all products secreted by the oocyte or embryo. Levels of these can be measured in a variety of ways to establish embryo viability (for review see Aydiner *et al.* 2010).

Analysis of spent culture media is an area already being explored as potential for a new indirect PGS platform. A recent study analysing uptake patterns of amino acids has shown that regulation of amino acid metabolism correlates with embryo aneuploidy. The study using FISH analysis of five chromosomes (13, 18, 21, X and Y) demonstrated altered amino acid turnover in embryos with grossly abnormal karyotypes when compared to genetically normal embryos (Picton *et al.* 2010). Although promising, these early data lack specificity and further work is needed to more accurately establish how embryo metabolism may be indicative of its chromosomal complement. Precise metabolic profiling of embryos with known copy number aberrations is proposed as a specific experiment to establish more meaningful correlations.

A further approach is based on the hypothesis of altered gene expression and protein synthesis of chromosomally abnormal embryos. One study, using a proteomic approach, has identified the first protein secreted by human blastocysts (Lipocalin-1) that is associated with generic chromosome aneuploidy (McReynolds *et al.* 2011) promising the biggest step to date towards a non-invasive PGS test.

9. Conclusion

PGS has proved to be one of the most controversial areas of reproductive medicine in recent times. The entire community is united in its collective will to improve IVF success, reduce miscarriage rates and ensure that couples avoid children with developmental abnormalities. The means by which this is achieved remains the subject of intense debate. What can be clear however is that the controversy will serve to increase the interest in PGS leading to new and radical future treatments.

10. List of abbreviations

aCGH	Array comparative genomic hybridisation
ADO	Allele dropout
AMA	Advanced maternal age
CGH	Comparative genomic hybridisation
DNA	Deoxyribonucleic acid
FISH	Fluorescence *in-situ* hybridization
ICM	Inner cell mass
IVF	*In-vitro* fertilisation
IVC	*In-vitro* culture
MDA	Multiple displacement amplification
MI	First meiotic division (Meiosis 1)
MII	Second meiotic division (Meiosis 2)
PB	Polar body
PB1	First polar body
PB2	Second polar body
PGS	Preimplantation genetic screening (for aneuploidy)
PS	Premature/precocious separation of sister chromatids
SNP	Single nucleotide polymorphism
TE	Trophectoderm
WGA	Whole genome amplification

11. References

(2008a) A long term analysis of the HFEA Register data (1991-2006). *HFEA Website* 1.

(2008b) Preimplantation genetic testing: a Practice Committee opinion. *Fertil Steril* 90, S136-43.

Alfarawati S., Fragouli E., Colls P., Stevens J., Gutierrez-Mateo C., Schoolcraft W.B., Katz-Jaffe M.G. & Wells D. (2011a) The relationship between blastocyst morphology, chromosomal abnormality, and embryo gender. *Fertil Steril* 95, 520-4.

Alfarawati S., Fragouli E., Colls P. & Wells D. (2011b) First births after preimplantation genetic diagnosis of structural chromosome abnormalities using comparative genomic hybridization and microarray analysis. *Hum Reprod* 26, 1560-74.

Almeida P.A. & Bolton V.N. (1996) The relationship between chromosomal abnormality in the human preimplantation embryo and development in vitro. *Reprod Fertil Dev* 8, 235-41.

Anderson R.A. & Pickering S. (2008) The current status of preimplantation genetic screening: British Fertility Society Policy and Practice Guidelines. *Hum Fertil (Camb)* 11, 71-5.

Angell R.R. (1991) Predivision in human oocytes at meiosis I: a mechanism for trisomy formation in man. *Hum.Genet.* 86, 383-7.

Angell R.R., Templeton A.A. & Aitken R.J. (1986) Chromosome studies in human in vitro fertilization. *Hum.Genet.* 72, 333-9.

Angell R.R., Xian J. & Keith J. (1993) Chromosome anomalies in human oocytes in relation to age. *Hum.Reprod* 8, 1047-54.

Angell R.R., Xian J., Keith J., Ledger W. & Baird D.T. (1994) First meiotic division abnormalities in human oocytes: mechanism of trisomy formation. *Cytogenet.Cell Genet.* 65, 194-202.

Aydiner F., Yetkin C.E. & Seli E. (2010) Perspectives on emerging biomarkers for non-invasive assessment of embryo viability in assisted reproduction. *Curr Mol Med* 10, 206-15.

Baart E.B., Martini E., Eijkemans M.J., Van Opstal D., Beckers N.G., Verhoeff A., Macklon N.S. & Fauser B.C. (2007) Milder ovarian stimulation for in-vitro fertilization reduces aneuploidy in the human preimplantation embryo: a randomized controlled trial. *Hum Reprod* 22, 980-8.

Banerjee I., Shevlin M., Taranissi M., Thornhill A., Abdalla H., Ozturk O., Barnes J. & Sutcliffe A. (2008) Health of children conceived after preimplantation genetic diagnosis: a preliminary outcome study. *Reprod Biomed Online* 16, 376-81.

Bean C.J., Hassold T.J., Judis L. & Hunt P.A. (2002) Fertilization in vitro increases non-disjunction during early cleavage divisions in a mouse model system. *Hum Reprod* 17, 2362-7.

Bean C.J., Hunt P.A., Millie E.A. & Hassold T.J. (2001) Analysis of a malsegregating mouse Y chromosome: evidence that the earliest cleavage divisions of the mammalian embryo are non-disjunction-prone. *Hum Mol Genet* 10, 963-72.

Bielanska M., Tan S.L. & Ao A. (2002) Chromosomal mosaicism throughout human preimplantation development in vitro: incidence, type, and relevance to embryo outcome. *Hum Reprod* 17, 413-9.

Blockeel C., Schutyser V., De Vos A., Verpoest W., De Vos M., Staessen C., Haentjens P., Van der Elst J. & Devroey P. (2008) Prospectively randomized controlled trial of PGS in IVF/ICSI patients with poor implantation. *Reprod Biomed Online* 17, 848-54.

Braude P., Bolton V. & Moore S. (1988) Human gene expression first occurs between the four- and eight-cell stages of preimplantation development. *Nature* 332, 459-61.

Brezina P.R., Benner A., Rechitsky S., Kuliev A., Pomerantseva E., Pauling D. & Kearns W.G. (2011) Single-gene testing combined with single nucleotide polymorphism microarray preimplantation genetic diagnosis for aneuploidy: a novel approach in optimizing pregnancy outcome. *Fertil Steril* 95, 1786 e5-8.

Carrell D.T., Liu L., Huang I. & Peterson C.M. (2005) Comparison of maturation, meiotic competence, and chromosome aneuploidy of oocytes derived from two protocols for in vitro culture of mouse secondary follicles. *J Assist Reprod Genet* 22, 347-54.

Chiang T., Duncan F.E., Schindler K., Schultz R.M. & Lampson M.A. (2010) Evidence that weakened centromere cohesion is a leading cause of age-related aneuploidy in oocytes. *Curr Biol* 20, 1522-8.

Cho C.K. & Diamandis E.P. (2011) Application of proteomics to prenatal screening and diagnosis for aneuploidies. *Clin Chem Lab Med* 49, 33-41.

Cieslak-Janzen J., Tur-Kaspa I., Ilkevitch Y., Bernal A., Morris R. & Verlinsky Y. (2006) Multiple micromanipulations for preimplantation genetic diagnosis do not affect embryo development to the blastocyst stage. *Fertil Steril* 85, 1826-9.

Cohen J. & Grifo J.A. (2007) Multicentre trial of preimplantation genetic screening reported in the New England Journal of Medicine: an in-depth look at the findings. *Reprod Biomed Online* 15, 365-6.

Cohen J., Wells D., Howles C.M. & Munne S. (2009) The role of preimplantation genetic diagnosis in diagnosing embryo aneuploidy. *Curr Opin Obstet Gynecol* 21, 442-9.

Cohen J., Wells D. & Munne S. (2007) Removal of 2 cells from cleavage stage embryos is likely to reduce the efficacy of chromosomal tests that are used to enhance implantation rates. *Fertil Steril* 87, 496-503.

Coonen E., Derhaag J.G., Dumoulin J.C., van Wissen L.C., Bras M., Janssen M., Evers J.L. & Geraedts J.P. (2004) Anaphase lagging mainly explains chromosomal mosaicism in human preimplantation embryos. *Hum Reprod* 19, 316-24.

Dailey T., Dale B., Cohen J. & Munne S. (1996a) Association between nondisjunction and maternal age in meiosis-II human oocytes. *Am.J.Hum.Genet.* 59, 176-84.

Dailey T., Dale B., Cohen J. & Munne S. (1996b) Association between nondisjunction and maternal age in meiosis-II human oocytes. *Am J Hum Genet* 59, 176-84.

Daphnis D.D., Delhanty J.D., Jerkovic S., Geyer J., Craft I. & Harper J.C. (2005) Detailed FISH analysis of day 5 human embryos reveals the mechanisms leading to mosaic aneuploidy. *Hum Reprod* 20, 129-37.

Debrock S., Melotte C., Spiessens C., Peeraer K., Vanneste E., Meeuwis L., Meuleman C., Frijns J.P., Vermeesch J.R. & D'Hooghe T.M. (2010) Preimplantation genetic screening for aneuploidy of embryos after in vitro fertilization in women aged at least 35 years: a prospective randomized trial. *Fertil Steril* 93, 364-73.

Delhanty J.D. (2005) Mechanisms of aneuploidy induction in human oogenesis and early embryogenesis. *Cytogenet Genome Res* 111, 237-44.

Egozcue S., Blanco J., Vidal F. & Egozcue J. (2002) Diploid sperm and the origin of triploidy. *Hum Reprod* 17, 5-7.

Findlay I., Ray P., Quirke P., Rutherford A. & Lilford R. (1995) Allelic drop-out and preferential amplification in single cells and human blastomeres: implications for preimplantation diagnosis of sex and cystic fibrosis. *Hum.Reprod.* 10, 1609-18.

Fragouli E., Alfarawati S., Goodall N.N., Sanchez-Garcia J.F., Colls P. & Wells D. (2011) The cytogenetics of polar bodies: insights into female meiosis and the diagnosis of aneuploidy. *Mol Hum Reprod.*

Fragouli E., Wells D., Thornhill A., Serhal P., Faed M.J., Harper J.C. & Delhanty J.D. (2006) Comparative genomic hybridization analysis of human oocytes and polar bodies. *Hum Reprod* 21, 2319-28.

Gabriel A.S., Hassold T.J., Thornhill A.R., Affara N.A., Handyside A.H. & Griffin D.K. (2011a) An algorithm for determining the origin of trisomy and the positions of chiasmata from SNP genotype data. *Chromosome Res* 19, 155-63.

Gabriel A.S., Thornhill A.R., Ottolini C.S., Gordon A., Brown A.P., Taylor J., Bennett K., Handyside A. & Griffin D.K. (2011b) Array comparative genomic hybridisation on first polar bodies suggests that non-disjunction is not the predominant mechanism leading to aneuploidy in humans. *J Med Genet* 48, 433-7.

Geraedts J., Montag M., Magli M.C., Repping S., Handyside A., Staessen C., Harper J., Schmutzler A., Collins J., Goossens V., van der Ven H., Vesela K. & Gianaroli L. (2011) Polar body array CGH for prediction of the status of the corresponding oocyte. Part I: clinical results. *Hum Reprod.*

Gianaroli L. (2000) Preimplantation genetic diagnosis: polar body and embryo biopsy. *Hum Reprod* 15 Suppl 4, 69-75.

Gianaroli L., Magli M.C., Ferraretti A.P., Lappi M., Borghi E. & Ermini B. (2007) Oocyte euploidy, pronuclear zygote morphology and embryo chromosomal complement. *Hum Reprod* 22, 241-9.

Griffin D.K., Abruzzo M.A., Millie E.A., Sheean L.A., Feingold E., Sherman S.L. & Hassold T.J. (1995) Non-disjunction in human sperm: evidence for an effect of increasing paternal age. *Hum Mol Genet* 4, 2227-32.

Griffin D.K., Wilton L.J., Handyside A.H., Winston R.M. & Delhanty J.D. (1992) Dual fluorescent in situ hybridisation for simultaneous detection of X and Y chromosome-specific probes for the sexing of human preimplantation embryonic nuclei. *Hum.Genet.* 89, 18-22.

Grossmann M., Calafell J.M., Brandy N., Vanrell J.A., Rubio C., Pellicer A., Egozcue J., Vidal F. & Santalo J. (1997) Origin of tripronucleate zygotes after intracytoplasmic sperm injection. *Hum Reprod* 12, 2762-5.

Gutierrez-Mateo C., Benet J., Wells D., Colls P., Bermudez M.G., Sanchez-Garcia J.F., Egozcue J., Navarro J. & Munne S. (2004) Aneuploidy study of human oocytes first polar body comparative genomic hybridization and metaphase II fluorescence in situ hybridization analysis. *Hum Reprod* 19, 2859-68.

Gutierrez-Mateo C., Colls P., Sanchez-Garcia J., Escudero T., Prates R., Ketterson K., Wells D. & Munne S. (2011) Validation of microarray comparative genomic hybridization for comprehensive chromosome analysis of embryos. *Fertil Steril* 95, 953-8.

Han T.S., Sagoskin A.W., Graham J.R., Tucker M.J. & Liebermann J. (2003) Laser-assisted human embryo biopsy on the third day of development for preimplantation genetic diagnosis: two successful case reports. *Fertil Steril* 80, 453-5.

Handyside A.H., Harton G.L., Mariani B., Thornhill A.R., Affara N., Shaw M.A. & Griffin D.K. (2010) Karyomapping: a universal method for genome wide analysis of genetic disease based on mapping crossovers between parental haplotypes. *J Med Genet* 47, 651-8.

Handyside A .H., Montag M., Magli M.C., Repping S., Harper J., Schmutzler A., Vesela K., Gianaroli L. & Geraedts J. (2012) Multiple meiotic errors caused by predivision of chromatids in women of advanced maternal age undergoing in vitro fertilisation. *European Journal of Human Genetics (In Press)*

Handyside A.H. & Thornhill A.R. (2007) In vitro fertilization with preimplantation genetic screening. *N Engl J Med* 357, 1770; author reply -1.

Hardarson T., Hanson C., Lundin K., Hillensjo T., Nilsson L., Stevic J., Reismer E., Borg K., Wikland M. & Bergh C. (2008) Preimplantation genetic screening in women of advanced maternal age caused a decrease in clinical pregnancy rate: a randomized controlled trial. *Hum Reprod* 23, 2806-12.

Hardy K., Martin K.L., Leese H.J., Winston R.M. & Handyside A.H. (1990) Human preimplantation development in vitro is not adversely affected by biopsy at the 8-cell stage. *Hum.Reprod.* 5, 708-14.

Harper J.C., Boelaert K., Geraedts J., Harton G., Kearns W.G., Moutou C., Muntjewerff N., Repping S., SenGupta S., Scriven P.N., Traeger-Synodinos J., Vesela K., Wilton L. & Sermon K.D. (2006) ESHRE PGD Consortium data collection V: cycles from January to December 2002 with pregnancy follow-up to October 2003. *Hum Reprod* 21, 3-21.

Harrison R.H., Kuo H.C., Scriven P.N., Handyside A.H. & Ogilvie C.M. (2000) Lack of cell cycle checkpoints in human cleavage stage embryos revealed by a clonal pattern of chromosomal mosaicism analysed by sequential multicolour FISH. *Zygote* 8, 217-24.

Hassold T., Hall H. & Hunt P. (2007) The origin of human aneuploidy: where we have been, where we are going. *Hum Mol Genet* 16 Spec No. 2, R203-8.

Hassold T. & Hunt P. (2001) To err (meiotically) is human: the genesis of human aneuploidy. *Nat Rev Genet* 2, 280-91.

Hassold T.J. (1986) Chromosome abnormalities in human reproductive wastage. *Trends Genet.* 2, 105-10.

Hellani A., Abu-Amero K., Azouri J. & El-Akoum S. (2008) Successful pregnancies after application of array-comparative genomic hybridization in PGS-aneuploidy screening. *Reprod Biomed Online* 17, 841-7.

Ioannou D., Meershoek E.J., Thornhill A.R., Ellis M. & Griffin D.K. (2011) Multicolour interphase cytogenetics: 24 chromosome probes, 6 colours, 4 layers. *Mol Cell Probes.*

Janny L. & Menezo Y.J. (1996) Maternal age effect on early human embryonic development and blastocyst formation. *Mol Reprod Dev* 45, 31-7.

Javed R. & Mukesh (2010) Current research status, databases and application of single nucleotide polymorphism. *Pak J Biol Sci* 13, 657-63.

Johnson D.S., Cinnioglu C., Ross R., Filby A., Gemelos G., Hill M., Ryan A., Smotrich D., Rabinowitz M. & Murray M.J. (2010a) Comprehensive analysis of karyotypic mosaicism between trophectoderm and inner cell mass. *Mol Hum Reprod* 16, 944-9.

Johnson D.S., Gemelos G., Baner J., Ryan A., Cinnioglu C., Banjevic M., Ross R., Alper M., Barrett B., Frederick J., Potter D., Behr B. & Rabinowitz M. (2010b) Preclinical validation of a microarray method for full molecular karyotyping of blastomeres in a 24-h protocol. *Hum Reprod* 25, 1066-75.

Johnson M.D. (1998) Genetic risks of intracytoplasmic sperm injection in the treatment of male infertility: recommendations for genetic counseling and screening. *Fertil Steril* 70, 397-411.

Kallioniemi A., Kallioniemi O.P., Sudar D., Rutovitz D., Gray J.W., Waldman F. & Pinkel D. (1992) Comparative genomic hybridization for molecular cytogenetic analysis of solid tumors. *Science* 258, 818-21.

Kallioniemi O.P., Kallioniemi A., Sudar D., Rutovitz D., Gray J.W., Waldman F. & Pinkel D. (1993) Comparative genomic hybridization: a rapid new method for detecting and mapping DNA amplification in tumors. *Semin Cancer Biol* 4, 41-6.

Kalousek D.K. & Vekemans M. (1996) Confined placental mosaicism. *J Med Genet* 33, 529-33.

Kokkali G., Traeger-Synodinos J., Vrettou C., Stavrou D., Jones G.M., Cram D.S., Makrakis E., Trounson A.O., Kanavakis E. & Pantos K. (2007) Blastocyst biopsy versus cleavage stage biopsy and blastocyst transfer for preimplantation genetic diagnosis of beta-thalassaemia: a pilot study. *Hum Reprod* 22, 1443-9.

Kolialexi A., Tounta G., Mavrou A. & Tsangaris G.T. (2011) Proteomic analysis of amniotic fluid for the diagnosis of fetal aneuploidies. *Expert Rev Proteomics* 8, 175-85.

Kuliev A., Cieslak J., Ilkevitch Y. & Verlinsky Y. (2003) Chromosomal abnormalities in a series of 6,733 human oocytes in preimplantation diagnosis for age-related aneuploidies. *Reprod Biomed Online* 6, 54-9.

Kuliev A., Cieslak J. & Verlinsky Y. (2005) Frequency and distribution of chromosome abnormalities in human oocytes. *Cytogenet Genome Res* 111, 193-8.

Lamb N.E., Feingold E., Savage A., Avramopoulos D., Freeman S., Gu Y., Hallberg A., Hersey J., Karadima G., Pettay D., Saker D., Shen J., Taft L., Mikkelsen M., Petersen M.B., Hassold T. & Sherman S.L. (1997) Characterization of susceptible chiasma configurations that increase the risk for maternal nondisjunction of chromosome 21. *Hum Mol Genet* 6, 1391-9.

Lamb N.E., Freeman S.B., Savage-Austin A., Pettay D., Taft L., Hersey J., Gu Y., Shen J., Saker D., May K.M., Avramopoulos D., Petersen M.B., Hallberg A., Mikkelsen M., Hassold T.J. & Sherman S.L. (1996) Susceptible chiasmate configurations of chromosome 21 predispose to non- disjunction in both maternal meiosis I and meiosis II. *Nat Genet* 14, 400-5.

Lasken R.S. (2007) Single-cell genomic sequencing using Multiple Displacement Amplification. *Curr Opin Microbiol* 10, 510-6.

Ling J., Zhuang G., Tazon-Vega B., Zhang C., Cao B., Rosenwaks Z. & Xu K. (2009) Evaluation of genome coverage and fidelity of multiple displacement amplification from single cells by SNP array. *Mol Hum Reprod* 15, 739-47.

Lister L.M., Kouznetsova A., Hyslop L.A., Kalleas D., Pace S.L., Barel J.C., Nathan A., Floros V., Adelfalk C., Watanabe Y., Jessberger R., Kirkwood T.B., Hoog C. & Herbert M. (2010) Age-related meiotic segregation errors in mammalian oocytes are preceded by depletion of cohesin and Sgo2. *Curr Biol* 20, 1511-21.

Liu J., Van den Abbeel E. & Van Steirteghem A. (1993) The in-vitro and in-vivo developmental potential of frozen and non-frozen biopsied 8-cell mouse embryos. *Hum Reprod* 8, 1481-6.

Magli M.C., Gianaroli L., Ferraretti A.P., Toschi M., Esposito F. & Fasolino M.C. (2004) The combination of polar body and embryo biopsy does not affect embryo viability. *Hum Reprod* 19, 1163-9.

Magli M.C., Montag M., Koster M., Muzi L., Geraedts J., Collins J., Goossens V., Handyside A.H., Harper J., Repping S., Schmutzler A., Vesela K. & Gianaroli L. (2011) Polar body array CGH for prediction of the status of the corresponding oocyte. Part II: technical aspects. *Hum Reprod.*

Mahmood R., Brierley C.H., Faed M.J., Mills J.A. & Delhanty J.D. (2000) Mechanisms of maternal aneuploidy: FISH analysis of oocytes and polar bodies in patients undergoing assisted conception. *Hum Genet* 106, 620-6.

Martin R.H., Ko E. & Rademaker A. (1991) Distribution of aneuploidy in human gametes: comparison between human sperm and oocytes. *Am J Med Genet* 39, 321-31.

Mastenbroek S., Twisk M., van Echten-Arends J., Sikkema-Raddatz B., Korevaar J.C., Verhoeve H.R., Vogel N.E., Arts E.G., de Vries J.W., Bossuyt P.M., Buys C.H., Heineman M.J., Repping S. & van der Veen F. (2007) In vitro fertilization with preimplantation genetic screening. *N Engl J Med* 357, 9-17.

McReynolds S., Vanderlinden L., Stevens J., Hansen K., Schoolcraft W.B. & Katz-Jaffe M.G. (2011) Lipocalin-1: a potential marker for noninvasive aneuploidy screening. *Fertil Steril* 95, 2631-3.

Mersereau J.E., Pergament E., Zhang X. & Milad M.P. (2008) Preimplantation genetic screening to improve in vitro fertilization pregnancy rates: a prospective randomized controlled trial. *Fertil Steril* 90, 1287-9.

Meseguer M., Herrero J., Tejera A., Hilligsoe K.M., Ramsing N.B. & Remohi J. (2011) The use of morphokinetics as a predictor of embryo implantation. *Hum Reprod* 26, 2658-71.

Montag M., van der Ven K., Delacretaz G., Rink K. & van der Ven H. (1998) Laser-assisted microdissection of the zona pellucida facilitates polar body biopsy. *Fertil Steril* 69, 539-42.

Munne S. (2006) Chromosome abnormalities and their relationship to morphology and development of human embryos. *Reprod Biomed Online* 12, 234-53.

Munne S., Bahce M., Sandalinas M., Escudero T., Marquez C., Velilla E., Colls P., Oter M., Alikani M. & Cohen J. (2004) Differences in chromosome susceptibility to aneuploidy and survival to first trimester. *Reprod Biomed Online* 8, 81-90.

Munne S., Magli C., Cohen J., Morton P., Sadowy S., Gianaroli L., Tucker M., Marquez C., Sable D., Ferraretti A.P., Massey J.B. & Scott R. (1999) Positive outcome after preimplantation diagnosis of aneuploidy in human embryos. *Hum Reprod* 14, 2191-9.

Munne S., Sandalinas M., Escudero T., Marquez C. & Cohen J. (2002) Chromosome mosaicism in cleavage-stage human embryos: evidence of a maternal age effect. *Reprod Biomed Online* 4, 223-32.

Munne S., Wells D. & Cohen J. (2010) Technology requirements for preimplantation genetic diagnosis to improve assisted reproduction outcomes. *Fertil Steril* 94, 408-30.

Nekkebroeck J., Bonduelle M., Desmyttere S., Van den Broeck W. & Ponjaert-Kristoffersen I. (2008) Mental and psychomotor development of 2-year-old children born after preimplantation genetic diagnosis/screening. *Hum Reprod* 23, 1560-6.

Northrop L.E., Treff N.R., Levy B. & Scott R.T., Jr. (2010) SNP microarray-based 24 chromosome aneuploidy screening demonstrates that cleavage-stage FISH poorly predicts aneuploidy in embryos that develop to morphologically normal blastocysts. *Mol Hum Reprod* 16, 590-600.

Pantos K., Athanasiou V., Stefanidis K., Stavrou D., Vaxevanoglou T. & Chronopoulou M. (1999) Influence of advanced age on the blastocyst development rate and pregnancy rate in assisted reproductive technology. *Fertil Steril* 71, 1144-6.

Papadopoulos G., Templeton A.A., Fisk N. & Randall J. (1989) The frequency of chromosome anomalies in human preimplantation embryos after in-vitro fertilization. *Hum.Reprod.* 4, 91-8.

Park S., Kim E.Y., Yoon S.H., Chung K.S. & Lim J.H. (1999) Enhanced hatching rate of bovine IVM/IVF/IVC blastocysts using a 1.48- micron diode laser beam. *J Assist Reprod Genet* 16, 97-101.

Pellestor F. (1995) The cytogenetic analysis of human zygotes and preimplantation embryos. *Hum Reprod Update* 1, 581-5.

Pellestor F., Andreo B., Arnal F., Humeau C. & Demaille J. (2002) Mechanisms of non-disjunction in human female meiosis: the co-existence of two modes of malsegregation evidenced by the karyotyping of 1397 in- vitro unfertilized oocytes. *Hum Reprod* 17, 2134-45.

Picton H.M., Elder K., Houghton F.D., Hawkhead J.A., Rutherford A.J., Hogg J.E., Leese H.J. & Harris S.E. (2010) Association between amino acid turnover and chromosome aneuploidy during human preimplantation embryo development in vitro. *Mol Hum Reprod* 16, 557-69.

Piyamongkol W., Bermudez M.G., Harper J.C. & Wells D. (2003) Detailed investigation of factors influencing amplification efficiency and allele drop-out in single cell PCR: implications for preimplantation genetic diagnosis. *Mol Hum Reprod* 9, 411-20.

Rabinowitz M., Beltsos A., Potter D., Bush M., Givens C. & Smortrich D. (2010) Effects of advanced maternal age are abrogated in 122 patients undergoing transfer of embryos with euploid microarray screening results at cleavage stage.

Robbins W.A., Baulch J.E., Moore D., 2nd, Weier H.U., Blakey D. & Wyrobek A.J. (1995) Three-probe fluorescence in situ hybridization to assess chromosome X, Y, and 8 aneuploidy in sperm of 14 men from two healthy groups: evidence for a paternal age effect on sperm aneuploidy. *Reprod Fertil Dev* 7, 799-809.

Sabhnani T.V., Elaimi A., Sultan H., Alduraihem A., Serhal P. & Harper J.C. (2011) Increased incidence of mosaicism detected by FISH in murine blastocyst cultured in vitro. *Reprod Biomed Online* 22, 621-31.

Schoolcraft W.B., Fragouli E., Stevens J., Munne S., Katz-Jaffe M.G. & Wells D. (2010) Clinical application of comprehensive chromosomal screening at the blastocyst stage. *Fertil Steril* 94, 1700-6.

Selva J., Martin Pont B., Hugues J.N., Rince P., Fillion C., Herve F., Tamboise A. & Tamboise E. (1991) Cytogenetic study of human oocytes uncleaved after in-vitro fertilization. *Hum.Reprod.* 6, 709-13.

Shi Q. & Martin R.H. (2000) Aneuploidy in human sperm: a review of the frequency and distribution of aneuploidy, effects of donor age and lifestyle factors. *Cytogenet Cell Genet* 90, 219-26.

Shi Q. & Martin R.H. (2001) Aneuploidy in human spermatozoa: FISH analysis in men with constitutional chromosomal abnormalities, and in infertile men. *Reproduction* 121, 655-66.

Simpson J.L. (2008) What next for preimplantation genetic screening? Randomized clinical trial in assessing PGS: necessary but not sufficient. *Hum Reprod* 23, 2179-81.

Staessen C., Platteau P., Van Assche E., Michiels A., Tournaye H., Camus M., Devroey P., Liebaers I. & Van Steirteghem A. (2004) Comparison of blastocyst transfer with or without preimplantation genetic diagnosis for aneuploidy screening in couples with advanced maternal age: a prospective randomized controlled trial. *Hum Reprod* 19, 2849-58.

Steptoe P.C. & Edwards R.G. (1978) Birth after the reimplantation of a human embryo [letter]. *Lancet* 2, 366.

Strom C.M., Levin R., Strom S., Masciangelo C., Kuliev A. & Verlinsky Y. (2000) Neonatal outcome of preimplantation genetic diagnosis by polar body removal: the first 109 infants. *Pediatrics* 106, 650-3.

Summers M.C. & Foland A.D. (2009) Quantitative decision-making in preimplantation genetic (aneuploidy) screening (PGS). *J Assist Reprod Genet* 26, 487-502.

Tesarik J., Kopecny V., Plachot M. & Mandelbaum J. (1988) Early morphological signs of embryonic genome expression in human preimplantation development as revealed by quantitative electron microscopy. *Dev.Biol.* 128, 15-20.

Treff N.R., Levy B., Su J., Northrop L.E., Tao X. & Scott R.T., Jr. (2010a) SNP microarray-based 24 chromosome aneuploidy screening is significantly more consistent than FISH. *Mol Hum Reprod* 16, 583-9.

Treff N.R., Northrop L.E., Kasabwala K., Su J., Levy B. & Scott R.T., Jr. (2011) Single nucleotide polymorphism microarray-based concurrent screening of 24-chromosome aneuploidy and unbalanced translocations in preimplantation human embryos. *Fertil Steril* 95, 1606-12 e1-2.

Treff N.R., Su J., Tao X., Levy B. & Scott R.T., Jr. (2010b) Accurate single cell 24 chromosome aneuploidy screening using whole genome amplification and single nucleotide polymorphism microarrays. *Fertil Steril* 94, 2017-21.

Twisk M., Mastenbroek S., Hoek A., Heineman M.J., van der Veen F., Bossuyt P.M., Repping S. & Korevaar J.C. (2008) No beneficial effect of preimplantation genetic screening in women of advanced maternal age with a high risk for embryonic aneuploidy. *Hum Reprod.*

Van Blerkom J. (1989) The origin and detection of chromosomal abnormalities in meiotically mature human oocytes obtained from stimulated follicles and after failed fertilization in vitro. *Prog.Clin.Biol.Res.* 296, 299-310.

Varrela J., Larjava H., Jarvelainen H., Penttinen R., Eerola E. & Alvesalo L. (1989) Effect of sex chromosome aneuploidy on growth of human skin fibroblasts in cell culture. *Ann Hum Biol* 16, 9-13.

Verlinsky Y., Cieslak J., Freidine M., Ivakhnenko V., Wolf G., Kovalinskaya L., White M., Lifchez A., Kaplan B., Moise J., Valle J., Ginsberg N., Strom C. & Kuliev A. (1996) Polar body diagnosis of common aneuploidies by FISH. *J Assist Reprod Genet* 13, 157-62.

Voullaire L., Slater H., Williamson R. & Wilton L. (2000) Chromosome analysis of blastomeres from human embryos by using comparative genomic hybridization. *Hum Genet* 106, 210-7.

Walsh P.S., Erlich H.A. & Higuchi R. (1992) Preferential PCR amplification of alleles: mechanisms and solutions. *PCR.Methods Appl.* 1, 241-50.

Wells D. & Delhanty J.D. (2000) Comprehensive chromosomal analysis of human preimplantation embryos using whole genome amplification and single cell comparative genomic hybridization. *Mol Hum Reprod* 6, 1055-62.

Wells D., Escudero T., Levy B., Hirschhorn K., Delhanty J.D. & Munne S. (2002) First clinical application of comparative genomic hybridization and polar body testing for preimplantation genetic diagnosis of aneuploidy. *Fertil Steril* 78, 543-9.

Xu Y.W., Peng Y.T., Wang B., Zeng Y.H., Zhuang G.L. & Zhou C.Q. (2011) High follicle-stimulating hormone increases aneuploidy in human oocytes matured in vitro. *Fertil Steril* 95, 99-104.

Zenzes M.T. & Casper R.F. (1992) Cytogenetics of human oocytes, zygotes, and embryos after in vitro fertilization. *Hum.Genet.* 88, 367-75.